WRITING DISSERTATION AND GRANT PROPOSALS
Epidemiology, Preventive Medicine and Biostatistics

WRITING DISSERTATION AND GRANT PROPOSALS

Epidemiology, Preventive Medicine and Biostatistics

Lisa Chasan-Taber

University of Massachusetts
Amherst, USA

CRC Press
Taylor & Francis Group
Boca Raton London New York

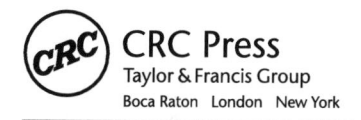

CRC Press is an imprint of the
Taylor & Francis Group, an **informa** business

A CHAPMAN & HALL BOOK

CRC Press
Taylor & Francis Group
6000 Broken Sound Parkway NW, Suite 300
Boca Raton, FL 33487-2742

© 2014 by Taylor & Francis Group, LLC
CRC Press is an imprint of Taylor & Francis Group, an Informa business

No claim to original U.S. Government works

Printed on acid-free paper
Version Date: 20140127

International Standard Book Number-13: 978-1-4665-1206-1 (Paperback)

This book contains information obtained from authentic and highly regarded sources. Reasonable efforts have been made to publish reliable data and information, but the author and publisher cannot assume responsibility for the validity of all materials or the consequences of their use. The authors and publishers have attempted to trace the copyright holders of all material reproduced in this publication and apologize to copyright holders if permission to publish in this form has not been obtained. If any copyright material has not been acknowledged please write and let us know so we may rectify in any future reprint.

Except as permitted under U.S. Copyright Law, no part of this book may be reprinted, reproduced, transmitted, or utilized in any form by any electronic, mechanical, or other means, now known or hereafter invented, including photocopying, microfilming, and recording, or in any information storage or retrieval system, without written permission from the publishers.

For permission to photocopy or use material electronically from this work, please access www.copyright.com (http://www.copyright.com/) or contact the Copyright Clearance Center, Inc. (CCC), 222 Rosewood Drive, Danvers, MA 01923, 978-750-8400. CCC is a not-for-profit organization that provides licenses and registration for a variety of users. For organizations that have been granted a photocopy license by the CCC, a separate system of payment has been arranged.

Trademark Notice: Product or corporate names may be trademarks or registered trademarks, and are used only for identification and explanation without intent to infringe.

Library of Congress Cataloging-in-Publication Data

Chasan-Taber, Lisa.
 Writing dissertation and grant proposals : epidemiology, preventive medicine and biostatistics / Lisa Chasan-Taber.
    pages cm
  Summary: "The scientific proposal-writing process can be a daunting experience for graduate students and young researchers. This book covers all aspects of the process, from structure and style to obtaining research grant funding. Organized much like a research proposal, the book covers identifying a research topic, drafting a hypothesis, conducting a literature review, describing methods for data collection and analysis, and presenting the proposal. The final section describes strategies for putting together a winning NIH proposal and responding to reviewer comments. Concepts are illustrated with examples, applications, exercises, and checklists of guidelines"-- Provided by publisher.
  Includes bibliographical references and index.
  ISBN 978-1-4665-1206-1 (paperback)
 1. Proposal writing in medicine. 2. Epidemiology--Research grants. 3. Public health--Statistical services--Research grants. 4. Proposal writing for grants. I. Title.

R853.P75C48 2014
808.06'661--dc23   2014001359

Visit the Taylor & Francis Web site at
http://www.taylorandfrancis.com

and the CRC Press Web site at
http://www.crcpress.com

Contents

Preface	xxi
Author	xxiii

1 Ten Top Tips for Successful Proposal Writing — 1
- 1.1 Tip #1: Start Early — 1
- 1.2 Tip #2: Create a Vision with the Help of a Mentor — 2
- 1.3 Tip #3: Look at Who and What They Funded before You — 3
- 1.4 Tip #4: Spend Half Your Time on the Abstract and Specific Aims — 4
- 1.5 Tip #5: Show That You Can Pull It Off — 6
- 1.6 Tip #6: Your Methods Should Match Your Aims and Vice Versa — 7
- 1.7 Tip #7: A Proposal Can Never Have Too Many Figures or Tables — 8
- 1.8 Tip #8: Seek External Review Prior to Submission — 9
- 1.9 Tip #9: Be Kind to Your Reviewers — 10
- 1.10 Tip #10: If at All Possible, Choose a Topic That You Find Interesting! — 11

PART ONE Preparing to Write the Proposal — 13

2 Starting a Dissertation Proposal — 15
- 2.1 Purpose of the Dissertation — 15
- 2.2 Purpose of the Dissertation Proposal — 16
- 2.3 Step #1: Preliminary Qualifying Exams — 16
- 2.4 Step #2: Selecting a Dissertation Topic — 17
  - 2.4.1 Ascertain If Original Data Collection Is Required — 18
  - 2.4.2 Pep Talk — 19
- 2.5 Step #3: Choosing a Chair — 19
- 2.6 Step #4: Choosing the Dissertation Committee Members — 19
  - 2.6.1 Role of the Dissertation Committee — 21
  - 2.6.2 Balance of Responsibilities between the Dissertation Chair and the Dissertation Committee — 22
- 2.7 Step #5: Writing the Dissertation Proposal — 22
  - 2.7.1 Structure of the Dissertation Proposal — 22
  - 2.7.2 Dissertation Proposal as a Contract — 23
  - 2.7.3 Format of the Dissertation Proposal — 23
- 2.8 Step #6: Proposal Defense — 24
- 2.9 Step #7: Submission of the Proposal to the Graduate School — 25
- 2.10 Step #8: Conduct the Dissertation Research — 25
- 2.11 Step #9: Dissertation Defense — 25
- 2.12 Step #10: Submit the Dissertation to the Graduate School — 26

	2.13	Suggested Timeline	26
	2.14	Examples	27
		2.14.1 Preproposal for a 3-Paper Model	27
		2.14.2 Dissertation Proposal Outline	29
3	**How to Develop and Write Hypotheses**		**31**
	3.1	Need for Hypotheses	31
	3.2	More about the Distinction between Hypotheses and Specific Aims	32
	3.3	Hypotheses Should Flow Logically from the Background and Significance Section	33
	3.4	How to Write Hypotheses If the Prior Literature Is Conflicting	34
	3.5	Guideline #1: A Research Hypothesis Should Name the Independent and Dependent Variables and Indicate the Type of Relationship Expected between Them	35
	3.6	Guideline #2: A Hypothesis Should Name the Exposure Prior to the Outcome	36
	3.7	Guideline #3: The Comparison Group Should Be Stated	37
	3.8	Guideline #4: When Your Study Is Limited to a Particular Population, Reference to the Population Should Be Made in the Hypothesis	38
	3.9	Guideline #5: Hypotheses Should Be as Concise as Possible and Use Measureable Terms	39
	3.10	Guideline #6: Avoid Making Precise Statistical Predictions in a Hypothesis	40
	3.11	Guideline #7: A Hypothesis Should Indicate What Will Actually Be Studied—Not the Possible Implications of the Study or Value Judgments of the Author	41
	3.12	Stylistic Tip #1: When a Number of Related Hypotheses Are to Be Stated, Consider Presenting Them in a Numbered or Lettered List	42
	3.13	Stylistic Tip #2: Because Most Hypotheses Deal with the Behavior of Groups, Plural Forms Should Usually Be Used	43
	3.14	Stylistic Tip #3: Avoid Using the Words *Significant* or *Significance* in a Hypothesis	43
	3.15	Stylistic Tip #4: Avoid Using the Word *Prove* in a Hypothesis	44
	3.16	Stylistic Tip #5: Avoid Using Two Different Terms to Refer to the Same Variable in a Hypothesis	45
	3.17	Stylistic Tip #6: Remove Any Unnecessary Words	46
	3.18	Stylistic Tip #7: Hypotheses May Be Written as Research Questions—But Use Caution	47
	3.19	Hypothesis Writing Checklist	47
4	**Conducting the Literature Search**		**49**
	4.1	How Do Literature Reviews for Grant Proposals Differ from Literature Reviews in Journal Articles or in Dissertation Proposals?	50
	4.2	Writing a Literature Review Is an Iterative Process	51

- 4.3 Step #1: Creating a Literature Review Outline … 51
- 4.4 Step #2: Searching for Literature (Do's and Don'ts) … 52
  - 4.4.1 Choosing a Relevant Database … 53
  - 4.4.2 What Type of Literature to Collect for Each Section of the Literature Review Outline … 53
    - 4.4.2.1 a. Introduction: public health impact of outcome (disease) … 53
    - 4.4.2.2 b. Physiology of exposure–outcome relationship … 54
    - 4.4.2.3 c. Epidemiology of exposure–outcome relationship … 54
  - 4.4.3 Should You Collect Epidemiologic Literature That Only Secondarily Evaluated Your Exposure–Outcome Relationship? … 55
  - 4.4.4 Collecting Literature for an Effect Modification Hypothesis … 56
  - 4.4.5 What to Do When Your Search Yields Thousands of *Hits* … 57
  - 4.4.6 What to Do If There Are Too Few Hits … 58
  - 4.4.7 How to Retrieve Articles (Hits) … 59
  - 4.4.8 How to Scan Articles for Relevance … 59
  - 4.4.9 Evaluating Your References for Completeness … 59
- 4.5 Step #3: Organizing the Epidemiologic Literature—Summary Tables … 60
  - 4.5.1 What Data Should I Include in a Summary Table? … 60
  - 4.5.2 Reviewing the Table to Identify Research Gaps … 62
  - 4.5.3 Should I Include the Summary Table in My Proposal? … 63
- 4.6 Examples … 64
  - 4.6.1 Example #1 … 64
  - 4.6.2 Example #2 … 64
  - 4.6.3 Example #3 … 65

5 Scientific Writing … 69
- 5.1 Tip #1: Consider Your Audience … 69
- 5.2 Tip #2: Avoid Using the First-Person Singular … 70
- 5.3 Tip #3: Use the Active Voice … 70
- 5.4 Tip #4: Use Transitions to Help Trace Your Argument … 71
- 5.5 Tip #5: Avoid Direct Quotations Both at the Beginning and within the Literature Review … 72
- 5.6 Tip #6: Avoid Saying *The Authors Concluded…* … 73
- 5.7 Tip #7: Omit Needless Words … 74
- 5.8 Tip #8: Avoid Professional Jargon … 75
- 5.9 Tip #9: Avoid Using Synonyms for Recurring Words … 76
- 5.10 Tip #10: Use the Positive Form … 77
- 5.11 Tip #11: Place Latin Abbreviations in Parentheses; Elsewhere Use English Translations … 77
- 5.12 Tip #12: Spell Out Acronyms When First Used; Keep Their Use to a Minimum … 78
- 5.13 Tip #13: Avoid the Use of Contractions … 78
- 5.14 Tip #14: Spell Out Numbers at the Beginning of a Sentence … 79
- 5.15 Tip #15: Placement of References … 79
- 5.16 Strive for a User-Friendly Draft … 80

5.17	Take Advantage of Writing Assistance Programs	81
5.18	Solicit Early *Informal* Feedback on Your Proposal	81
5.19	Who Must Read Your Proposal	82
5.20	Incorporating Feedback	82
5.21	How to Reconcile Contradictory Feedback	83
5.22	Annotated Example	84

PART TWO The Proposal: Section by Section 87

6 Specific Aims 89
- 6.1 Purpose of the Specific Aims Page 89
- 6.2 A Word of Caution 90
- 6.3 Outline for the Specific Aims Page 90
  - 6.3.1 Paragraph #1: Study Background and Research Gap 91
  - 6.3.2 Paragraph #2: Synopsis of the Study Methods 93
  - 6.3.3 Paragraph #3: Your Aims and Corresponding Hypotheses 94
  - 6.3.4 Paragraph #4: Summary of Significance and Innovation 95
- 6.4 Tip #1: How to Deal with the One-Page Limitation for the Specific Aims Page 97
- 6.5 Tip #2: Avoid Interdependent Aims 97
- 6.6 Tip #3: Aims Involving the Use of an Existing Dataset—Pros and Cons 98
- 6.7 Tip #4: Should You Aim to Conduct Analytic or Descriptive Studies? 99
- 6.8 Tip #5: How to Decide Whether to Include Exploratory or Secondary Aims 100
- 6.9 Tip #6: Don't Be Too Ambitious 100
- 6.10 Tip #7: Remember That All Aims Should Be Accompanied by Hypotheses 101
- 6.11 Tip #8: If You Plan to Evaluate Effect Modification in Your Methods, Then Include This as a Specific Aim 102
- 6.12 When to Consider Discarding Your Original Aims and Hypotheses 103
- 6.13 Annotated Examples 103
  - 6.13.1 Example #1: Needs Improvement 103
  - 6.13.2 Example #2: Does Not Need Improvement 105

7 Background and Significance Section 109
- 7.1 Refer Back to Your Literature Review Outline 109
- 7.2 Background and Significance Should Be Made Up of Subsections Corresponding to Each Hypothesis 110
- 7.3 Section a: Summarize the Public Health Impact of Outcome (Disease) 110
- 7.4 Section b: Summarize the Physiology of Exposure–Outcome Relationship 111

	7.5	Section c: Summarize the Epidemiology of Exposure–Outcome Relationship (Describe Studies in Groups)	113
		7.5.1 In Summarizing the Epidemiologic Literature, Note the Relationships between Study Methods and Their Corresponding Findings	114
		7.5.2 Finding the Research Gap in the Prior Epidemiologic Literature	115
		7.5.3 How Big a Research Gap Do I Need to Fill?	115
		7.5.4 Highlight the Limitations of Prior Studies That Your Proposal Will Be Able to Address	116
		7.5.5 What Should You Do If the Prior Literature Is Conflicting?	117
		7.5.5.1 Let reviewers know that you are aware of controversies	117
		7.5.5.2 Give clear reasons for taking a side	117
		7.5.6 Highlight Key Studies	118
	7.6	Section d: Summarize the Significance and Innovation	119
	7.7	Tip #1: Should You Have One Consolidated Background and Significance Section?	120
	7.8	Tip #2: Be Sure to Express Your Own Opinions about a Prior Study's Limitations	121
	7.9	Tip #3: You May Refer to Comments from a Review Article	121
	7.10	Tip #4: Occasionally You May Provide the Historical Context	122
	7.11	Tip #5: Summarize at the End of Each Section in the Background and Significance Section	122
	7.12	Tip #6: Avoid Broad and Global Statements in the Background and Significance Section	123
	7.13	Tip #7: Be Comprehensive and Complete in Citations	123
	7.14	Tip #8: References Should Directly Follow the Studies That They Relate To	124
	7.15	Tip #9: If You Are Commenting on a Time Frame, Be Specific	125
	7.16	Annotated Examples	125
		7.16.1 Example #1: Needs Improvement	125
		7.16.2 Example #2a: Grant Proposal Version *Not* in Need of Improvement	128
		7.16.3 Example #2b: Dissertation Proposal Version *Not* in Need of Improvement	128
8	**Summarizing Preliminary Studies**		**133**
	8.1	What Are Preliminary Studies?	133
	8.2	Do Preliminary Data Need to Be Previously Published?	134
	8.3	How to Describe Preliminary Data	135
	8.4	Use the Preliminary Studies Section to Demonstrate Established Relationships with Your Coinvestigators	136
	8.5	What If You Do Not Have Preliminary Data?	137

	8.6	What If Your Preliminary Data Contradict Your Proposed Hypotheses?	138
	8.7	Double-Check That All Your Preliminary Findings Relate to One or More of Your Proposed Hypotheses	139
	8.8	Pitfalls of Preliminary Data	140
	8.9	Where to Place Preliminary Studies in an NIH Grant Proposal?	140
	8.10	Should I Include Preliminary Results Even If the Grant Does Not Require Them?	140
	8.11	Preliminary Studies within Proposals Based upon Existing Datasets	141
	8.12	Tip #1: Include Tables and Figures in the Preliminary Studies Section	142
	8.13	Tip #2: When Describing Results in a Table or Figure, Point Out the Highlights for the Reviewer	143
	8.14	Tip #3: Include Descriptive Tables of the Study Population	144
	8.15	Tip #4: Describe Preliminary Findings in Layperson's Terms	145
		8.15.1 How to Describe a Relative Risk in Layperson's Terms	146
		8.15.2 How to Describe a Beta Coefficient in Layperson's Terms	146
		8.15.3 How to Describe Effect Modification in Layperson's Terms	147
	8.16	Stylistic Tip #1: Describe Tables in Numeric Order	147
	8.17	Stylistic Tip #2: Try to Describe Tables from Top to Bottom	147
	8.18	Stylistic Tip #3: Spell Out Numbers That Start Sentences	148
	8.19	Stylistic Tip #4: Avoid Presenting Confidence Intervals and p-Values	148
	8.20	Stylistic Tip #5: Avoid Referring to Your Tables as Active Beings	149
	8.21	Stylistic Tip #6: Tips for Table Titles	150
	8.22	Preliminary Study Examples	150
		8.22.1 Preliminary Study #1	151
		8.22.2 Preliminary Study #2	151

9 Study Design and Methods — 153

	9.1	Goals of the Study Design and Methods Section	154
	9.2	Overall Strategy	154
	9.3	Identify Benchmarks for Success	155
	9.4	Section a: What Is Your Study Design?	156
		9.4.1 Consider a Study Design Figure	157
	9.5	Section b: Study Population (Setting, Subject Ascertainment, and Eligibility)	159
		9.5.1 How to Describe Subject Ascertainment	160
		9.5.2 How to Describe Eligibility Criteria	160
	9.6	Section c: Exposure Assessment	161
		9.6.1 How Your Exposure Data Will Be Collected	161
		9.6.2 Exposure Parameterization	163
		9.6.3 How to Parameterize Your Variable	163
		9.6.4 Validity of Exposure Assessment	164
		9.6.5 What to Do If There Are No Prior Validation Studies	166

9.7	Section d: Outcome Assessment	167
9.8	Section e: Covariate Assessment	168
9.9	Section f: Variable Categorization Table	169
9.10	Pitfalls to Avoid	173
9.11	Examples	174
	9.11.1 Example #1	174
	9.11.2 Example #2	176

10 Data Analysis Plan 179
10.1	Part I: Framework for the Proposed Data Analysis Plan	179
	10.1.1 Start the Data Analysis Plan by Repeating Your Specific Aims Verbatim	179
	10.1.2 What If All Your Aims Require the Identical Data Analysis Plan?	180
10.2	Part II: Scope and Depth of Proposed Analyses	181
	10.2.1 Step #1: Are Your Specific Aims Descriptive or Analytic?	181
	10.2.2 Step #2: How Will You Parameterize Your Variables?	182
10.3	Outline for a Basic Data Analysis Plan	183
	10.3.1 Univariate Analysis Plan	183
	10.3.2 Bivariate Analysis Plan	185
	10.3.3 Multivariable Analysis Plan	187
	10.3.3.1 A. Select an appropriate model	187
	10.3.3.2 B. Specify how the model will adjust for potential confounding factors (i.e., covariates)	188
	10.3.3.3 C. Specify how you will evaluate potential effect modifiers	190
	10.3.4 Exploratory Data Analyses	191
	10.3.5 Mock Tables	192
10.4	Part III: Best Practices	192
10.5	Example Data Analysis Plan for a Dissertation Proposal	195

11 Power and Sample Size 203
11.1	Timeline	203
11.2	What Is Power?	204
11.3	Key Characteristics of Power	204
11.4	When Is It OK Not to Include a Power or Sample Size Calculation?	205
11.5	Step #1: Estimate Your Sample Size	206
	11.5.1 Basis for Sample Size Estimation	206
11.6	Step #2: Choose User-Friendly Software to Calculate Power	207
11.7	Step #3: Remind Yourself of Your Measure of Association	208
11.8	Step #4: Calculate and Present Your Power for Ratio Measures of Association (i.e., Relative Risks)	209
	11.8.1 A. For Cohort and Cross-Sectional Studies	209
	11.8.2 B. For *Unmatched* Case–Control Studies	211
	11.8.3 C. How to Display Your Power in the Proposal	212

11.9	Step #5: Calculate and Present Your Power for Difference Measures of Association (i.e., Continuous Outcome Variables)	214
	11.9.1 A. For Cohort and Cross-Sectional Studies	215
	11.9.2 B. How to Display Your Power in the Proposal	215
11.10	What If Your Power Is Not Adequate?	216
11.11	Other Factors That Influence Power	217
11.12	Final Pep Talk	217

12 Review of Bias and Confounding 219

12.1	First: A Pep Talk	220
12.2	Study Limitations: Chance, Bias, and Confounding	220
12.3	Chance	221
12.4	Bias	222
12.5	Nondifferential Misclassification	222
	12.5.1 Nondifferential Misclassification of Exposure	222
	12.5.2 Nondifferential Misclassification of Outcome	223
12.6	Selection Bias	225
	12.6.1 Selection Bias in a Case–Control Study	225
	12.6.2 Selection Bias in a Cohort Study	226
12.7	Information Bias	226
	12.7.1 Information Bias in a Case–Control or Cross-Sectional Study	227
	12.7.2 Information Bias in a Cohort Study	228
12.8	Confounding	229
	12.8.1 Confounding in Randomized Trials	231
	12.8.2 Difference between Confounding and Effect Modification	231
	12.8.3 Will You Be Missing Information on Any Potential Confounding Factors?	232
12.9	Other Limitations Specific to Cross-Sectional and Case–Control Studies	234
12.10	Generalizability	234
	12.10.1 Reasons to Limit Generalizability	236
12.11	Exercises	237
12.12	Issues for Critical Reading	239
	12.12.1 Cohort Studies	239
	12.12.2 Randomized Trials	240
	12.12.3 Case–Control and Cross-Sectional Studies	241
12.13	Examples	242
	12.13.1 Example #1	242
	12.13.2 Example #2	244

13 How to Present Limitations and Alternatives — 245
13.1 Which Limitations to Highlight? — 245
13.2 Part I: How to Strategically Present Limitations—a Fourfold Approach — 246
13.2.1 Step #1: Describe the Potential Limitation — 246
13.2.2 Step #2: Describe the Potential Impact of the Limitation on Your Study Findings — 247
13.2.3 Step #3: Discuss Alternatives — 249
13.2.4 Step #4: Describe Methods to Minimize the Limitation — 249
13.2.5 Conclusion to Fourfold Approach to Address Limitations — 250
13.2.6 Where to Place Your Study Limitations in a Grant Proposal — 250
13.2.6.1 Limitations section at the end of the approach section — 251
13.2.6.2 Intermingled limitations sections — 251
13.3 Part II: Methods to Minimize Classic Limitations—Design and Analysis Techniques — 252
13.3.1 How to Present Nondifferential Misclassification — 252
13.3.1.1 Design techniques to minimize nondifferential misclassification — 252
13.3.1.2 Analysis techniques to minimize nondifferential misclassification — 253
13.3.2 How to Present Selection Bias — 253
13.3.2.1 Study design techniques to minimize selection bias — 254
13.3.2.2 Analysis techniques to minimize selection bias — 254
13.3.3 How to Present Information Bias — 254
13.3.3.1 Study design techniques to minimize information bias — 254
13.3.3.2 Analysis techniques to minimize information bias — 255
13.3.4 How to Present Confounding — 256
13.3.4.1 Study design techniques to minimize confounding — 256
13.3.4.2 Analysis techniques to minimize confounding — 258
13.3.4.3 Techniques to minimize lack of data on a confounder — 259
13.3.5 How to Present Survivor Bias — 260
13.3.6 How to Present Temporal Bias — 260
13.3.7 How to Present Generalizability — 261
13.4 Examples — 262
13.4.1 Example #1 — 262
13.4.2 Example #2 — 264

14 Reproducibility and Validity Studies — 267
- 14.1 Why Conduct a Reproducibility or Validity Study? — 267
- 14.2 What Is Reproducibility and Validity? — 268
- 14.3 Relationship between Reproducibility and Validity — 269
- 14.4 Both Subjective and Objective Measurement Tools Require Evidence of Reproducibility and Validity — 270
  - 14.4.1 Questionnaires — 270
  - 14.4.2 Particular Challenge of Behavioral Questionnaires — 271
  - 14.4.3 Objective Measures Also Require Reproducibility and Validity Studies — 272
- 14.5 Study Design of Reproducibility Studies — 273
- 14.6 Study Design of Validity Studies — 274
  - 14.6.1 Subjective Comparison Measures — 274
  - 14.6.2 Objective Comparison Measures — 275
  - 14.6.3 Number of Administrations of the Comparison Method — 276
- 14.7 Writing Data Analysis Sections for Reproducibility/Validity Studies — 277
- 14.8 Writing Limitations Sections for Reproducibility/Validity Studies — 278
  - 14.8.1 Threats to Observed Reproducibility Scores — 279
  - 14.8.2 Threats to Observed Validity Scores — 281
  - 14.8.3 Threats to Generalizability — 282
- 14.9 How to Interpret Findings from Reproducibility/Validity Studies — 283
- 14.10 Issues of Sample Size and Power for a Reproducibility and Validity Study — 284
- 14.11 Summary — 284
- 14.12 Example — 285

15 Abstracts and Titles — 287
- 15.1 Outline for Proposal Abstract — 287
- 15.2 How to Get Started Writing an Abstract — 288
- 15.3 When to Finalize the Abstract — 289
- 15.4 NIH Review of an Abstract — 290
- 15.5 Examples of Funded Abstracts — 290
- 15.6 Strategies for Meeting the Word Count/Line Limitations — 291
- 15.7 Abstract: Step by Step — 291
  - 15.7.1 Background Section — 291
    - 15.7.1.1 Public health impact of outcome (disease) — 292
    - 15.7.1.2 Physiology of exposure–outcome relationship — 292
    - 15.7.1.3 Epidemiology of exposure–outcome relationship — 293
  - 15.7.2 II. Research Aims — 294
  - 15.7.3 III. Highlights of the Methodology — 295
  - 15.7.4 IV. Summary of the Significance and Innovation — 297
- 15.8 How to Write a Title for Your Proposal — 299
  - 15.8.1 Tip #1: Use Agency-Friendly Keywords — 300
  - 15.8.2 Tip #2: Titles Should Include the Key Variables Being Evaluated — 301

		15.8.3 Tip #3: The Title Should Not State the Expected Results of the Proposed Study	301
		15.8.4 Tip #4: Titles Should Mention the Study Design If a Strength	302
		15.8.5 Tip #5: The Title Should Mention the Study Population When Important	302
		15.8.6 Tip #6: Titles Should Mention Any Other Unique Features of the Study	303
		15.8.7 Tip #7: A Title Should Be Consistent with the Overall Study Goal	303
		15.8.8 Stylistic Tip #1: Avoid Clever Titles	304
		15.8.9 Stylistic Tip #2: Avoid Writing Titles as Questions	304
	15.9	Examples	305
		15.9.1 Example #1	305
		15.9.2 Example #2: Needs Improvement	306
		15.9.3 Example #3: Needs Improvement	307
16	**Presenting Your Proposal Orally**		**309**
	16.1	How to Get Started	309
	16.2	General Guidelines	310
		16.2.1 Guideline #1: Organize the Presentation Based on Your Proposal Outline	310
		16.2.2 Guideline #2: How to Allocate Presentation Time	310
		16.2.3 Guideline #3: A Presentation Cannot Have Too Many Figures or Tables	311
		16.2.4 Guideline #4: How to Create User-Friendly Text Slides	314
		16.2.5 Guideline #5: Recommended Slide Aesthetics	315
	16.3	Presenting Background and Significance	315
	16.4	Presenting Preliminary Studies or Findings from the Prior Literature	318
		16.4.1 Keep Results Tables Simple	319
		16.4.2 Presenting *Mock Tables* for a Dissertation Proposal	321
	16.5	Include *Backup* Slides	321
	16.6	Guidelines for Your Speech	322
		16.6.1 Guideline #1: Consider How Your Words Will Supplement Your Slides	322
		16.6.2 Guideline #2: How to Discuss Tables/Figures	322
		16.6.3 Importance of Rehearsing Your Speech	324
		16.6.4 Cultivating a Relationship with the Audience	324
		16.6.5 Tip #1: Don't Undercut Your Message	325
		16.6.6 Tip #2: Try Not to Talk Too Quickly	325
		16.6.7 Tip #3: Try Not to Spend Too Much Time on Each Slide	325
	16.7	Consider How the Presentation Will Be Evaluated	325
	16.8	Proposal Presentation Critique	326

PART THREE Grantsmanship — 329

17 Choosing the Right Funding Source — 331
- 17.1 Part I: Developing Your Grant-Funding Plan — 331
  - 17.1.1 Step #1: Locate a Mentor for Grantsmanship — 331
    - 17.1.1.1 How to identify a mentor — 332
  - 17.1.2 Step #2: Develop Your Overall Grantsmanship Goal — 332
    - 17.1.2.1 Plan for a steady trajectory of grants from small to large — 333
    - 17.1.2.2 Avoid classic pitfall #1: Don't skip straight to large funding mechanisms — 334
  - 17.1.3 Plan for More Than One Potential Funding Pipeline — 335
  - 17.1.4 Serve as a Coinvestigator on Established Teams — 335
  - 17.1.5 Avoid Classic Pitfall #2: Do Not Propose Overly Ambitious Specific Aims — 336
  - 17.1.6 Avoid Classic Pitfall #3: Do Not Embed Pilot or Validity Studies within a Larger Proposal — 336
- 17.2 Part II: Choosing the Appropriate Funding Mechanism for Your Early Grants — 337
  - 17.2.1 Focus on Grants Targeted to Early-Career Faculty and Postdoctoral Fellows — 337
  - 17.2.2 Internal University Funding — 337
  - 17.2.3 Foundation Grants — 338
  - 17.2.4 Resources for Selecting the Right Funding Source — 338
  - 17.2.5 Look at Who and What They Funded before You — 339
  - 17.2.6 Look at Who Serves as Reviewers — 339
- 17.3 Part III: Step-by-Step Advice for Finding the Right Funding Source at NIH — 340
  - 17.3.1 Step #1: Determine Which NIH Institute's Mission Encompasses Your Topic — 340
  - 17.3.2 Step #2: Choose a Funding Mechanism Sponsored by Your Selected NIH Institute — 340
    - 17.3.2.1 Doctoral and postdoctoral fellowships (F series) "Ruth L. Kirschstein Individual National Research Service Award" (NRSA) — 342
    - 17.3.2.2 Training grants (T series) "Ruth L. Kirschstein Individual National Research Service Award" — 343
    - 17.3.2.3 Career development awards (K series) — 343
    - 17.3.2.4 Loan repayment programs — 345
    - 17.3.2.5 Research supplements — 345
    - 17.3.2.6 Research awards (R series) — 346
    - 17.3.2.7 New investigator advantages — 347
  - 17.3.3 Step #3: Choose the Corresponding Funding Opportunity Announcement Number — 347
    - 17.3.3.1 Read the FOA carefully! — 349

	17.4	Examples of Choosing the Right Funding Sources	349
		17.4.1 Example #1: A Postdoctoral Researcher Transitioning to Early-Career Faculty	349
		17.4.2 Example #2: An Early-Career Faculty Member	351

18 Submission of the Grant Proposal — 353

18.1 How to View the Submission Process Overall — 353
18.2 Part I: Getting Started — 354
    18.2.1 How Far Ahead to Start the Grant Preparation Process — 354
    18.2.2 Begin to Assemble the Research Team Early — 355
        18.2.2.1 How to choose collaborators — 355
        18.2.2.2 Establish working relationships with coinvestigators before submission — 356
        18.2.2.3 Consider a multiple principal investigator model — 356
    18.2.3 Spend Half Your Time on the Specific Aims and Project Summary (Abstract) — 357
    18.2.4 Allow Time for External Review Prior to Submission — 358
    18.2.5 External Review: *Chalk-Talk Forums* — 359
    18.2.6 External Review: Mock NIH Study Sections — 359
18.3 Part II: Strategic Tips for Each Component of the Grant Submission — 360
    18.3.1 Section I: Scientific Component — 361
        18.3.1.1 I.a. Title — 361
        18.3.1.2 I.b. Project summary (abstract) — 362
        18.3.1.3 I.c. Specific aims — 363
        18.3.1.4 I.d. Project narrative — 363
        18.3.1.5 I.e. Research strategy — 363
        18.3.1.6 I.f. Training information for doctoral and postdoctoral fellowships (F series) — 365
        18.3.1.7 I.g. Candidate information for career development awards (K series) — 367
        18.3.1.8 I.h. Bibliography and references cited — 369
        18.3.1.9 I.i. Human subjects protection/responsible conduct of research — 369
        18.3.1.10 I.j. Inclusion of women, minorities, and children; Targeted/planned enrollment — 370
    18.3.2 Section II: Nonscientific Forms — 371
        18.3.2.1 II.a. Cover letter — 371
        18.3.2.2 II.b. Facilities and other resources — 372
        18.3.2.3 II.c. Equipment — 372
        18.3.2.4 II.d. Biosketch — 373
        18.3.2.5 II.e. Budget and budget justification — 374
        18.3.2.6 II.f. Resource sharing plan — 376
        18.3.2.7 II.g. Appendices and supplemental materials — 377
        18.3.2.8 II.h. Other pages — 377

	18.3.3	Section III: Items Needed from Others	377
		18.3.3.1 III.a. Letters of support	377
		18.3.3.2 III.b. Biosketches	378
		18.3.3.3 III.c. Consortium/contractual arrangements	379
18.4	Part III: Timeline for Submission of an NIH Grant		379

19 Review Process 381
19.1	Part I: Review Process		381
	19.1.1	Scientific Review Group (*Study Section*)	381
	19.1.2	Role of the Scientific Review Officer	382
	19.1.3	Study Section Reviewers	383
	19.1.4	How the Study Section Members Review Your Grant Application	384
	19.1.5	Review Criteria for Research Grants (R Series)	384
		19.1.5.1 Overall impact	384
		19.1.5.2 1. Significance	385
		19.1.5.3 2. Investigator(s)	385
		19.1.5.4 3. Innovation	386
		19.1.5.5 4. Approach	386
		19.1.5.6 5. Environment	386
	19.1.6	Review Criteria for Career Development Awards (K Series)	387
		19.1.6.1 Overall impact for a career award	387
		19.1.6.2 1. Candidate	388
		19.1.6.3 2. Career development plan/career goals and objectives	388
		19.1.6.4 3. Research plan	388
		19.1.6.5 4. Mentor(s), co-mentor(s), consultant(s), and collaborator(s)	389
		19.1.6.6 5. Environment and institutional commitment to the candidate	389
	19.1.7	Review Criteria for Fellowship Awards (F Series)	389
		19.1.7.1 Overall impact/merit for a fellowship award	389
		19.1.7.2 1. Fellowship applicant	390
		19.1.7.3 2. Sponsors, collaborators, and consultants	390
		19.1.7.4 3. Research training plan	390
		19.1.7.5 4. Training potential	391
		19.1.7.6 5. Institutional environment and commitment to training	391
	19.1.8	During the Study Section Meeting	391
	19.1.9	Common Reasons for Low Scores	392
	19.1.10	Tips for a Successful Review	392
19.2	Part II: After Your Application Is Reviewed		393
	19.2.1	Step #1: Read the Summary Statement	393
	19.2.2	If Your Application Was Streamlined (Unscored)	394
	19.2.3	Step #2: Contact Your Program Official	394

	19.2.4	Appeal	395
	19.2.5	Funding: What Determines Which Awards Are Made?	395

20 Resubmission of the Grant Proposal — 397
20.1 Part I: Pathway to Resubmitting — 397
- 20.1.1 Whether to Resubmit — 398
- 20.1.2 Contact Your Program Official — 398
- 20.1.3 Timing of a Resubmission — 398
- 20.1.4 Not All Reviewer Comments Are Equal — 399
- 20.1.5 How Much Revision Is Necessary — 400
- 20.1.6 Study Section Review of Resubmissions — 400

20.2 Part II: Introduction to the Resubmission — 400
- 20.2.1 General Format of the Introduction Page — 401
- 20.2.2 Tip #1: Clearly Connect Your Responses to Specific Reviewer Concerns — 402
- 20.2.3 Tip #2: Resist the Urge to Defend Yourself — 402
- 20.2.4 Tip #3: Avoid Disagreeing with a Reviewer — 403
- 20.2.5 Tip #4: If You Must Disagree with a Reviewer, Focus on the Science — 404
- 20.2.6 Tip #5: Avoid Using Cost or Logistics as a Rationale for Not Being Responsive to a Reviewer Comment — 404
- 20.2.7 Tip #6: Multiple-Bullet-Point Response to Major Concerns Is Highly Responsive — 405
- 20.2.8 Tip #7: Acknowledge Your Mistakes or Lack of Clarity — 406
- 20.2.9 Tip #8: Don't Skip Any Reviewer Comments — 406
- 20.2.10 Tip #9: Avoid Collapsing Too Many Reviewer Concerns into One Bullet Point — 407
- 20.2.11 Tip #10: Be Sure to Make Changes to the Body of the Proposal — 407
- 20.2.12 Stylistic Tip #1: Use Active (Not Passive) Voice — 408
- 20.2.13 Stylistic Tip #2: Avoid Use of the First Person — 408
- 20.2.14 Stylistic Tip #3: Don't Waste Too Much Space Apologizing — 409

20.3 Part III: Body of the Resubmission — 409
- 20.3.1 How to Identify Revisions to a Grant Proposal — 409
- 20.3.2 Rereview the Published Literature to Check for Recent Relevant Publications — 410
- 20.3.3 Obtain Revised Letters of Collaboration — 410
- 20.3.4 Update Biosketches: Both Your Own and Those of Your Coinvestigators — 410

20.4 Examples — 411
- 20.4.1 Proposal to Conduct a Randomized Trial of a Postpartum Diabetes Prevention Program — 411
- 20.4.2 K Award Proposal to Conduct a Web-Based Intervention Study to Prevent Weight Gain in Men — 413

Index — 415

Preface

For more than 15 years, I have taught a graduate course on grant proposal writing for students in the School of Public Health and Health Sciences at the University of Massachusetts at Amherst. With their encouragement and suggestions, this textbook has come to be a reality. Competition for research funds has never been more intense and, at the same time, the grant application and review process at such agencies as the National Institutes of Health (NIH) are undergoing significant transformation. *Writing Dissertation and Grant Proposals: Epidemiology, Preventive Medicine, and Biostatistics* is unique in representing an up-to-date textbook targeting effective grant proposal writing in this growing and important field.

The text covers all aspects of the proposal-writing process from *soup to nuts*. Step-by-step tips address grant structure and style alongside broader strategies for developing a research funding portfolio. Throughout, concepts are illustrated with annotated examples from successfully funded proposals in the field. Strategies to avoid common errors and pitfalls (e.g., *do's and don'ts*) and summary checklists of guidelines are provided. Essentially, the text can be viewed as a virtual *cookbook* of the appropriate ingredients needed to construct a successful grant proposal.

Therefore, this text is not only highly relevant for early-stage investigators including graduate students, medical students/residents, and postdoctoral fellows, but also valuable for more experienced faculty, clinicians, epidemiologists, and other health professionals who cannot seem to break the barrier to NIH-funded research. This book can serve as the primary text for courses in grant and proposal writing and as an accompanying text to courses in research methods, epidemiology, preventive medicine, statistics, and population health, as well as a personal resource.

Chapter 1, *Ten Top Tips for Successful Proposal Writing*, reviews what I believe are the ten most important factors in developing a grant proposal. The text is then divided into three parts. Part One, Preparing to Write the Proposal, begins with Chapter 2, *Starting a Dissertation Proposal*, which provides tips on selecting a dissertation topic, strategies for selecting and interacting with a dissertation committee, and a plan of action with suggested timelines. Chapter 3, *How to Develop and Write Hypotheses*, outlines strategies for developing your ideas into effective hypotheses. The often daunting task of conducting the literature search is made manageable through the step-by-step approach provided in Chapter 4, *Conducting the Literature Search*. Guidelines for writing with clarity and precision are provided in Chapter 5, *Scientific Writing*.

Part Two, The Proposal: Section by Section, follows the structure of a research proposal beginning with crafting your *Specific Aims* (Chapter 6) to leverage a research gap that your proposal will address and then continuing through *Background and Significance Section* (Chapter 7), *Summarizing Preliminary Studies* (Chapter 8), *Study Design and Methods* (Chapter 9), *Data Analysis Plan* (Chapter 10), and *Power and Sample Size* (Chapter 11).

Potential study limitations and a fourfold approach to strategically present and minimize these limitations are reviewed in Chapter 12, *Review of Bias and Confounding*, and Chapter 13, *How to Present Limitations and Alternatives*. Issues specific to pilot and feasibility studies, often excellent topics for early grant proposals, are described in Chapter 14, *Reproducibility and Validity Studies*. Techniques for crafting your abstract, potentially the most critical component of a grant proposal, are discussed in Chapter 15, *Abstracts and Titles*. Chapter 16, *Presenting Your Proposal Orally*, covers preparing the visual and oral content of a proposal presentation.

Part Three, Grantsmanship, provides strategies for putting together a winning NIH proposal and is kicked off by Chapter 17, *Choosing the Right Funding Source*, which outlines how to develop a grant funding plan. Chapter 18, *Submission of the Grant Proposal*, continues by providing strategic tips for each component of the grant application. Chapter 19, *Review Process*, describes the review criteria for research, career, and fellowship awards; ways to maximize your chances for a successful review; and potential reasons for rejection. Finally, Chapter 20, *Resubmission of the Grant Proposal*, goes on to describe the pathway to resubmitting your grant proposal along with strategic tips for how to be highly responsive to reviewer concerns—the key criteria in a successful resubmission.

Throughout the chapters, examples from successfully funded proposals in the field appear in shaded boxes. These excerpts have been edited to remove reference to specific investigators and study sites; details of the study design have often been modified. Therefore, superscripts in the text demonstrate where references should be placed, but actual references are not included. In this manner, the examples focus on the structure and techniques used in scientific writing and can be broadly applied to a variety of grant topics.

While the focus of the text is on principles to guide the pursuit of funding primarily from NIH, these principles also apply to other federal and state agencies as well as foundations. NIH, however, remains the largest funder of biomedical research in the world, and NIH funds research in just about every area that is remotely related to human health and disease. It is also important to note that this book is not designed to teach you research methodology or statistics; readers without exposure to these areas would profit by referring to an introductory text. Instead, the focus of the text is on how to convert your research ideas into a successful grant proposal. Keep in mind that in science, if one is to make an impact, it is not sufficient to reach the truth; you must persuade your colleagues of it.

Finally, I would like to acknowledge the help I received in bringing this book to completion. The concepts in this book owe much to the work and ideas of my mentors, colleagues, and former students and were greatly informed by the grant review panels on which I have served. This book is also in debt to earlier courses that I took at Harvard and is a tribute to my mentor Dr. Meir Stampfer. In addition, crucial input on specific chapters has been provided by Drs. Michael D. Schmidt, Amy E. Haskins, Sarah Goff, Larissa R. Brunner Huber, Scott Chasan-Taber, Renée Turzanski Fortner, and Tiffany A. Moore Simas. JCT contributed her formidable formatting skills. The support of my indomitable daughters, Adina and Jessie, has been unwavering. Lastly, this book is dedicated to my husband Scott, the composer of the best proposal I have ever heard.

Author

Dr. Lisa Chasan-Taber is a professor of epidemiology and the former associate dean for research in the School of Public Health and Health Sciences at the University of Massachusetts Amherst. She is a reproductive epidemiologist and a nationally and internationally recognized expert on physical activity during pregnancy. Early in her career, Dr. Chasan-Taber received the American Diabetes Association Career Development Award, and she has consistently been funded by the National Institutes of Health (NIH) as a principal investigator for the last 15 years. Dr. Chasan-Taber was a standing member of the NIH Infectious Disease, Reproductive Health, Asthma, and Pulmonary Epidemiology (IRAP) Study Section and has served on multiple national review panels, as a mentor on NIH Research Career Development Awards, and as the principal investigator of Mentoring Grants designed to provide early-career faculty with successful grant-writing strategies. For more than 15 years, she has taught a class on proposal and grant writing for epidemiology graduate students, which serves as the basis for this book. She has been recognized for her research through the Chancellor's Medal, the highest recognition bestowed to faculty by the university, and for her teaching excellence and innovative approaches to instruction through the College Outstanding Teacher Award. Chasan-Taber received her postdoctoral and doctoral training in epidemiology at the Harvard School of Public Health, a master's in public health from the University of Massachusetts, and a bachelor of arts from the University of Pennsylvania.

Ten Top Tips for Successful Proposal Writing

If I were asked to distill my proposal writing advice down to the 10 most important tips, the following would be my list. These best practices in grantsmanship also apply to any type of proposal writing.

1.1 TIP #1: START EARLY

These days, funding is more difficult to obtain than it has ever been before. However, graduate students and early-career faculty have certain advantages upon which they can capitalize. In fact, given the current challenging economic climate, making the most of these advantages is now more important than ever.

Doctoral and postdoctoral granting mechanisms as well as early-career awards provide the highest chances for success. A primary advantage of these mechanisms is that they typically do not require significant preliminary data. This is fortuitous, as you are unlikely to have preliminary data at this point in your career. Instead, funding decisions for these awards rely most heavily on your promise and potential as a candidate.

This potential is indicated by three items:

- Your education to date (including prior publications and project-related experience)
- The mentors with which you have surrounded yourself
- The public health importance of your topic

A key advantage of these funding mechanisms is that, unlike larger grant awards, you will be competing in a smaller pool of investigators all of whom will be at a comparable stage in their careers as yourself. This advantage should not be minimized, as it avoids the risk of competing against senior investigators who already have established track records. As a senior investigator once said, "Avoid competing against the 'big boys and girls' as long as you can!" This advantage that you now have will quickly be over after several years pass by and you find yourself no longer eligible for these early-career investigator awards.

Therefore, if you are a graduate student, seek out grant mechanisms designed for graduate students. Such grants include National Institutes of Health (NIH) predoctoral (F31) and postdoctoral (F32) fellowship awards. If you are an early-career faculty member, look for grants designed for early-career faculty members. These may include small seed-money grants provided by your university (e.g., Faculty Research Grants) or foundation grants targeted for career development (e.g., the American Diabetes Association Career Award, the March of Dimes Starter Scholar Award). In addition, NIH offers career development awards such as the K series awards. At the same time, always be on the lookout for opportunities to collaborate as a coinvestigator on other applications where the principal investigator (PI) is a senior, established investigator. If you need help identifying these programs, most universities have resources to help you find grants relevant to your interest area and level. Online services are available as well. Chapter 17, *Choosing the Right Funding Source*, provides an in-depth discussion of how to locate these opportunities.

1.2 TIP #2: CREATE A VISION WITH THE HELP OF A MENTOR

In spite of my advice in Tip #1 to start small, this does not mean that you should not have a vision. Indeed, it is critical that postdoctoral fellows and early-career faculty have a big vision. Each small grant—be it a seed grant, a postdoctoral fellowship, or an early-career award—should be viewed as providing preliminary data for one or two of the specific aims of your ultimate larger grant. Typically, large grants are funded by the NIH R01 mechanism.

Therefore, early on in the process, it is critical to try to envision your ultimate large project. For example, let's assume that a typical R01 contains three to five specific aims. Once you are able to envision these aims, your next steps become clear: Step by step, you start *biting off* small chunks of this larger grant through writing small grants designed to support *one or two* of these ultimate aims. These small grants should not be designed to provide the definitive answer to these aims but instead to show that the aims are feasible and/or provide preliminary data in thier support. These small grants will be limited by smaller sample sizes and budgets, but will be able to show proof of principal—that you can *pull it off* (see Tip #5).

Seek the advice of your mentor A key factor in developing a vision of your ultimate large project is the advice of your mentor(s). If you do not currently have a mentor, speak to your department chair and ask if they can provide you with a mentor. If not, it is usually considered acceptable to seek out your own mentor. Indeed, many early-career faculty will assemble a *mentorship team*, each member of which can provide guidance in different career aspects (e.g., a teaching mentor, a research mentor). Consider both on-site and off-site faculty as potential mentors. In this age of teleconferencing and e-mail, I often find that I communicate more with my off-site mentors than with those directly down the hall. You can use web-based resources such as Community of Science (COS) (http://pivot.cos.com/) and NIH Reporter (http://projectreporter.nih.gov/reporter.cfm) to help locate a potential mentor by searching on your topic and identifying a list of PI names. Then view the grant track record by which these investigators achieved their aims. Ask yourself if it matches up with where you want to be in your grantmaking career.

Key pitfalls to avoid Early-career faculty want to be successful and, as such, are often tempted by the wish to immediately make a big impact and *land a big grant*.

Others are under pressure from their institutions and department chairs to immediately apply for a large grant (e.g., an NIH R01) without a track record of smaller grant funding. In my experience as an NIH review panel member, this approach is almost certainly destined to fail. Review panels often see a large grant as the culmination of a growing body of work. They want to see evidence of this stairway to success and it's your job to demonstrate that you have been on this stairway. You do this by showing your successful procurement and management of previous smaller grants, as well as the translation of these grants into publications. A desirable grant-funding history starts from small seed grants progressing to larger and larger awards in a cumulative fashion. Chapter 17, *Choosing the Right Funding Source*, provides example plans for a steady trajectory of grants from small to large. While it is always tempting to skip to the last page of a novel to see what happens, one needs to earn one's way there.

There are certainly some exceptions to this rule. For example, you may be an early-career faculty member within a research team that already has a track record in your area. If so, you could take advantage of their expertise by including them as coinvestigator(s) or even as a co-PI on your proposal. In addition, because they are participating on the grant, you gain the advantage of including their preliminary data in your application. However, as described in Chapter 19, *Review Process*, and Chapter 20, *Resubmission of the Grant Proposal*, one of the key criteria upon which a grant is scored is the expertise of the PI. Regardless of your investigative team, if you are the PI, the reviewers will be looking for your track record in managing a large grant. It is unlikely you will be able to provide this assurance of feasibility at an early stage in your career.

1.3 TIP #3: LOOK AT WHO AND WHAT THEY FUNDED BEFORE YOU

Funding agencies will often make publically available a list of prior grant awardees. These lists may include the grant title, recipient name, amount awarded, and institution. If the granting agency does not provide a list of past grant recipients, your own institution's grants and contracts office may have a list of investigators on your campus who have obtained these same grants. Look over this list and see if you or your mentors know any of these investigators.

This is useful for several reasons. First, it shows the interest of the funding agency in funding research in epidemiology and preventive medicine. Some funding agencies simply don't have the interest or track record in funding population-based research and instead limit their funding to laboratory studies (*bench science*). Second, it is reasonable to consider asking successful fundees to share their applications with you, particularly if you, or your mentors, recognize any names on the fundee list or see that they are from your institution. Reassure these successfully funded investigators that you are simply seeking a model for the appropriate scope and depth of the research plan, not the actual content of their aims. When framed in this manner, people are typically willing to share.

Funding websites are a rich source of information
In addition to posting prior grant awardees on their website, funding agencies may also post a list of prior and current grant reviewers and their affiliations. Go through this list and review the expertise of these investigators. Ask yourself if their expertise overlaps with your study aims and methodology. For example, are any of these investigators population health researchers? Are any from similar departments/divisions to yours? It would be a high-risk proposition to write a proposal for a foundation that does not include investigators in epidemiology and preventive medicine on their review panels.

1.4 TIP #4: SPEND HALF YOUR TIME ON THE ABSTRACT AND SPECIFIC AIMS

The bulk of your writing time should be spent refining your abstract and specific aims. Indeed, writers of successful grant applications typically report that 50% of their time was spent on revising and rewriting their specific aims (Figure 1.1). The specific aims should be the first item that you write when you *set pen to paper*, prior to writing a literature review or methodology section. Early in the process, send a one-page sketch of your study design and aims—in the manner of an NIH grant—to your mentor and coinvestigators with the goal of kicking off an iterative process of rewriting, revising, and rereviewing. In addition, it is critical that these aims be understandable by anyone with a scientific background. Chapter 3, *How to Develop and Write Hypotheses*, discusses strategies and writing conventions for developing hypotheses and specific aims including exercises and annotated examples and tips.

Another excellent resource is the NIH Reporter (http://projectreporter.nih.gov/reporter.cfm). This site can be invaluable in helping you to formulate the scope of

Steps
Draft aims
Calculate power
Calculate budget

FIGURE 1.1 The first 3 steps in proposal writing.

your grant. This site lists abstracts of both active and prior NIH awards. Because these awards have all successfully been funded, they serve as excellent examples. Viewing funded abstracts can help you answer the following questions: "How many aims did the investigators include?" "What was their sample size?" You can limit your search to particular key terms as well as particular grant mechanisms (e.g., smaller and larger awards). The output, in addition to listing the abstract, will also provide the name of the review panel and the NIH institute. Therefore, *surfing* the NIH Reporter is not only useful for both the smaller grant mechanisms but also for envisioning the ultimate larger grant. More on NIH is included in Part Three "Grantsmanship."

One reason that specific aims are so critical is the nature of the peer review process, described in more detail in Chapter 19, *Review Process*. Briefly, because only three to four reviewers are assigned as primary and secondary reviewers of your grant, the majority of reviewers on the review panel may only read your abstract and/or specific aims during the 10–20 min time period that the grant is discussed. Therefore, it is critical that the aims not only provide a snapshot of the entire study but also convey what is novel. Chapter 15, *Abstracts and Titles*, provides tips and strategies for how to write, and what merits inclusion, in your abstract. See Figure 1.1.

After drafting your aims, the second step in this process is to calculate your statistical power to achieve these aims. This will help you to answer the question, "Will your sample size provide you with sufficient power to detect a difference between groups, if there is truly a difference?" If you are basing your grant upon a preexisting dataset, your sample size is typically fixed, and the question of whether or not you have adequate power can be answered quickly. A negative answer, while disappointing, can quickly and efficiently result in a change in study aims.

If instead you are proposing to launch a new study and recruit participants, you can choose the sample size you need to achieve sufficient power. However, in this case, progressing to Step #3 of calculating the budget will be critical. A common pitfall of new investigators is to be too ambitious—proposing a larger sample size than they have the budget and experience to handle. Chapter 11, *Power and Sample Size*, provides user-friendly approaches to power and sample size calculations, available software, and annotated examples with strategies and tips.

Therefore, the third step is to evaluate if your budget can afford your required sample size. The number of participants will have an immediate impact on the costs of conducting your study. Such costs include the number of assays, interviewer time for recruitment and follow-up, as well as the cost of participant incentives. Also, ask yourself whether your study site can feasibly provide this number of participants. For example, does the hospital actually see that number of patients per day/week/year? Are that many patients likely to be eligible *and* agree to participate? Such questions of feasibility can be answered by your own preliminary work, by that of your coinvestigators, or by other investigators at your proposed study site. Alternatively, if you are proposing a pilot grant, you can clearly state that the goal of your pilot is to assess recruitment and eligibility rates to calculate power for a larger grant submission. Chapter 8, *Summarizing Preliminary Studies*, describes this approach in greater detail.

Now, in light of everything you have learned from Steps 1, 2, and 3, and incorporating your mentors' and colleagues' feedback, go back and refine the aims and start the process over again. Once you have settled on the aims, you will find that writing the rest of the application will flow easily. As described in Part Two of this text, "The Proposal: Section by Section," each section of a well-written grant proposal flows directly from and mirrors components of the specific aims.

1.5 TIP #5: SHOW THAT YOU CAN PULL IT OFF

Showing that you can logistically and feasibly conduct the proposed grant is critical if you are a graduate student or early-career faculty. Assurance that you can *pull it off* is a key factor for which the reviewer is seeking reassurance and can be accomplished through several techniques. First, if possible, collaborate with senior investigators who have conducted similar grants in similar populations. Their involvement on your proposal will be a critical factor supporting your potential for success.

Capitalize upon your coinvestigators It is important that these coinvestigators do not appear in name only. Show established working relationships with these investigators via either coauthored publications (or submitted publications under review), copresentations, or an established mentoring relationship (e.g., as part of a training grant). Another way to show an ongoing relationship with coinvestigators is to list grants on which you are both investigators or consultants. Of course, much of this information will appear in your biosketches, but you cannot rely upon the reviewers to connect the dots between you and your coinvestigators. Instead, make it easy for the reviewers by pointing out this prior collaboration in your Preliminary Studies Section. Specific examples of this grantsmanship strategy as well as others are discussed in detail in Chapter 8, *Summarizing Preliminary Studies*.

A second way to show that you can *pull it off* is to present evidence that you have conducted smaller feasibility studies as mentioned in Tip #1. Such feasibility studies can provide key data on a number of factors. They can provide evidence that you, as a PI, are able to recruit subjects and collect data. Such preliminary data have the added benefit of providing key figures necessary for calculating power and sample size for your larger grants. Participant satisfaction surveys administered in a feasibility study can provide data on the acceptability of your methods. Validation studies of your proposed methods (as described in Chapter 14, *Reproducibility and Validity Studies*) can provide assurance that a study based upon these methods will work. In summary, ideally, the goal is to show proof of principal.

Avoid interdependent aims It is important to acknowledge here that in earlier, more economically advantaged times, it was considered acceptable for a large NIH R01 grant to include pilot studies within its aims. However, in the current climate, reviewers do not look favorably upon this approach. They naturally ask, "What if the pilot study finds that the methods are not successful? How would the investigator accomplish the subsequent aims of the project?" For example, imagine if aim 1 proposes to conduct a validation study of the questionnaire to be used in aims 2 and 3. If aim 1 subsequently fails to find that the questionnaire is valid, then how can the remainder of the project proceed? These are termed interdependent aims and reviewers often consider such aims to be a fatal flaw of a proposal. In Chapter 6, *Specific Aims*, I describe how to create a strong set of study aims, avoiding this as well as other pitfalls.

1.6 TIP #6: YOUR METHODS SHOULD MATCH YOUR AIMS AND VICE VERSA

A typical pitfall that early-career investigators fall into is to fail to include methods to address each of their study aims or, alternatively, to include additional methods that do not correspond to any study aims. These scenarios can simply be summed up as (1) proposing to study A and B, but only including methods for A, or (2) proposing to study A, but including methods designed to measure A and B.

The former situation will be viewed by reviewers as an important omission. For mentored career award applications, in particular, this mistake may be attributed to the mentor, which in some ways is even worse than having the error attributed to you. That is, this mistake can be interpreted as an indicator of poor mentorship either due to minimal effort by the mentor (e.g., in failure to spend time to adequately review your proposal) or due to the inability of the mentor to detect this problem at all. It may be viewed as reflective of the future amount and content of mentorship that you would be receiving over the course of the grant period if awarded.

Avoid being overly ambitious
The latter situation, in which the grant describes more analyses than are necessary to conduct the stated aims, is a great temptation of early-career investigators who are often driven to demonstrate to the reviewers how rich the dataset will be and therefore how many questions they can answer. However, this approach can be viewed as overly ambitious. An *ambitious* application is one of the most common reason for reviewers to give an application a poor score (or to triage the application, as described in Chapter 19, *Review Process*). Instead, it is much more impressive to exercise restraint and have a focused plan with a data analysis section directly tied to the specific aims.

However, there are some specific situations where it is reasonable to mention additional methods that do not correspond to the proposed aims. For example, in a small grant proposal (e.g., a seed grant), it is often reasonable to state that some data will be collected solely to support subsequent grant applications. However, this is only considered appropriate when it is highly efficient both in terms of study design and participant burden to collect this information in real time, as opposed to returning to participants at a later point in time. The application could state,

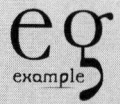

> *e.g.* example
> While we are not including genetic aims within this proposal, these stored samples will be available to support the investigation of future hypotheses. Similarly, placentas will be collected and stored for future hypotheses.

In this example, it is clear that trying to collect this information at a later point in time would not be feasible, either because the samples would no longer be available or because disease may have already occurred and thereby influenced levels of these samples. In these situations, a data analysis plan would not be included for these proposed future aims.

So, moving forward, there are several ways to ensure that your methods match up with your aims and vice versa. The most traditional approach (and the approach that is most kind to your reviewer) is to copy your aims verbatim from the specific aims page and repeat them, in italics, in the data analysis section. Below each italicized aim, you will insert the relevant statistical analysis designed to achieve this aim. Alternatively, another acceptable approach is to format the structure of the proposal sequentially such that aim #1 is immediately followed by the methods to achieve aim #1; aim #2 follows, and is immediately followed with the methods to achieve aim #2, etc. This approach tends to only be efficient when each aim has a distinct methodologic and data analysis plan. Otherwise, you run the risk of repetition of similar methods and wasteful use of precious space. In Chapter 9, *Study Design and Methods*, and Chapter 10, *Data Analysis Plan*, I describe tips for efficient writing of methods and data analyses sections corresponding to study aims.

1.7 TIP #7: A PROPOSAL CAN NEVER HAVE TOO MANY FIGURES OR TABLES

In general, the more figures and tables in a grant application, the better. Not only does the process of creating these figures and tables help you to crystallize your specific aims and study methods, but they are also kinder to the reviewers. As compared to dense text, tables and figures are easier for the reviewer to digest and help them more quickly grasp your methods. This fact should not be underestimated given how pressed the reviewer is for time. Figures and tables also demonstrate your grasp of your proposal and your organizational skills. They can save space by reducing the text—critical for the page limitations of most proposals.

Indeed, the inclusion of figures and tables is relevant for every section of a grant application. For example, in the specific aims section, a figure showing how the specific aims interrelate is always appreciated by reviewers (Chapter 6, *Specific Aims*). Another key figure displaying your anticipated results can be placed in the Background and Significance section (see Chapter 7, *Background and Significance Section*). Some reviewers feel that this latter figure is essential. Other examples include study design figures, tables listing study variables, and statistical power displays. The grant application often ends with a timeline figure—showing each study activity and the quarters during which it will be conducted. Chapter 9, *Study Design and Methods* shows examples of key tables and figures that can be used throughout the proposal, ranging from specific aims tables and study design figures to tables for the data analysis and power/sample size sections.

1.8 TIP #8: SEEK EXTERNAL REVIEW PRIOR TO SUBMISSION

It is generally acknowledged that a local mock study section review almost doubles your chances of funding. A *study section* is defined as the NIH review panel that conducts the initial scientific merit review of research applications. *Mock* study sections simulate a real study section by following the grant review process as closely as possible.

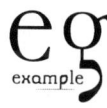

Example procedures for conducting a mock study section:

Early-career faculty will submit a proposal for review using the NIH submission guidelines. The review panel will be made up of senior faculty who have served on NIH study sections, are familiar with the area of study, and have a track record of mentorship. Each proposal will be reviewed by 3 section members. Faculty will receive the written reviews of their proposals and the NIH scoring system will be applied (1–9).

To provide even greater mentorship, a mock NIH study section can be modified in a few key ways from a true NIH study section. For example, early-career faculty can be invited to sit in on mock study sections as silent observers. While it may be stressful to watch the reviewers discuss your proposal, you will experience first-hand the dynamics of study section deliberations and the proposal review process becomes demystified. After the session is over, many mock sessions schedule a short debriefing period to allow early-career faculty to ask questions and talk directly with the reviewers. This differs substantively from a true study section after which you will only receive written comments from the reviewers. NIH posts video tapes of mock study sections on their website. These are invaluable to watch.

Another useful way to get constructive feedback on your proposal is to participate in a *chalk-talk* forum. These consist of informal seminars to discuss your research ideas and/or specific aims early in the process—prior to writing a full proposal. If your department does not currently offer such a forum, suggest that they start one. Chapter 16, *Presenting Your Proposal Orally*, provides a step-by-step guide for creating an oral and visual presentation of your proposal.

Some departments will fund early-career faculty to attend local and national grant-writing workshops and will compensate outside scientists, with expertise on the proposed topic, to review and critique your grant proposals. Your office of grants and contracts may sponsor a grantsmanship seminar series or brown bag lunch session in which you can participate. Lastly, many departments will enlist the services of a grant writer. By encouraging you to concisely convey your aims and methods as clearly as possible, the best grant writers will help you to further refine your specific aims and convey the potential impact of your findings.

Real-world (not mock) submission and resubmission processes are carefully described in a step-by-step manner with accompanying strategic tips in Chapter 18, *Submission of the Grant Proposal*, Chapter 19, *Review Process*, and Chapter 20, *Resubmission of the Grant Proposal*.

1.9 TIP #9: BE KIND TO YOUR REVIEWERS

Reviewers are assigned a large number of applications to read and discuss. This task is in addition to their own responsibilities as a researcher themselves. So, a happy reviewer should be one of your top goals.

Subheadings should match review criteria
The most effective way to make a reviewer happy is to help them complete their review forms. Every reviewer, regardless of funding agency, is required to use a structured critique form. For example, NIH reviewers are required to write bullet points on the strengths and weaknesses of overall impact, significance, investigators, innovation, approach, and environment. However, the formatting requirements of NIH grant applications do not require clearly labeled sections for each of these criteria. Therefore, the first way to be *kind* to your reviewers is by using these key terms as subheadings in your application.

For example, the reviewer must describe whether they believe your grant is innovative. You may have thought that the innovative aspects of your application were obvious and therefore failed to include a specific subsection on *innovation*. This is risky. Not only may the reviewer fail to see all the innovative aspects of your proposal, but you run the risk that they may not deduce any innovation at all. Simply including a clearly labeled subsection on innovation will save the reviewer time. It does not guarantee that they will agree with you but provides a basis for their draft of that section in their critique. In Chapter 7, *Background and Significance Section*, I describe tips for writing the innovation section.

Highlight key sentences
A second key kindness is to bold, or otherwise highlight, one key sentence in each paragraph of the Background and Significance section. Indeed, the act of searching for this key sentence provides the added benefit of ensuring that each paragraph does indeed have a key point. With space at a premium in grant proposals (e.g., current limits for the research strategy for smaller NIH grants can be as low as six pages), each paragraph needs to count.

Another way to be kind to the reviewers is in the Preliminary Studies section. The description of each preliminary study should end with a sentence specifying the rationale for why it is relevant to the current proposal. This summary sentence removes the burden on the reviewer. It is your job to connect the dots between your preliminary work and how it relates to or supports your proposed aims. The act of creating these sentences also serves a dual purpose of ensuring that you are not including extraneous preliminary findings not directly relevant to your aims. Examples of such summaries are provided in Chapter 8, *Summarizing Preliminary Studies*.

Another way of being kind to the reviewer is by inserting a brief summary paragraph at the very beginning of the Methods section that encapsulates all the key features of the study design. This paragraph would give the sample size, study population, study design (e.g., prospective cohort case–control study, cross-sectional study), the key assessment tools to be used (e.g., self-reported questionnaire, plasma samples, medical record data), and any other key features of your study methods. This will help the reviewer to concisely present your study to the review panel. Examples of such summaries are provided in Chapter 9, *Study Design and Methods*.

The same person cannot write a proposal *and* review it for clarity

Regardless of how carefully you reread your grant, and no matter how conscientious you are, simply by virtue of your familiarity with the material, you will not be able to review it for final clarity. One common approach is to ask your colleagues to read the application. It is well accepted that a well-written application should be readable and understandable by anyone with scientific knowledge. Therefore, it is not necessary that your readers have expertise in your area of interest and perhaps even preferable if they do not.

While this is often surprising to hear, it is important to note that some of your assigned grant reviewers may not have expertise in your area of interest. That is, while one reviewer may have a specific background in your area, others are assigned based on their expertise in the proposed methodology (e.g., epidemiology), and others are assigned to review the statistical analysis section. For example, a grant designed to identify risk factors for infertility may be assigned to the following three reviewers: (1) a physician who has a track record of publications on *in vitro* fertilization techniques, (2) an epidemiologist who has conducted prospective cohort studies among infertile women, and (3) a statistician. It is even possible that the physician or the epidemiologist will not have direct experience with infertility but are instead more generalist reproductive or perinatal epidemiologists.

However, it is reassuring to note that, if your proposal is well written, even a generalist reviewer will be able to assess (1) whether your goals are clearly stated, (2) whether your proposal clearly justifies how it extends prior work in the field, (3) what is innovative about your proposal, as well as (4) the impact of your potential findings on public health and clinical practice. In recent years, the last point has become a critical factor in funding decisions. With the recent revision in the NIH grant review process, reviewers now prioritize the overall impact. This aspect alone is often the most critical in the assigned score for an application. In Chapter 7, *Background and Significance Section*, I outline tips for writing this section. Chapter 19, *Review Process*, describes how these sections are considered in the review process.

In summary, the underpinning of all of these kindnesses is to remember that it is not the job of the reviewer to justify the importance of your proposal but instead your job to lay out your rationale and give the reviewers the opportunity to critique it. You do the work; they conduct the critique. This is the recipe for a happy reviewer.

1.10 TIP #10: IF AT ALL POSSIBLE, CHOOSE A TOPIC THAT YOU FIND INTERESTING!

There is nothing less conducive to your future success and day-to-day productivity than choosing a topic that you do not find interesting. However, given today's difficult grant-funding climate, the only way to ensure grant success is to have several proposals in the pipeline and/or under review at once. In this way, even if all the initiatives are not the most interesting to you, at least one of them will likely be. It is even more preferable if these initiatives fit within an overall research theme (as discussed in Tip #2: Create a Vision) so that, in the wonderful event that all are funded, they can all serve as pilot data for your larger R01-type grant.

Another way to ensure success is to also serve as a coinvestigator on a grant led by one of your senior colleagues while you are beginning your own independent research track. The advantages of serving as a coinvestigator on ongoing or new proposals submitted by your more established colleagues should not be underestimated. These grants will require a somewhat reduced effort on your part (in comparison to being PI). In addition, because ongoing projects were underway before you joined, you can also anticipate an earlier payoff in terms of timing of published manuscripts. Joining an established research project also provides you with the opportunity to apply for supplementary funding that builds upon the aims (and the established methods and successes) of these ongoing grants.

All this being said, developing your own independent line of research proposals is important. Indeed, one criterion for tenure and promotion at many research institutes is movement away from the area of your dissertation work and development of independence in your own research aims. If the work of your departmental colleagues does not relate to your area, then other collegial relationships and sources of grant data can be found in many locations—be they across campus or even across the state or country (see Chapter 17, *Choosing the Right Funding Source*). Luckily, in these days of electronic communication, Skype, and other electronic media, it has become increasingly easy to communicate with colleagues at other institutions electronically.

In summary, these 10 top tips for successful proposal writing should help to launch you on your proposal writing journey!

PART ONE

Preparing to Write the Proposal

Starting a Dissertation Proposal

2

A dissertation proposal and a grant proposal share many factors in common. Indeed, a strategic approach taken by many graduate schools is to have the development of a dissertation proposal mimic the process of developing a grant proposal. In this manner, the graduate student obtains experience with grant writing within the supportive context of his or her graduate education.

Using this approach, the dissertation committee serves as a proxy for your coinvestigators and mentors on your future grants. The proposal defense serves as a proxy for a grant proposal presentation. Input from the committee can be considered similar to receiving reviewer comments. Responding to such comments will give the graduate student valuable experience with the most challenging task that they will face in the future as grant writers.

This chapter reviews guidelines relevant to the **graduate student** including tips on selecting a topic and strategies for selecting and interacting with your committee chair and members. The chapter continues to walk through each step in the dissertation process, providing an overall timeline for completion. Note that these functions are to be carried out in conformity with the guidelines of your own graduate school.

It is important to note that Chapter 17, *Choosing the Right Funding Source*, provides similar guidance for postdoctoral fellows and early career faculty but tailored to the goal of seeking and obtaining grant funding.

2.1 PURPOSE OF THE DISSERTATION

A dissertation proposal represents the onset of the culmination of the PhD degree program. The dissertation itself provides the graduate student with an opportunity to:

- Develop an individual research project under the guidance of a faculty committee
- Gain experience in problem identification, data analysis, and interpretation
- Develop methodological and technical skills

- Demonstrate competence in applying theory and appropriate methodology to investigating a problem
- Establish professional working relationships with the members of the dissertation committee

2.2 PURPOSE OF THE DISSERTATION PROPOSAL

At most institutions, the **written dissertation proposal** defines an area of interest, describes the research problem and method of investigation, and outlines anticipated limitations and the significance of the inquiry. The dissertation proposal essentially represents a demonstrated readiness to conduct research on a specific topic.

The **oral presentation of the dissertation proposal**, if required, provides a collegial forum within which to present the major points of the proposal and defend the planned approaches. At this time, the student is expected to demonstrate considerable skill in communicating the importance of the research and the validity of their research plan.

Some institutions offer a **course** designed to help doctoral students create and develop their dissertation proposal. Indeed, it was such a course that led to the development of this text. At best, such a course standardizes expectations and gives students tools for how to achieve them. The presence of such a course greatly increases the probability that students will complete their dissertation and graduate in a timely manner. See the suggested timeline at the end of the chapter.

2.3 STEP #1: PRELIMINARY QUALIFYING EXAMS

At most institutions, the dissertation proposal process cannot start until the graduate student passes a preliminary comprehensive examination consisting of a written and oral component. If dissertation work is begun prior to that time, the student is *at risk* for any investment of time or resources.

The format of the written examination varies from institution to institution as well as from department to department. It may be an open- or closed-book examination consisting of questions prepared by each member of the dissertation committee, a take-home exam designed as a mini-grant proposal, a series of questions requiring a literature search, or other variations of the above as long as it is a written exam of a quality generally accepted as sufficient for the degree of PhD.

The intent of the examination is not only to determine the extent of knowledge that the student possesses but to be a learning experience and, even more importantly, to indicate to the student the limitations of her/his knowledge.

At some institutions, an oral qualifying exam, not related to the dissertation proposal topic, follows completion of the written component. The timing of this oral qualifying exam is also specific to the institution.

Regardless, the outcome of the qualifying exam is typically communicated by the major professor to the graduate program director or department head who in turn communicates it to the graduate school. Then the dissertation proposal process can begin!

2.4 STEP #2: SELECTING A DISSERTATION TOPIC

The process of coming up with a topic for their dissertation is often quite daunting for students. Planning for dissertation research usually begins with the informal exploration of topics that are of interest to the student and to a faculty member who is likely to be named as chair of the dissertation committee.

Consider possible topics based upon areas of personal interest and discussions with your academic advisor and other faculty. Such a brainstorm session could begin by answering the following questions:

- Where do you hope to obtain your data?
- What is your exposure of interest?
- What is your outcome of interest?

A review of theses and dissertations recently completed by other students will help give you an idea of the range, scope, and depth of proposal topics consistent with your department's expectations.

An important caveat It is important to note that while the topic should be of interest to you, your dissertation does not have to be identical to the topic of your future career. Often, practicality in the form of what data are available takes precedence over the perfect fit of the dissertation topic with your interests. It is reassuring to note that one criterion for tenure and promotion at many research institutes is movement away from the area of your dissertation work and development of independence in terms of your own research aims. So, be careful not to take the choice of dissertation topic so seriously that you fail to take the plunge and select one!

2.4.1 Ascertain If Original Data Collection Is Required

Typically, for students in epidemiology and preventive medicine, the selection of a dissertation topic relies on access to data.

Sources of data for dissertations range from:

- Original data collection
- Secondary datasets
  - Publically available datasets
  - Datasets assembled via faculty grant-funded research in your department
- Internships or practica in the field

Early in the process, ascertain whether your institution requires that the dissertation involve the collection, on your part, of **original data**. Historically, it was feasible for doctoral students to design and conduct their own small studies to collect original data upon which their dissertation would be based. In more recent times, however, this is often not feasible due to several barriers. The most important barrier is the decrease in availability of funds for dissertation work given the overall decrease in NIH funding. As described in Chapter 17, *Choosing the Right Funding Source*, doctoral students are eligible for training grants, fellowships, and loan repayment programs, which may provide funding for their dissertation work. However, for doctoral students, the time to submit a proposal to a funding agency and then revise and resubmit the application is often prohibitive. Similarly, the time lag required for IRB review of a dissertation designed to collect original data from human participants may also significantly extend the time to completion of the degree.

Some institutions provide internal funding for doctoral students to collect original data. However, the sample size required by most studies in epidemiology and preventive medicine to detect a statistically significant/clinically significant difference, as well as the need for follow-up time in the case of a prospective study, typically requires a budget that is prohibitively large.

Therefore, a second source of data for doctoral dissertations is **secondary datasets**. These datasets could be publically available datasets such as the Behavioral Risk Factor Surveillance Survey (BRFSS). Sometimes, such datasets also require a proposal and approval process that should be factored into your timeline. However, in general, use of such datasets is fairly straightforward. Other datasets available to you could be from ongoing grant-funded studies run by the faculty in your department. Therefore, it is important to explore the option of participating in ongoing funded research early in the dissertation proposal process.

A third source of dissertation data is via an **internship or practicum program**. Many programs in epidemiology and preventive medicine require that their students participate in a practicum. Data from such programs could serve as the basis of the dissertation with the permission of the practicum advisor. This typically requires that the dissertation hypothesis address a question that does not overlap with the main hypothesis for which the data were already collected. Analysis of such a question may also require IRB approval, but again the process should not be as lengthy as the data will have already been collected.

2.4.2 Pep Talk

Given the constraints on data sources and funding mentioned above, the dataset available to a doctoral student may be limited in size and/or scope. I always advise my graduate students that they will be fortunate if their doctoral dissertation is fraught with limitations. In this way, they have the *opportunity* to face these limitations in the context of a supportive environment of dissertation committee members and senior advisors. What better place to practice these skills than surrounded by mentors? Once students graduate, and have embarked on their own career, they may never again have this level of support.

Imagine a student who had a simple dissertation with few, if any, study limitations. Let's say they had access to a large prospective dataset with thousands of participants and comprehensive objective data on both exposures and outcomes of interest. Once this student graduates, and finds themselves in the field creating their own line of research, they will be facing the challenging issues of bias and confounding—perhaps for the first time!

Understanding the strengths and limitations of the methodology selected should be emphasized in the dissertation proposal process and will serve the student well in their future as a grant writer. Indeed, the best grant proposals delineate limitations and alternatives should problems arise (as described in Chapter 13, *How to Present Limitations and Alternatives*). Thus, the faculty considers the process of carrying out the dissertation, and the integration of knowledge by the student, to be just as, or more, important than the study findings.

2.5 STEP #3: CHOOSING A CHAIR

Once a specific topic or problem has been defined, the next step is to obtain a formal commitment from a faculty member in the major area of concentration to chair the committee. The dissertation committee chair is typically the faculty member with particular expertise on your selected topic and/or the PI of the dataset that you will be utilizing. The dissertation chair is expected to assume the major role in guiding the student through the project.

In many institutions, this chair may or may not be the graduate advisor assigned to the student for academic advice at the time the student commenced her/his program. Most typically, the chair takes over the role of academic advisor at the time they take on the role of dissertation chair.

2.6 STEP #4: CHOOSING THE DISSERTATION COMMITTEE MEMBERS

Once you have identified a dissertation committee chair, the next step is to recruit other committee members who can provide the expertise to help you carry out the research project. The formulation of the dissertation committee must meet your graduate school guidelines, and your specific program may have additional regulations as to who can or should serve on a dissertation committee. Therefore, these rules should be considered early in the process.

Use a preproposal as a recruitment tool In many institutions, a preproposal or *dissertation outline* is the first step in recruiting the dissertation committee. With the help of the chair, the student drafts a brief one- or two-page *preproposal* synopsis of the project. This preproposal describes the overall dissertation topic(s) and serves as a blueprint for the development of the dissertation proposal. See the end of this chapter for an example preproposal.

Ideally, dissertation committee members have expertise in different aspects of your proposed dissertation. Indeed, similar considerations come into play when choosing committee members as when choosing coinvestigators for a grant proposal (as described in Chapter 18, *Submission of the Grant Proposal*.)

The main theme is to enlist committee members who have expertise in your **exposure** or **outcome** of interest. It is also generally expected that dissertation committees in epidemiology and preventive medicine will include an **epidemiologist and/or statistician**.

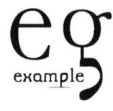

example — Imagine that you are planning to write a dissertation proposal designed to identify genetic and environmental risk factors for prostate cancer using a nationally available dataset. Your committee members should ideally include (1) an **oncologist** who has a track record of publications on prostate cancer, (2) an **epidemiologist** who has designed and led studies on prostate cancer or a related cancer, and (3) a **statistician** with expertise in genetic analyses, ideally in the cancer field.

If there is no one at your institution with expertise in the particular area that you have selected, some schools will allow you to invite **outside members** to serve on your committee. These outside members could be related professionals such as graduate faculty from other campuses, departments, or health agencies. Often, these faculty are termed *consultants* to the dissertation committee and have no vote at the time of the defense even though they are expected to contribute to the dissertation and attend the defense.

Adjunct faculty, if they have a graduate level appointment, may be eligible to serve as voting members of a committee but typically may not serve as chair of the committee.

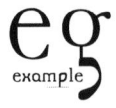

example — Example graduate school requirements for a dissertation committee:

- Be composed of no less than three (3) full-time *graduate* faculty from your institution.
    - The chair must be from the academic major and must be a full-time faculty at the primary institution.
    - At least two members must have their primary appointment in your school.

- Include an *outside* faculty member who must be:
  - A graduate faculty member from another department at your institution
  - Someone who may also serve as the minor faculty advisor
- Include one or more additional faculty or adjunct faculty from other specialties as appropriate:
  - If these additional faculty are not graduate faculty at your institution or are adjunct graduate faculty from outside the university, they may be appointed only as (nonvoting) consultants.

Recommendation for committee members is typically made by the committee chair and is communicated to the graduate program director and then the graduate school. The appointment of the committee is officially made by the dean of the graduate school. In some programs, this committee is formed prior to the qualifying exam and plays a role in guiding the student toward the preliminary comprehensive examination. At others, it occurs at the same time as the proposal submission.

A potential pitfall to avoid While the advantage of including members with expertise in the topic of your dissertation is clear, care should be taken not to assemble too large a committee. The old adage **"too many cooks spoil the soup"** is certainly true here. All committee members will want to feel that they are contributing to your proposal. You will find that the number of comments and suggestions will increase proportionately with the addition of each new member. The other downside of a large committee can be conflicting advice by committee members and the subsequent challenge of obtaining consensus to the satisfaction of all members.

2.6.1 Role of the Dissertation Committee

While the dissertation committee chair is expected to assume the major role in guiding the student through the project, the committee members generally contribute to selected aspects of the project. The committee is responsible for guiding and supervising the dissertation research and is often responsible for conducting the oral defense. Typically, the dissertation committee will meet as a whole several times throughout the dissertation process:

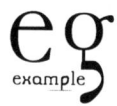

Example Dissertation meetings:

1. An initial committee meeting to review the preproposal (e.g., overall scope and timeline)
2. A second meeting to review the draft proposal in its entirety
3. At the dissertation proposal defense
4. A meeting to review preliminary findings from the dissertation
5. At the dissertation defense

Note that the example above includes two dissertation committee meetings prior to the dissertation proposal defense. These ensure that the entire committee is *on board* with your research plan and that you are not faced with any surprises during your defense.

2.6.2 Balance of Responsibilities between the Dissertation Chair and the Dissertation Committee

The balance of responsibilities between the dissertation chair and committee vary according to institutions. Several approaches can be taken. Below, I describe a recommended approach.

After the dissertation scope and the timeline is approved by the dissertation committee (meeting #1 above), the doctoral student should primarily work with the chair to develop the preproposal into a reasonably polished full proposal. Exceptions would be for specific advice in areas of expertise of the committee members. Only after the chair and the student are satisfied with this draft of the full proposal should it be circulated to the committee members for their input.

In this way, one avoids having all committee members correct the same typo. This saves the committee members time, avoids replication of advice, but does put the burden of work on the committee chair.

It is generally accepted that any written drafts be submitted to faculty at least 10 days to 2 weeks in advance of a committee meeting or deadline. In this manner, the committee is given adequate time to comment on the draft(s).

How to resolve conflicting demands from the committee It is important that the student keep each of the committee members up to date on significant aspects of the project. In the case of conflicting or extreme demands from the committee, the student should inform the chair and request a committee meeting to resolve any issues. Any substantial change in the proposed project should trigger a meeting of the full committee.

2.7 STEP #5: WRITING THE DISSERTATION PROPOSAL

2.7.1 Structure of the Dissertation Proposal

As mentioned earlier, a strategic approach taken by many graduate schools is to have the dissertation proposal match the format of a grant proposal. In this manner, the graduate student obtains experience with grant writing within the supportive context of his or her graduate education. Some programs require the student to write three such grant proposals for the dissertation as it quickly leads to three publishable papers after the dissertation is defended—this is often called a *3-paper model*. The proposal outline at the end of this chapter provides a detailed outline of a sample dissertation proposal.

2.7.2 Dissertation Proposal as a Contract

It is useful to view the dissertation proposal as a **contract** between you and your dissertation committee. The more your research is tied to your specific aims as outlined in your proposal, the greater protection you will have from committee members who may ask you to conduct additional ad hoc analyses late in the stages of your dissertation.

In this vein, Chapter 10, *Data Analysis Plan*, provides specific suggestions for detailed creation of *mock tables* (sometimes known as *dummy tables*) as part of the proposal. *Mock tables* are tables that do not contain data but are otherwise complete with titles, row, and column headings. Mock tables provide a *home* for all the results generated by your proposed data analysis, within a table. By tying your data analysis plan to your aims up front, you will have clearly indicated how all of your proposed analyses will have direct relevance to your aims.

Creating mock tables as part of the proposal writing process will not only save you time after your proposal has been approved and you have conducted your data analysis but will serve as a type of *contract* between you and your committee. More importantly, simply the process of creating mock tables will crystallize your understanding of your data analysis plan—making it concrete. You will be able to visualize the statistics that your data analysis plan will generate and whether it is feasible. The process of creating mock tables, therefore, may lead you to revise and refine your specific aims.

For example, if you find yourself generating multiple tables to house the data for one aim, you may decide that this aim is too broad. Broadly defined aims are one of the most common pitfalls faced by doctoral students. On the other hand, having too little data to present in a table might indicate that your aims are too narrow. Seeing the tables will allow both you and your dissertation committee to consider the appropriateness and relevance of your anticipated study findings. By having the committee *sign off* on these tables, you help to reduce the risk of requests for additional ad hoc analyses.

2.7.3 Format of the Dissertation Proposal

Typically, a graduate school's Office of Degree Requirements has specific rules for proposal style and formatting. These rules contain detailed guidelines for preparing the dissertation in the proper format and include requirements for tables, figures, and bibliography. To facilitate compliance with these guidelines, many graduate schools post a Word template with such formatting on their website.

Typically, requirements must be followed exactly in order to ensure acceptance and approval of the dissertation proposal by the graduate school. By complying with these guidelines in the proposal writing stage, you will avoid a lot of unnecessary hassle at the last minute when you need it the least.

In the absence of such guidelines, you could consult a current and appropriate style manual recommended by your department and used by your discipline for issues of form and content. However, it is important to note that regulations from your graduate school take precedence over rules found in style manuals. Other approaches are to use the table format, reference format, and reference citation method of the *American Journal of Epidemiology* or *Preventive Medicine* or other widely accepted journal in the field. Use of such guidelines will also facilitate ultimately submitting your dissertation findings as a manuscript for publication.

The proposal should be written using the future tense. More details on scientific writing style for proposals can be found in Chapter 5, *Scientific Writing*. In this vein, review several recent dissertation proposals submitted by other doctoral students in your department. These are often available as electronic resources in the university library, in the department library, or from faculty members.

2.8 STEP #6: PROPOSAL DEFENSE

At many universities, a dissertation proposal defense is required and, if so, is conducted by the dissertation committee. One of the most useful parts of the defense process is the professional evaluation by the committee of the presentation itself.

Each committee member should receive a *final* polished version of the proposal at least 2 weeks before the proposal defense. Note that the graduate school may require that all members of the committee be present for the defense to be held. The proposal defense is also typically open to any departmental faculty member or graduate student who wishes to attend. Other persons may often only attend the defense with advance approval by the committee chair.

The dissertation committee chair oversees the proceedings of the defense. The student is expected to present, generally in about 40 min, a synopsis of the key elements of the project, emphasizing the methods, analytical approach, limitations, and the potential significance of the results in terms of their public health importance and impact on clinical practice. See Chapter 16, *Presenting Your Proposal Orally*, for step-by-step tips on creating a presentation of your proposal.

Ideally, the committee chair should review your proposal defense slides prior to the presentation. Asking your chair to also review a draft of your **speaking points** to accompany the slides is highly recommended.

Usually, questions of information or clarification are asked during the presentations, but matters of substance are held for the question period that is directed by the chair at the end of the presentation. After questions from the general audience are addressed, the general audience may be dismissed and the dissertation committee itself poses questions to the student. Questions focus predominantly on the proposal itself but may also encompass course material learned over the student's program.

Upon completion of this question period, the committee then meets in private to discuss the student's performance and votes for a pass or not. To pass, the candidate must usually receive a unanimous vote. Committee members may recommend minor changes to the dissertation proposal. If major changes are required, then the defense was held prematurely.

2.9 STEP #7: SUBMISSION OF THE PROPOSAL TO THE GRADUATE SCHOOL

Once the dissertation proposal is approved and signed by the dissertation committee, it is submitted (usually by graduate program director) to the graduate school. At many universities, the graduate school requires that the dissertation proposal be submitted at least 7 months prior to the scheduling of the final dissertation defense. This time lag is designed to give the student adequate time to complete the dissertation before defending the final results. In other words, it is designed for the student's protection.

It is often expected that the student will provide the members of the committee with a final copy of the proposal. When appropriate, the proposal should be submitted to the school's Human Subject Review Committee.

2.10 STEP #8: CONDUCT THE DISSERTATION RESEARCH

A well-written proposal will greatly facilitate the conduct of the dissertation research. If, as part of the proposal, you have carefully outlined your study methods as well as created *mock tables* (see Chapters 6 through 13), then conducting the dissertation should be akin to following your own cookbook—with yourself and your committee as the cookbook writers!

Many fine texts have been published providing tips for **conducting** dissertation research, and this topic is beyond the scope of this text on proposal writing.

2.11 STEP #9: DISSERTATION DEFENSE

The final dissertation defense (oral) is scheduled when the committee chair affirms a consensus among the committee members that the dissertation research is completed and the manuscript is approved by all the committee members.

Typically, the graduate program director announces the time and place of the defense at least 2 weeks prior to allow public notification of the defense. The graduate school requires that every member of the dissertation committee be present for the defense. Any graduate faculty from within the university as well as from the school may attend the dissertation defense. Students from the school may attend as well. Other guests may attend only at the request of the examinee and with the permission of the committee chair.

Only members of the dissertation committee vote as to whether the defense was satisfactory or not, and this vote must typically be unanimous for the student to pass the dissertation defense. In the case of failure, many departments allow the exam to be retaken from 1 to 6 months later. If the second attempt results in failure, the student is usually dismissed from the doctoral program. The results of the exam are communicated by the dissertation chair to the graduate program director who communicates it to the graduate school.

Be sure to build into your timeline at least 1 week after the dissertation defense **to allow for final revisions** or changes to the dissertation and the submission of the final copy to the graduate school.

It is important to be aware that at many universities, the faculty have 9-month appointments and are not obligated to be available during June, July, or August. Also, in your planning, you should query the faculty about any sabbatical or leave of absence plans.

2.12 STEP #10: SUBMIT THE DISSERTATION TO THE GRADUATE SCHOOL

You will typically be required to submit your manuscript electronically. Doctoral dissertations may also be available to the public as circulating copies shelved in the library or appropriate branch.

2.13 SUGGESTED TIMELINE

All institutions have their own specific guidelines regarding the timing of events to ensure a successful dissertation proposal submission and defense. Below is one sample timeline that can serve as a general model (Table 2.1).

TABLE 2.1 Timeline for dissertation proposal and completion

PROPOSAL PROCESS

Step #1: Preliminary qualifying exams
Step #2: Select a dissertation topic
Step #3: Choose a chair of the committee
    Meet with chair
    Write preproposal
Step #4: Choose the dissertation committee members
    Committee meeting #1: Review scope and timeline
    Committee meeting #2: Review research plan
Step #5: Write the dissertation proposal
    Submit draft sections to chair
    Submit draft to committee at least 2 weeks prior to proposal defense
Step #6: Defend the dissertation proposal
Step #7: Submit the proposal to the graduate school
    Submit proposal to IRB (if appropriate)

Conduct of the Dissertation

Step #8: Conduct the dissertation research
Step #9: Committee meeting to review preliminary findings.
Step #10: Submit final dissertation to committee at least 2 weeks prior to defense
Step #11: The dissertation defense
    Make any requested revisions to dissertation
Step #12: Submit the dissertation to the graduate school
    Graduation!
Final step: Submit dissertation to a journal(s) for publication

2.14 EXAMPLES

2.14.1 Preproposal for a 3-Paper Model

Modifiable Risk Factors for Hypertensive Disorders of Pregnancy in Latina Women

Introduction

Subgroups of Latina women are at a twofold increased risk of preeclampsia relative to non-Hispanic white women. However, there is little research on risk factors for hypertensive disorders of pregnancy, including gestational hypertension and preeclampsia, in this population. Both gestational hypertension and preeclampsia have serious implications for both mother and child, including fetal death and future development of cardiovascular disease in the mother. This dissertation will analyze data from the Latina Gestational Diabetes Mellitus (GDM) Study, a prospective cohort study of 1231 Latina women, primarily of Puerto Rican descent. Data from this study include data from two interviewer-administered interviews and postdelivery medical record abstraction. The proposed analyses will focus on modifiable risk factors for hypertensive disorders of pregnancy.

Paper #1. Gestational Weight Gain, Prepregnancy BMI, and Hypertensive Disorders of Pregnancy
The Institute of Medicine (IOM) has issued guidelines for weight gain during pregnancy based on women's prepregnancy BMI. However, there is virtually no data on the implication of excessive or inadequate weight gain on the hypertensive disorders of pregnancy. Additionally, while there are data on prepregnancy BMI as a risk factor for hypertensive disorders of pregnancy, there are little data in a Latina population. Therefore, the proposed study will evaluate the association between gestational weight gain (inadequate, adequate, or excessive gain as defined by the IOM), prepregnancy adiposity as measured through BMI, and hypertensive disorders of pregnancy.

Paper #2. Pre- and Early Pregnancy Physical Activity and Hypertensive Disorders of Pregnancy
The American College of Obstetrics and Gynecology (ACOG) recommends that pregnant women without contraindications participate in moderate physical activity on most days and there is evidence that physical activity reduces the risk of preeclampsia. However, there is limited research in this area and no studies to date have included a sufficient number of Latina women. This study will assess the association between physical activity in four domains (occupational, household/caregiving, sports/exercise, and active living) and total physical activity and risk of hypertensive disorders of pregnancy.

Paper #3. Early Pregnancy Stress and Hypertensive Disorders of Pregnancy
There is no previous research evaluating perceived stress and hypertensive disorders of pregnancy, although studies in nonpregnant populations have suggested that decreased stress may decrease blood pressure. The proposed study will evaluate perceived stress in early pregnancy as measured through the Perceived Stress Scale, as well as the Modified Life Events Inventory. Previous research in pregnant populations has been limited to job-related stress, which restricts generalizability to women who are employed. This study will add to the limited research looking at psychosocial risk factors for hypertensive disorders of pregnancy.

2.14.2 Dissertation Proposal Outline (Table 2.2)

TABLE 2.2 Brief outline

I. Title and Abstract
II. Abstract (Project Summary)
III. Specific Aims and Hypotheses
IV. Background and Significance
    a. Introduction: Public Health Impact of Outcome (Disease)
    b. Physiology of Exposure–Outcome Relationship
    c. Epidemiology of Exposure–Outcome Relationship
    d. Summary of Significance and Innovation
V. Study Design and Methods
    a. Study Design
    b. Study Population
        i. Setting
        ii. Subject ascertainment
        iii. Eligibility criteria/Exclusion criteria
    c. Exposure Assessment
        i. How exposure data will be collected
        ii. Exposure parameterization
        iii. Validity of exposure assessment
    d. Outcome Assessment
        i. How outcome data will be collected
        ii. Outcome parameterization
        iii. Validity of outcome assessment
    e. Covariate Assessment
        i. How covariate data will be collected
        ii. Covariate parameterization
        iii. Validity of covariate assessment
    f. Variable Categorization Table
VI. Data Analysis Plan
    a. Univariate Analysis
    b. Bivariate Analysis
    c. Multivariate Analysis
    d. Sensitivity Analyses (if relevant)

(continued)

TABLE 2.2 (continued) Brief outline

VII. Sample Size and Power Calculations
VIII. Alternatives and Limitations
    a. Threats to Internal Validity
        i. Chance
        ii. Bias
            1. Nondifferential
                a. Nondifferential misclassification of exposure
                b. Nondifferential misclassification of outcome
            2. Differential misclassification
                a. Selection bias
                b. Information bias
        iii. Confounding
    b. Threats to External Validity
        i. Generalizability
IX. Human Subject Protection
    a. Informed Consent
    b. Confidentiality
    c. Risks
    d. Benefits

How to Develop and Write Hypotheses

3

The importance of writing hypotheses cannot be underestimated. A well-written research hypothesis describes the results that a researcher expects to find. In effect, it is a prediction. The process of crafting hypotheses should kick off the start of your proposal-writing endeavor.

3.1 NEED FOR HYPOTHESES

With few exceptions, all proposals considered compelling by a doctoral committee or fundable by granting agencies must include hypotheses. As shown in the accompanying Figure 3.1, these hypotheses should be nested within specific aims. In a grant application, this is one of the first sections of your proposal to be read by reviewers. The maxim that *first impressions matter* is particularly true in this case.

While most graduate students and early-career faculty know that they need to include specific aims in their proposals, they often omit or have trouble articulating hypotheses. This omission is even true at the senior faculty level. Indeed, in my experience serving as an NIH reviewer, I saw many grants that were scored poorly simply due to the fact that they failed to include hypotheses and instead only listed specific aims.

The guidelines and stylistic tips described in this chapter will walk you through the hypothesis writing process. At first, these guidelines and tips might appear deceptively simple. But, almost without exception, once you try your hand at writing your own hypotheses, you will find that more often than not one or more guidelines are not being followed!

Typical format
Specific aim #1
Hypothesis #1
Specific aim #2
Hypothesis #2

FIGURE 3.1 Typical format for specific aims and corresponding hypotheses.

3.2 MORE ABOUT THE DISTINCTION BETWEEN HYPOTHESES AND SPECIFIC AIMS

Specific aims are a list of tasks that you, as an investigator, propose to accomplish. Essentially, specific aims outline what you propose to *do* in the project; they are a *to-do list* of tasks. In contrast, hypotheses state the relationship that you expect to observe, your anticipated findings. This may sound difficult, and it is. Indeed, the formulation of hypotheses can only occur after a comprehensive review of the prior literature on your proposed topic. Hypotheses must extend logically from this prior research and be a reasonable expectation by anyone who has read this prior work. Thus, writing and including hypotheses indicates that you have a clear grasp of the literature.

As you can see in the example below, if one views the specific aims without the hypotheses, the proposal is simply listing tasks to be accomplished. In contrast, with the addition of hypotheses, it becomes clear that the investigator has assimilated the prior literature and, more importantly, has an educated hunch as to what they will find.

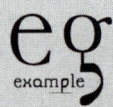

> **Original Version**
> Specific Aim #1: To evaluate the association between pregnancy stress and risk of adverse birth outcomes
> Specific Aim #2: To evaluate the association between pregnancy stress and risk of hypertensive disorders of pregnancy
>
> **Improved Version**
> Specific Aim #1: To evaluate the association between pregnancy stress and risk of adverse birth outcomes
> Hypothesis #1: There will be a positive association between pregnancy stress and preterm birth and low birth weight.
> Specific Aim #2: To evaluate the association between pregnancy stress and risk of hypertensive disorders of pregnancy.
> Hypothesis #2: There will be a positive association between pregnancy stress and hypertensive disorders of pregnancy.

Hypotheses indicate your overall impact

A key advantage to including hypotheses is that they indirectly show off the *overall impact* of your proposal. In other words, by articulating what you anticipate to be the potential results of your study, the reviewer can begin to envision how your findings might influence public health and clinical practice. In the example above, discovering that stress during pregnancy increases risk of adverse birth outcomes might inform future prenatal intervention programs that would help to reduce low birth weight. As discussed in Chapter 19, *Review Process*, the *overall impact* score is one of the most important factors in NIH funding decisions.

3.3 HYPOTHESES SHOULD FLOW LOGICALLY FROM THE BACKGROUND AND SIGNIFICANCE SECTION

Hypotheses are the climax of your proposal

The placement of the specific aims/hypotheses in your proposal depends on whether you are writing a dissertation proposal or a grant proposal (and your institutions' guidelines). Regardless, the principle remains the same that the hypotheses should flow logically from the Background and Significance sections (see Chapter 7, *Background and Significance Section*). In other words, the literature review presented in the background section sets the stage. It points out the limitations of the current research and highlights the research gap. In this way, by the time the reader gets to the hypotheses, they should be craving for someone to fill this research gap. The hypotheses serve to fulfill this desire. In this manner, the hypotheses can be viewed as the *climax* of the proposal.

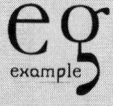

> *example*
>
> Imagine a dissertation proposal to evaluate the long-term impact of a vitamin D supplementation program. In the background/significance section, you described the prior studies of vitamin D supplementation. In particular, you highlighted the point that the prior literature was limited to evaluating the short-term impact (e.g., 6 months) of these programs and that no investigators had evaluated the long-term impact of such programs. This was your "research gap."
>
> **End of Background and Significance section:**
>
> These findings suggest that vitamin D supplementation programs for reproductive aged women are likely to yield short-term improvements in depression. It is not clear, however, if such improvements can be maintained over time.

> **Specific Aims and Hypotheses:**
> Specific aim #1: We propose to conduct a randomized controlled trial of a vitamin D supplementation program for reproductive aged women.
> Hypothesis #1: We hypothesize that after 5 years, women randomized to a vitamin D supplementation program will report fewer depressive symptoms as compared to women randomized to the placebo group.

3.4 HOW TO WRITE HYPOTHESES IF THE PRIOR LITERATURE IS CONFLICTING

Often, prior studies are contradictory. For example, some prior vitamin D supplementation programs may have shown no impact on depression, while others showed some improvement. Or, even more extreme, some studies may have shown an adverse impact. In these situations you, as a proposal writer, will be faced with choosing a hypothesized direction of effect. This task can be daunting at first. However, it may be a relief to hear that the most persuasive approach is for you to be as transparent as possible regarding your decision-making process. That is, include the thought process behind this choice in your proposal. This process is described in detail in Chapter 7, *Background and Significance Section*.

In brief, the first step is to acknowledge that you are aware that the prior literature is conflicting. This reassures the reviewer that you are knowledgeable about the state of the research in this field. Then, proceed to describe the studies. Consider which studies might be methodologically stronger; a review article in this area, if available, will be particularly helpful to cite. Then, lastly, state why you feel that the evidence is more persuasive in one direction (e.g., a protective effect) as opposed to another direction (e.g., an adverse effect or a null effect). This is the direction that you will then hypothesize.

Your rationale should be based upon the quality of the prior studies. For example, you may more heavily weigh the prior studies that used a validated measurement tool or were conducted in a study population similar to your own. Other criteria to consider are strength of study design (e.g., case–control vs. prospective study) or sample size and power. There are a large number of factors that can be considered.

Key pitfalls to avoid With this approach, you avoid the pitfall of appearing unaware of prior work—which would not be viewed favorably by reviewers. Indeed, some of the reviewers may have been the authors of studies that reported alternative findings. Reviewers would rather have you acknowledge the complexity of the situation, and then clarify your thought process, rather than gloss over contradictory findings.

In the situation where prior studies have been null, and did not indicate an effect in either one direction or another, formulating a hypothesis can be even more challenging. Highlight for the reviewer why your study will be more likely to observe an effect (e.g., by nature of your larger sample size and therefore enhanced power) as compared to those prior null studies. Other reasons for why you might have an advantage over prior studies could include your use of improved measurement tools, a stronger study design, or your focus on a high-risk population.

Finally, there may be very few, or no, prior studies in your area. In this situation, it is best to rely upon the proposed physiologic association between your exposure and your outcome in formulating your hypotheses. The plus side of this challenging situation is that, with no prior studies, the need for your study should be even clearer. Highlight this dearth of research to the reviewer.

3.5 GUIDELINE #1: A RESEARCH HYPOTHESIS SHOULD NAME THE INDEPENDENT AND DEPENDENT VARIABLES AND INDICATE THE TYPE OF RELATIONSHIP EXPECTED BETWEEN THEM

In epidemiology and preventive medicine, the independent variable can be viewed as the *exposure variable*. This term is used broadly to encompass both risk factors and protective factors for some type of outcome (typically a disease). A common misperception is to view *exposures* as referring to adverse factors (e.g., cigarette smoking, drug use), but the definition is actually more broad. Specifically, the independent variable is any factor that may lead to a health outcome. It is also important to note that dependent variables or *outcomes* in epidemiology and preventive medicine are often diseases but can also be positive outcomes such as psychological well-being.

Below is a simple example of a hypothesis that contains an independent and dependent variable and describes their relationship.

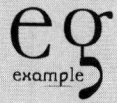

> *eg example* There will be a positive relationship between level of coffee intake and risk of Parkinson's disease.

In this example, the level of coffee intake is the independent variable (i.e., the exposure variable) and Parkinson's disease is the dependent variable (i.e., the outcome variable). Note that this example also clarifies the direction of effect. In other words, that coffee increases risk of Parkinson's disease.

> **Original Version**
> Elderly adults will differ in their acid blocker use and they also will differ in their vitamin B12 levels.
>
> **Improved Version**
> Among elderly adults, there will be an inverse relationship between their acid blocker use and their vitamin B12 levels.

The improved version clarifies the direction of effect between the exposure (acid blocker use) and the outcome (vitamin B12 levels).

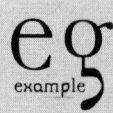

3.6 GUIDELINE #2: A HYPOTHESIS SHOULD NAME THE EXPOSURE PRIOR TO THE OUTCOME

This guideline may appear intuitive but is not often followed in practice. Remember that reviewers are reading your proposal for the first time. While you are thoroughly familiar with which variable is your exposure variable and which variable is your outcome variable, the reviewer is just learning this. Therefore, consistently ordering the exposure variable prior to the outcome variable will result in a proposal that is easier to read and understand. This is a kindness to the reviewer that can save them precious time, and its importance should not be underestimated. In contrast, a hypothesis that lists the outcome variable first can often lead to reviewer confusion as to which is the exposure and which is the outcome variable.

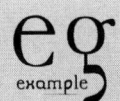

> **Original Version**
> There will be a positive relationship between depression and diagnosis of diabetes.
>
> **Improved Version**
> There will be a positive relationship between diagnosis of diabetes and depression.

This version is improved because it lists the exposure (diabetes) before the outcome (depression). You can see from this example that it would have been very easy for confusion to arise. The reviewer could have mistakenly assumed that depression was the exposure and that the proposal was hypothesizing that depression may physiologically lead to an increased risk of diabetes. Indeed, there is a body of research that has proposed such an association. However, the proposal was hypothesizing the reverse: that those diagnosed with diabetes are more likely to become depressed. It is only by a consistent ordering of exposure prior to disease that such confusion can be avoided.

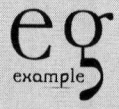

> **Original Version**
> More physical activity will be observed among children who watch less television.
> **Improved Version**
> Children who watch less television will participate in more physical activity than those who watch more television.

This improved version lists the exposure (television) before the outcome (physical activity) and also states the comparison group (see Guideline #3).

3.7 GUIDELINE #3: THE COMPARISON GROUP SHOULD BE STATED

Hypotheses for study designs in epidemiology and preventive medicine usually involve the comparison of two or more groups, typically termed the *exposed* and *unexposed*. The general structure of a hypothesis therefore tends to follow the format "Do exposed people have a greater risk of disease than unexposed people?" In the following original version, you will see that the comparison group is not stated.

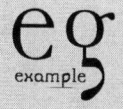

> **Original Version**
> Overweight adults will have an increased risk of hypertension.
> **Improved Version**
> Overweight adults will have an increased risk of hypertension as compared to normal-weight adults.

In the original example, failure to state the comparison group could lead the reader to believe that the comparison group might be *underweight adults* or perhaps *obese adults*. In other words, failure to specify the comparison group gives the reviewer more work to do (spending time trying to determine who is your comparison group), and may result in a misidentification of this comparison group.

38 Writing Dissertation and Grant Proposals

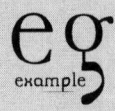

> **example**
>
> **Original Version**
> Among endometrial cancer patients, there will be a high level of talc use.
>
> **Improved Version**
> Talc users will have an increased risk of endometrial cancer as compared to those who do not use talc.

The improved version not only specifies the comparison group (*those who do not use talc*) but also lists the exposure before the outcome.

A caveat You may be interested in evaluating the impact of your exposure both as a categorical variable (e.g., exposed vs. unexposed) and a continuous variable. In the latter case, you may be hypothesizing a dose–response relationship between your exposure and outcome variable. In this situation, it is appropriate to include several hypotheses, one specifying your comparison group (for your categorical exposure) and one hypothesizing your dose–response relationship (for your continuous exposure variable).

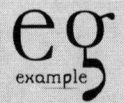

> **example**
>
> **Hypothesis for a Categorical Exposure**
> Hypothesis #1a. Children exposed to formaldehyde will have an increased risk of asthma as compared to those not exposed to formaldehyde.
>
> **Hypothesis for a Continuous Exposure**
> Hypothesis #1b. Dose of formaldehyde exposure will be positively associated with asthma risk.

Note that the hypothesis for the continuous version of the exposure variable (hypothesis #1b) does not specify a comparison *unexposed* group because the idea is that risk of the outcome increases with increasing level of the exposure.

3.8 GUIDELINE #4: WHEN YOUR STUDY IS LIMITED TO A PARTICULAR POPULATION, REFERENCE TO THE POPULATION SHOULD BE MADE IN THE HYPOTHESIS

This guideline is particularly critical to follow when one of the key aspects of your proposal is your particular study population. For example, if you will be the first investigator to examine an association within a high-risk group, highlight this key feature in the hypothesis—it will certainly increase your chances of having the proposal funded. Another reason to highlight your study population is when that population is a relatively understudied group. In other words, your proposal fills a *research gap* by focusing on this particular population.

On the flip side, if your study will be very large and/or use national data, this is also a key strength to highlight through making reference to the population in the hypothesis. For example, proposing to use data from a national surveillance study (e.g., the Behavioral Risk Factor Surveillance System [BRFSS]) improves your ability to observe an effect (via the large sample size) and the representative nature of the sample greatly enhances the generalizability of your potential findings.

In terms of readability, it is preferable to highlight the study population in an introductory parenthetical phrase followed by a comma as is done in the improved example below.

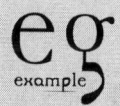

> **Original Version**
> Elderly adults differ in their levels of mobility and they differ in their self-reported quality of life.
>
> **Improved Version**
> Among elderly adults, there is a positive relationship between level of mobility and self-reported quality of life scores.

This improved example, aside from now highlighting the population of interest in an introductory clause (*Among elderly adults...*), is also improved because it shows the hypothesized direction of effect of the exposure on the outcome (e.g., a positive relationship).

While highlighting the study population can be important, there are also occasions when it would not be useful, for example, if your study population is a convenience sample and/or is not significantly different from the population used by prior studies in the area. In this case, highlighting the study population could actually reduce the impact of your hypotheses and add unnecessary wordiness. At worst, it could detract from the real novelty of your proposal, which, for example, might be a new assessment methodology. It is important to remember that, regardless of whether you mention your study population in your hypotheses, you will still have plenty of time to describe your study population in the methods section.

3.9 GUIDELINE #5: HYPOTHESES SHOULD BE AS CONCISE AS POSSIBLE AND USE MEASUREABLE TERMS

Ultimately, hypothesis writing is a balancing act in which you weigh the benefits of being more specific with the risk of wordiness. Always keep in mind, that you will be able to provide more details in the methods section.

A potential pitfall is the use of simple terms to save space at the expense of clarity. In other words, a simple term for the exposure or outcome variable is not useful if the reviewer cannot envision how this variable will be measured.

> **Original Version**
> There will be a positive relationship between patients' social class and their health literacy.
>
> **Improved Version**
> Among patients, there will be a positive relationship between income level and performance on a cardiovascular risk factor awareness test.

The improved version could have been written in a variety of ways. But, regardless the improvement is due to the use of measureable terms in place of *social class* and *health literacy*. The improved version indicates that *social class* will be measured in terms of income level and that *health literacy* will be measured as performance on a cardiovascular risk factor awareness test.

As with any advice, however, it is possible to take this too far. For example, it would be an ineffective use of space, as well as a distraction, to become too detailed in the hypotheses. For example, the following includes details that are better left to the methods section: "Among patients, there will be a positive relationship between gross annual income in 2012 and their performance on the Smith 5-level Likert cardiovascular risk factor awareness scale."

This decision to mention the assessment tool in the hypotheses depends upon whether the assessment tool is an advance in the field or somehow reflects a strength of the study. For example, if you are the first to use a specific questionnaire and this is the key advance of your study, then mention this questionnaire in the hypothesis. Or, if the majority of prior studies were based on self-report and you will be using an objective measure.

3.10 GUIDELINE #6: AVOID MAKING PRECISE STATISTICAL PREDICTIONS IN A HYPOTHESIS

Precise statistical predictions can rarely be justified by the prior literature. For example, imagine that you are proposing to conduct a study of antidepressant use on attempted suicide risk. You hypothesize that risk would be reduced by 50% but instead you find that risk is reduced by 52%. In this case, your hypothesis would not be supported. Indeed, findings for any other percentile other than 50% would result in the rejection of your hypothesis. Even providing a range of predictions (e.g., a 10%–20% reduction) is generally not acceptable in a hypothesis.

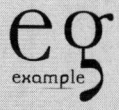

> **example**
> **Original Version**
> Cigarette smokers will have a 35% higher risk of influenza as compared to nonsmokers.
> **Improved Version**
> Cigarette smokers will have a higher risk of influenza as compared to nonsmokers.

The improved version of the example gives the direction of effect but does not give a precise amount.

3.11 GUIDELINE #7: A HYPOTHESIS SHOULD INDICATE WHAT WILL ACTUALLY BE STUDIED—NOT THE POSSIBLE IMPLICATIONS OF THE STUDY OR VALUE JUDGMENTS OF THE AUTHOR

There will be plenty of time in your background and significance section to justify the importance of your proposed research as well as its possible implications.

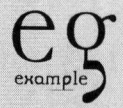

> **example**
> **Original Version**
> Good diets will have a dramatic benefit among older adults.
> **Improved Version**
> Among older adults, those who have a Mediterranean-style dietary pattern will have a lower risk of heart disease as compared to those who eat a diet high in carbohydrates.

The improved example removes the term *dramatic* which could be viewed as reflecting the value judgments of the writer. The second advantage of the improved example is that it follows Guideline #5 by removing vague terms, such as *good diets* and *benefit*, and instead clarifies how the exposure (diet) and the outcome will be measured (i.e., as dietary pattern and heart disease risk, respectively). The improved example also follows Guideline #3 by specifying the comparison group (e.g., diet high in carbohydrates).

3.12 STYLISTIC TIP #1: WHEN A NUMBER OF RELATED HYPOTHESES ARE TO BE STATED, CONSIDER PRESENTING THEM IN A NUMBERED OR LETTERED LIST

Often, hypotheses may be stated for a group of related exposure or outcome variables. In this situation, consider a numbered or lettered list.

> **eg** *example*
>
> Females taking the alcohol awareness course will
>
> 1. Be less likely to engage in binge drinking
> 2. Be more committed to alcohol abstinence
> 3. Obtain a higher grade point average
>
> as compared to those not taking the course.

This approach is most useful when you have one exposure variable and several outcome variables. In this example, the exposure is taking the alcohol awareness course, and the outcomes are the impact of the course on three factors. This approach is also only feasible when the comparison group is identical for all three hypotheses (i.e. those not taking the course).

When to use a single hypothesis for multiple factors

In contrast, it is also permissible to include more than one hypothesis in a single sentence as long as the sentence is reasonably concise and its meaning clear. The more connected the hypotheses are, the more desirable this approach is.

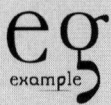

> **eg** *example*
>
> Premenopausal women who take oral contraceptives will experience higher rates of cardiovascular risk factors (i.e. HDL, LDL, triglycerides) as compared to those who do not take oral contraceptives.

In this example, the use of one sentence encompassing several subhypotheses is preferable due to the fact that there is a standardly accepted umbrella term that encompasses cardiovascular risk factors. It would be lengthy and somewhat unwieldy to include multiple hypotheses for each of the cardiovascular risk factors.

3.13 STYLISTIC TIP #2: BECAUSE MOST HYPOTHESES DEAL WITH THE BEHAVIOR OF GROUPS, PLURAL FORMS SHOULD USUALLY BE USED

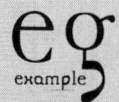

e.g. example

Original Version
There will be a positive association between a midwife's years in practice and her rate of episiotomy use.

First Improved Version
There will be a positive association between midwives' years in practice and their rate of episiotomy use.

Second Improved Version
Among midwives, there will be a positive association between years in practice and rate of episiotomy use.

The first improved example replaces the term *her* with *their*. This assumption could be viewed as offensive as not all midwives are women. The second improved example has the additional benefit of removing the possessive apostrophe.

3.14 STYLISTIC TIP #3: AVOID USING THE WORDS *SIGNIFICANT* OR *SIGNIFICANCE* IN A HYPOTHESIS

The terms *significant* and *significance* refer to tests of statistical significance used by most empirical studies. Statistical significance refers to the probability that the observed findings occurred by chance alone and is typically set at $p < 0.05$. Statistical significance has a number of limitations. For example, it can be influenced by the sample size of your study (i.e., the larger the sample, the more likely that the findings will be statistically significant). In addition, even if you observe statistically significant results (i.e., $p < 0.05$), this does not rule out that your results might be due to bias (e.g., confounding, selection bias).

Another limitation to the use of the term *significance* is that it can refer to clinical significance (as opposed to statistical significance). Clinical significance is a more subjective term and is based on the expert opinion of key leaders in the field and/or upon the prior literature. For example, imagine that you conducted a study of the impact of prenatal exercise on birth weight. Let's assume that you found a 50 g difference in birth weight between exercisers (exposed group) and nonexercisers (unexposed group), which was **statistically significant** at p = 0.01. However, obstetricians may not consider a 50 g difference in birth weight to be **clinically significant**; that is, such a small difference in birth weight may not impact the current or future health of the baby. On the flip side, let's assume that you found a 200 g difference in birth weight that was not statistically significant (e.g., p = 0.25). Such a difference may be viewed as clinically significant but, due to your small sample size, was not statistically significant.

Therefore, it is always best to avoid the use of the terms *significant* or *significance* in hypotheses. Instead, describe the techniques that you will use to assess statistical significance, clinical significance, as well as the role of bias and confounding in the methods section of the proposal.

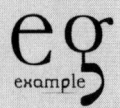

> **example**
>
> **Original Version**
> Obese women will have a significantly greater risk of premenstrual syndrome as compared to normal-weight women.
>
> **Improved Version**
> Obese women will have a greater risk of premenstrual syndrome as compared to normal-weight women.

3.15 STYLISTIC TIP #4: AVOID USING THE WORD *PROVE* IN A HYPOTHESIS

Epidemiologic and biostatistical research is almost always conducted among study samples drawn from larger populations. The corresponding statistical techniques are designed to take into account this sampling variability and yield findings with observed probabilities and confidence intervals. Thus, it is critical to remember that we, as investigators, gather data that offer varying degrees of confidence regarding various conclusions. We are therefore not able to *prove* a hypothesis in our proposed study. In addition, our observed findings may not only be due to chance, but they may also be due to biases such as confounding, selection bias, information bias, and misclassification. Because of these realities, it is never appropriate to use the word *prove* in a hypothesis.

Consider the example of a case–control study that found that exercise increased the risk of preterm birth. This finding could be due to bias. That is, women who had a preterm birth may be more likely to attribute their poor pregnancy outcome to their prenatal behaviors and therefore inadvertently overreport their exercise. This type of recall bias is particularly a concern when participants are aware of a potential association between the exposure and disease of interest.

Consider the **Bradford Hill criteria**, otherwise known as **Hill's Criteria for Causation**, which are a group of minimal conditions necessary to provide adequate evidence of a causal relationship between an exposure and disease in epidemiology and preventive medicine. Among such factors as *strength of association* and *biologic plausibility*, these criteria also include *consistency*. Consistency refers to repeated observations of a similar association across different study populations using different study designs. Clearly, your one proposed study is not going to be sufficient to meet the condition of *consistency*.

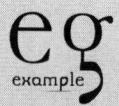

> **Original Version**
> Our hypothesis is to prove that birth weight will be positively associated with bone density among children.
>
> **Improved Version**
> Birth weight will be positively associated with bone density among children.

3.16 STYLISTIC TIP #5: AVOID USING TWO DIFFERENT TERMS TO REFER TO THE SAME VARIABLE IN A HYPOTHESIS

This guideline fits under the general theme of being kind to the reader. Many recall their college English classes where they were told to avoid using the same term over and over again and instead to make their writing interesting by using synonyms for terms. While this suggestion may be appropriate for creative writing, this practice is discouraged for scientific writing. Instead, be as clear as possible by consistently using the same terms for your exposure and outcome variables throughout the proposal. While you as the proposal writer may be very familiar with your topic of interest, your reviewer may not be. Synonyms will make it difficult for a first-time reviewer of your proposal to become familiar with your key variables.

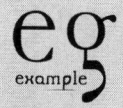

> **Original Version**
> Students who receive courses in stress reduction plus training in healthy dietary behaviors will have better attitudes toward their school work than those who receive only the new approach to stress reduction.
>
> **Improved Version**
> Students who receive courses in stress reduction plus training in healthy dietary behaviors will have better attitudes toward their school work than those who receive only courses in stress reduction.

In the original example, it is unclear if *the new approach to stress reduction* refers to the *courses in stress reduction* alone, or to some new approach which the writer mistakenly forgot to mention. At worst, the reader may decide that you inadvertently failed to describe the new approach. In contrast, while the improved version may appear repetitive to those with a creative writing bent—it is the ideal approach for scientific writing.

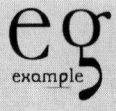

> **Original Version**
> Students who take the AIDS awareness course will report fewer risk-taking behaviors than those who do not take the introductory health course.
>
> **Improved Version**
> Students who take the AIDS awareness course will report fewer risk-taking behaviors than those who do not take the AIDS awareness course.

3.17 STYLISTIC TIP #6: REMOVE ANY UNNECESSARY WORDS

A hypothesis should be free of terms and phrases that do not add to its meaning. This guideline again fits under the goal of being kind to your reviewer. Removing unnecessary words helps you to clearly and efficiently make your point. You will find that it actually takes much longer to write a short hypothesis than a longer hypothesis. The hypothesis should be reread several times to make sure that every word counts. Avoid the pitfall of believing that longer hypotheses make your work appear more sophisticated; a targeted, precise hypothesis is always more impactful.

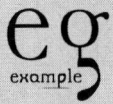

> **Original Version**
> Among naval shipyard workers, those who are working on seasonal schedules will report having more occupational injuries than those who are working in naval shipyards that follow a more traditional year-round schedule.
>
> **Improved Version**
> Naval shipyard workers who work on seasonal schedules will have higher injury rates than those who work on year-round schedules.

The improved version of the example is shorter, yet its meaning is clearer. Words such as *will report* and *more traditional* as well as the second repetition of *naval shipyards* are removed.

3.18 STYLISTIC TIP #7: HYPOTHESES MAY BE WRITTEN AS RESEARCH QUESTIONS—BUT USE CAUTION

Stating a hypothesis in the form of a question may, at first glance, make the hypothesis sound more compelling and potentially interesting. The question form also has the advantage of clearly pointing out to the reader the research gap (i.e., the question) that the hypothesis will address. However, the wording of a hypothesis as a question can be cumbersome. The other disadvantage of this approach could be a perceived lack of scientific rigor. Many reviewers may view the question form as more typical of a newspaper or magazine article.

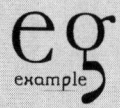

> **Original version**
> Do older men with high dietary glycemic load have higher levels of high-sensitivity CRP as compared to older men with low dietary glycemic load?
>
> **Improved version**
> Among older men those with high dietary glycemic load willl have higher levels of high-sensitivity CRP as compared to those with low dietary glycemic load.

3.19 HYPOTHESIS WRITING CHECKLIST

- A research hypothesis should name the independent and dependent variables and indicate the type of relationship expected between them.
- A hypothesis should name the exposure prior to the outcome.
- The comparison group should be stated.
- When your study is limited to a particular population, reference to the population should be made in the hypothesis.
- Hypothesis should be as concise as possible and use measurable terms.
- Avoid making precise statistical predictions in a hypothesis.

- A hypothesis should indicate what will actually be studied—not the possible implications of the study or value judgments of the author.
- When a number of related hypotheses are to be stated, consider presenting them in a numbered or lettered list.
- Because most hypotheses deal with the behavior of groups, plural forms should usually be used.
- Avoid using the words *significant* or *significance* in a hypothesis.
- Avoid using the word *prove* in a hypothesis.
- Avoid using two different terms to refer to the same variable in a hypothesis.
- Remove any unnecessary words.
- Hypotheses may be written as research questions—but use caution.

Conducting the Literature Search

4

The importance of a focused literature review cannot be understated and is a key skill in proposal writing. You likely have already had experience conducting literature searches as part of your undergraduate or graduate training.

However, unlike literature reviews that you may have conducted in the past, the literature review for a proposal is your opportunity to not only clarify the gap in the prior research for yourself but also to clarify it for the reviewer. Showing that your proposal will extend this prior literature by filling, at least in part, this **research gap** will be a critical feature in justifying your research and improving your chances of funding.

Therefore, in this chapter, I describe a three-step process for conducting a literature search designed to best justify the need for your study. This process begins with drafting a literature review outline, which in turn drives the collection of literature. The process then culminates with the completion of a summary table—a critical component to have in place before writing. These methods will not only be useful for a dissertation but are key for grant proposals and even journal articles. To this day, I follow the process as outlined below whenever I write a grant proposal.

The first step—creating a literature review outline—describes the process of going from your hypotheses to an outline that will serve as a roadmap for your literature search.

The second step—conducting the literature search—describes techniques for the collection of literature and goes over how to locate relevant research articles.

The third step—organizing the literature: summary tables—describes how to analyze, synthesize, and evaluate the articles in an efficient manner with the goal of clarifying and/or further refining the **research gap**. The summary tables assimilate all the literature you have collected into a final form that prepares you for the next step of writing the literature review, which is described in Chapter 7, *Background and Significance Section*.

4.1 HOW DO LITERATURE REVIEWS FOR GRANT PROPOSALS DIFFER FROM LITERATURE REVIEWS IN JOURNAL ARTICLES OR IN DISSERTATION PROPOSALS?

The process of conducting the literature review for a grant or dissertation proposal is essentially the same as the process of conducting the literature review for a journal article.

Literature reviews for journal articles For a journal article, the literature review is found in the Introduction section of the article. It is typically brief and usually consists of the first *one to two paragraphs* of the article. The Introduction of a journal article is designed to provide the rationale for the research questions; that is, to describe the current state of literature in the topic area and clarify how the article is designed to extend this prior research.

Literature reviews for dissertation proposals Literature reviews for dissertation proposals are designed to provide a comprehensive and up-to-date review of the topic and demonstrate to the dissertation committee that the student has a thorough command of the area. In contrast to a journal article or grant proposal, literature reviews for dissertation proposals may be substantively longer. However, in my experience, this generous allowance for length can lead to a common pitfall: the *laundry list* approach to writing a literature review. Such an approach involves describing each study, one after another, without organizing the material for the reader, critically reviewing the studies, or identifying the research gap. I would therefore argue that, even for a dissertation proposal, following the techniques below will result in a targeted review that will give you hands-on practice for writing a grant proposal—the ultimate direction of your career.

Literature reviews for grant proposals Literature reviews for a grant proposal fall within the Background and Significance section of a grant (see Chapter 7). The space for this section is usually limited but may be longer than a journal article depending upon the granting agency's requirements (one to two paragraphs to one to two pages). It is through this section that you assure the reviewer that the proposed study will fill a research gap and extend prior research in the area.

In summary, all literature reviews, whether written for a journal article, dissertation proposal, or grant proposal, are designed to fill a **research gap**. The size of this research gap will vary according to the type of proposal—smaller for a pilot or feasibility study and largest for an R01 award (see Chapter 17, *Choosing the Right Funding Source*, for details on size of awards).

In summary, writing a literature review for a proposal has two main goals:

1. Provide a comprehensive and up-to-date **review of the topic**.
2. Provide a **basic rationale** for your research.

4.2 WRITING A LITERATURE REVIEW IS AN ITERATIVE PROCESS

Writing the literature review should be viewed as iterative. In other words, after searching for and reviewing the literature in the area, you may find that the overall aims and hypotheses need to be revised in order to persuasively achieve a basic rationale for your proposal. That is, the process of the literature search will most likely lead to a refining or even, at times, a redefining of your topic and research questions.

The key point to keep in mind, therefore, when conducting your search is that it is best to not become too wedded to your initial aims and hypotheses and to be flexible in response to what you learn in the literature search.

4.3 STEP #1: CREATING A LITERATURE REVIEW OUTLINE

The process of conducting a literature search starts with creating an outline of the literature review. The outline will directly relate to and be driven by your specific aims and hypotheses. Having an outline in hand when you start to search the literature will be invaluable in keeping you focused and avoid the common pitfall of becoming overwhelmed by the literature. Without an outline, much time can be misspent collecting literature that does not directly relate to an aspect of the proposal; or alternatively, omitting to collect literature that does relate to an aspect of the proposal. In general, all the literature collected should directly support one of the specific aims/hypotheses.

For proposals in epidemiology and preventive medicine (and following the overall proposal outline in Chapter 2, *Starting a Dissertation Proposal*), the literature that you will collect will address four major themes relevant to the Background and Significance Section of the proposal

IV. Background and Significance
    a. Introduction: Public Health Impact of Outcome (Disease)
    b. Physiology of Exposure–Outcome Relationship
    c. Epidemiology of Exposure–Outcome Relationship
    d. Summary of Significance and Innovation

Your first step is to create an outline. Let's use the example specific aims and hypotheses below to demonstrate how to create a literature review outline:

> *eg example* Specific aim #1: We propose to assess the relationship between postmenopausal hormone use, antioxidants, and Alzheimer's disease in the Phoenix Health Study.
> Hypothesis #1a: Postmenopausal hormone will be inversely associated with Alzheimer's disease.
> Hypothesis #1b: Antioxidant use will be inversely associated with Alzheimer's disease.

Using this example, the literature review outline would be as follows:

a. Introduction: Public Health Impact of Outcome (Disease)
   i. Prevalence and incidence of Alzheimer's disease
   ii. Sequelae of Alzheimer's disease
   iii. Established risk factors for Alzheimer's disease
b. Physiology of Exposure–Outcome Relationship
   i. The physiologic relationship between postmenopausal hormone use and Alzheimer's disease
   ii. The physiologic relationship between antioxidants and Alzheimer's disease
c. Epidemiology of Exposure–Outcome Relationship
   i. The prior epidemiologic studies on the relationship between postmenopausal hormone use and Alzheimer's disease
   ii. The prior epidemiologic studies on the relationship between antioxidants and Alzheimer's disease
d. Summary of Significance and Innovation

Below, at the end of this chapter, you will find three examples of literature review outlines.

4.4 STEP #2: SEARCHING FOR LITERATURE (DO'S AND DON'TS)

Now that you have your outline in hand, you are ready to start searching for literature. Remember that you will only be searching for articles that directly relate to Section a (Public Health Impact), Section b (Physiology of Exposure–Outcome Relationship), and Section c (Epidemiology of Exposure–Outcome Relationship). As you retrieve articles, group them in these categories—either using file folders (for hard copies) or electronic folders (for electronic copies). Within each section, you may want to additionally organize by topics, subtopics, and in chronological order.

4.4.1 Choosing a Relevant Database

For proposal writing in epidemiology and preventive medicine, the literature review will focus on empirical research reports. These are original reports of research found in academic journals and constitute the primary sources of published information. As such, these articles provide detailed methods, results, and discussion of findings. These details will be critical in helping you justify the research gap. In contrast, secondary sources of data (e.g., textbooks, newspaper articles) provide global description of results with few details on methods and should be avoided or used as a source of last resort.

The first step is identifying the correct database to search. Typically, for proposals in epidemiology and preventive medicine, PubMed which encompasses the MEDLINE database, is the primary choice. For some epidemiologic studies that involve a psychosocial exposure or outcome, the database PsycINFO may also be relevant. Google Scholar or Lexus/Nexus may also be useful. Refer to your library's website for a description of the searchable databases to which your institution has access or contact a reference librarian for further assistance.

4.4.2 What Type of Literature to Collect for Each Section of the Literature Review Outline

Using the example above, I will describe the type of literature to collect for each section of the literature review outline.

4.4.2.1 a. Introduction: public health impact of outcome (disease)

First, the proposal needs to support the public health significance of your outcome of interest (Alzheimer's disease). Search for literature that shows the current **prevalence and incidence rates** of Alzheimer's disease, changes in incidence rates over time, and how many people are affected by this disorder. If the study will be conducted among a particular subpopulation, collect literature that not only provides national rates but also provides specific rates in the subpopulation (e.g., Hispanics) or the geographic region where the study will be conducted, if these rates are available.

Another important way to support the public health importance of your outcome of interest is to mention any **sequelae of your outcome/disease**. Does it lead to significant future morbidity and/or mortality? Literature should be collected to support such statements.

Collect literature that demonstrates the **established risk factors** for your outcome of interest. In terms of our example, cite studies (or a review article) that describes established risk factors for Alzheimer's disease.

Finally, the public health impact of your proposal can be further enhanced by citing literature that supports the public health impact of your exposure. In terms of the example above, literature showing a high and/or increasing prevalence of postmenopausal

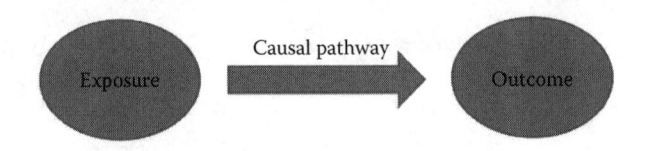

FIGURE 4.1 The causal pathway between an exposure and an outcome.

hormone use would be relevant. In other words, the more people exposed, the greater the potential public health impact of your proposal.

4.4.2.2 b. Physiology of exposure–outcome relationship

Secondly, the proposal needs to support the physiologic or behavioral rationale for a potential relationship between your exposure and your outcome (Figure 4.1). In other words, your job in this section is to demonstrate that there is a feasible mechanism by which your exposure may impact your disease. In terms of our example, search for literature that supports the physiologic mechanisms by which postmenopausal hormone use could impact Alzheimer's disease.

A pitfall to avoid In my experience, students tend go astray when writing this section. That is, they become tempted to spend their time describing the physiology of their outcome in isolation. In doing so, they fail to describe the potential mechanism by which their exposure may influence their disease. In the example above, instead of describing the mechanism by which hormones may impact Alzheimer's disease, they instead dedicate this section to describing the physiology of Alzheimer's disease—its symptoms, signs, and impact on the body. Now certainly a basic knowledge of how Alzheimer's disease develops is key to understanding how it could be impacted by exposures such as hormones. However, failure to cite literature which addresses the **link** between postmenopausal hormone use and Alzheimer's disease is failure to justify your specific aim.

An alternative trap to avoid is to dedicate this section to a description of the physiology of the exposure variable in isolation. The general impact of postmenopausal hormone use on the body is not sufficient. Instead, after a brief description of how hormones function, locate literature that shows how postmenopausal hormone use could influence the occurrence of Alzheimer's disease.

These potential mechanisms will be the thrust of the physiology section. Remember that reviewers are expected to have a general scientific knowledge. So, in light of your page limitations, focus on your causal mechanism (see Figure 4.1).

4.4.2.3 c. Epidemiology of exposure–outcome relationship

The goal of this section is to summarize the findings of prior epidemiologic studies that evaluated the association between your exposure and outcome. Therefore, for this section, collect literature (i.e., published epidemiologic studies) that included an evaluation of the relationship between postmenopausal hormones and risk of Alzheimer's disease regardless of whether the studies found positive, negative, or null results.

A pitfall to avoid When searching through the prior epidemiologic literature, articles that only provide information on the prevalence of your exposure without also evaluating the relationship between your exposure and your outcome would not merit inclusion in this section. For example, a paper that just gave incidence rates of Alzheimer's disease would be very useful for the Introduction (Section a), but unless it also gave measures of association between postmenopausal hormone use and Alzheimer's disease, it would not be relevant for this epidemiology section. Instead, you will be looking for studies that presented measures of association (e.g., relative risks [RRs], odds ratios, correlation coefficients, or mean differences in levels of the outcome) between the exposed and unexposed groups.

In my experience, students and early-career faculty often become discouraged when searching through the prior epidemiologic literature. If they see one prior published study on their exposure–outcome relationship of interest, they worry that there is no longer a research gap and that their hypothesis of interest has already been answered. Recall that, the **Bradford Hill criteria** (i.e., the group of minimal conditions necessary to provide adequate evidence of a causal relationship between an exposure and disease) include *consistency*. Consistency refers to repeated observations of a similar association across different study populations using different study designs. Clearly, one prior study is not going to be sufficient to conclude *consistency*.

4.4.3 Should You Collect Epidemiologic Literature That Only Secondarily Evaluated Your Exposure–Outcome Relationship?

Sometimes an epidemiologic study will have evaluated your exposure and outcome relationship but only as an ancillary analysis in the context of a larger topic on which they are primarily focused. Using our example above, let's imagine that a prior published study focused on stress and its impact on Alzheimer's disease. However, in their tables, the authors may also have included findings on the impact of postmenopausal hormone use on Alzheimer's disease. Perhaps they conducted this *sidebar* analysis to assess postmenopausal hormone use as a potential confounder of stress. You will typically find these ancillary findings in descriptive or bivariate tables.

Even though your exposure–outcome relationship of interest was not the prior publication's relationship of interest, it may still be relevant to cite this article. In other words, because this article still includes an assessment of your exposure and outcome, it is relevant for your epidemiology section. At the same time, it is also important to note that these findings are often unadjusted for potential confounding factors and may simply show the unadjusted relationship between your exposure (e.g., postmenopausal hormone use) and your outcome (Alzheimer's disease). Most likely, you will be improving upon these prior findings!

4.4.4 Collecting Literature for an Effect Modification Hypothesis

You may also wish to evaluate whether the relationship between your exposure and disease of interest differs within strata of your population. In other words, you might hypothesize that the relationship will be different among one particular subgroup of people as compared to another. Subgroups could be groups of differing genders, races, ethnicities, ages, or other factors. This is classically termed effect modification or interaction. If this is of interest, it is typically required that this question be included as a hypothesis. By including this hypothesis *a priori* (i.e., before the research has been initiated), you will also minimize reviewer concerns that you are simply *data dredging*.

In the example above, let's say that the proposal writer, in conducting their literature search, found physiologic studies for Section b that suggested that the impact of postmenopausal hormone use on Alzheimer's disease might be enhanced among obese women. In other words, there might be some synergistic effect between postmenopausal use and obesity, in terms of their impact on Alzheimer's disease. Their corresponding hypothesis would state the following:

> Hypothesis #1c: There will be a stronger inverse association between postmenopausal hormone use and Alzheimer's disease among obese women as compared to nonobese women.

This hypothesis must also be addressed in the outline.

Using the example above, the revised literature review outline would look as follows:

a. Introduction: Public Health Impact of Outcome (Disease)
   i. Prevalence and incidence of Alzheimer's disease
   ii. Sequelae of Alzheimer's disease
   iii. Established risk factors for Alzheimer's disease
b. Physiology of Exposure–Outcome Relationship
   i. The physiologic relationship between postmenopausal hormone use and Alzheimer's disease
   ii. The physiologic relationship between antioxidants and Alzheimer's disease
   iii. *The physiologic relationship between postmenopausal hormone use and Alzheimer's disease among obese women and among nonobese women*
c. Epidemiology of Exposure–Outcome Relationship
   i. The prior epidemiologic studies on the relationship between postmenopausal hormone use and Alzheimer's disease
   ii. The prior epidemiologic studies on the relationship between antioxidants and Alzheimer's disease

      iii. *The prior epidemiologic studies on the relationship between postmenopausal hormone use and Alzheimer's disease among obese women and among nonobese women*
   d. Summary of Significance and Innovation

The addition of this hypothesis would influence the search in the following way. You would now want to locate literature suggesting that there is a different physiologic association between postmenopausal hormone use and Alzheimer's disease in obese women. Then, second, each of the epidemiologic studies collected as part of Section c above would need to be carefully examined to see whether those authors also evaluated the same effect modification/interaction hypothesis.

4.4.5 What to Do When Your Search Yields Thousands of *Hits*

Search engines such as PubMed make the search process easier but have the associated hazards of retrieving too many *hits*. Imagine the shock faced by a student proposing to evaluate the association between coffee and bladder cancer when they find 30,000 hits after entering the key terms *coffee* and *bladder cancer*.

    Therefore, the first step is learning how to carefully limit the search. Consider your choice of key search terms. As noted in the example above, just using the name of your exposure and your outcome variables may yield an overwhelming number of hits. Tips to limit this search depend on which section of the outline that your search is aiming to fill (e.g., Section a, b, or c). For example, for the epidemiology section, adding the key term *epidemiology* will limit your search. In addition, setting a limit on where the search term must appear (e.g., title or title/abstract) will also limit the search. In PubMed, such a limit can be set using the *filter* option.

    Other tips to limit the search include searching within a key journal in your field. For example, a search limited to *American Journal of Epidemiology* will ensure that you start out with some key epidemiology articles in your area. To do this in PubMed, enter the standard journal abbreviation *Am J Epidemiol* in the search box along with your key terms. Once you become familiar with the research in your area, you may also find it helpful to limit the search to a key author in that field.

    Another way to limit search *hits* is to limit the search to journal articles within the past 5 years. Or start with the most recent article and work backward using the reference list of each article.

    In a similar vein, starting with a review article on your topic, if available, is also a good first step. This can be done by limiting the search to review articles. However, caution should still be taken. Although review articles provide you with a comprehensive reference list, you will still need to search for articles published since the review. In addition, often the review article is on a similar, but not identical, topic to yours—therefore requiring more searching on your part. Also, I cannot emphasize enough that it is not sufficient to abstract data on the individual studies from the review article. Instead, you must obtain copies of each article referenced in the review. This is true for two reasons. First, often the key data that you will need for your literature review will not be provided with adequate detail in the review article. Second, you do not want to rely on the author of the review article for the accuracy of their abstracted information.

4.4.6 What to Do If There Are Too Few Hits

This can be a particular concern for Section c (Epidemiology of Exposure–Outcome Relationship): If you have entered your key exposure and outcome variable names together in the search box and received less than 5–10 relevant papers, it may be useful to expand your search. One approach is to use noncurrent articles. First, consider expanding the search to the past 10 years or longer. Even if a study is older, if it is the only evidence available on a given topic, then it is important to include. It is also reasonable to include a landmark or classic study in the area whose inclusion helps to understand the evolution of a research technique.

If you determine that there is no literature with a direct bearing on one or more aspects of your topic, this should be cautiously viewed as good news. That is, you may have identified a research gap given that no one has evaluated your proposed association of interest. However, on the other hand, you want to assure the reader that your proposed association is reasonable to hypothesize. In other words, perhaps there are no papers on your topic because there is no physiologic rationale for why your proposed exposure may be associated with your proposed outcome.

In this case, your goal will be to assure the reader that your hypothesis is reasonable. Search for studies with same exposure as yours, but a different, albeit physiologically related, outcome. The concept is to choose an outcome similar to your own, so that a reasonable reader would consider it possible that a similar mechanism might link your exposure to your outcome.

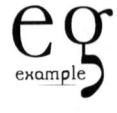

e.g. example Imagine that you are interested in the association between depression during pregnancy and risk of gestational diabetes mellitus (defined as diabetes that develops during pregnancy). You conduct a search for epidemiologic studies on this topic using PubMed but find no studies. Or, you only identify two studies that evaluated this association. This amount of evidence may not be sufficient to reassure reviewers that your proposed association is plausible. However, when you search on the association between depression and type 2 diabetes outside of pregnancy, you find a plethora of studies. The presence of these studies and the strength of their findings bolster up the rationale for examining this association in pregnancy.

The second approach if there are too few *hits* is to abstract articles on a different exposure but the same outcome. Again, the idea is to select an exposure similar in nature to your exposure. For our example, you could search for studies on anxiety or stress during pregnancy and risk of gestational diabetes. The argument is that if these other psychosocial factors impact risk of gestational diabetes, then it might be reasonable to assume that depression also impacts risk of gestational diabetes. Again, the criteria for including such studies should be to bolster up a reasonable physiologic mechanism for your proposed, but clearly novel, association.

4.4.7 How to Retrieve Articles (Hits)

Once you identify an article, there are several ways to retrieve it—for example, electronically or via interlibrary loan or at the library. These days, most universities have subscriptions to online versions of most manuscripts. Some journals provide electronic access to complete versions of their published articles.

4.4.8 How to Scan Articles for Relevance

Once you retrieve articles, the first step is to quickly scan them. This involves a quick look at the:

- Abstract
- Last paragraph of the Introduction
- Tables
- First and last paragraphs of the Conclusion

In scanning the article, your goal is simply to identify whether this article will provide key substantive (e.g., numerical) findings that will support Sections a, b, or c of your literature search outline as delineated above. The **Abstract** will, in 200–250 words, encapsulate the key aspects of the paper including the goals/purpose, study design, study methods, highlights of the results, and primary conclusions. The last paragraph of the **Introduction** is important as this is where the author will have articulated the relevant prior literature, the research gap, and their specific aims and hypotheses. The *tables* should be searched to see if they provide relevant measures of association between your exposure and your outcome. Remember not to get distracted by findings for other exposure–outcome relationships found within the tables. Later, in Chapter 12, *Review of Bias and Confounding*, we will address the issue of potential confounding by these factors. The first and last paragraphs of the **Conclusion** are also key because this is where the author will reiterate the major findings of the article.

4.4.9 Evaluating Your References for Completeness

At this point, you should now have collected articles that relate to Section a (Introduction), Section b (Physiology of Exposure–Outcome Relationship), and Section c (Epidemiology of Exposure–Outcome Relationship). Ensure that your list is complete and up to date. Remember that a literature review should demonstrate that it represents the latest work done in the subject area. Often, grant reviewers or journal reviewers are selected from experts in the field; that is, those authors who have also evaluated your exposure or outcome of interest. Imagine their concern if they are assigned to review your proposal and see that you did not cite their directly relevant published paper in the field.

4.5 STEP #3: ORGANIZING THE EPIDEMIOLOGIC LITERATURE— SUMMARY TABLES

A summary table is an invaluable tool for organizing the epidemiologic literature collected for Section a (Epidemiology of Exposure–Outcome Relationship). Indeed, you are probably familiar with such summary tables as they are often included in review articles as an efficient way to present the key aspects of the published studies in an area. Having one of these summary tables in hand will make the writing process smooth and efficient (see Chapter 7, *Background and Significance Section*).

Indeed, the process of creating a summary table will be one of the most valuable activities in helping you to identify the major trends or patterns in the literature and thereby identifying the **research gap**.

4.5.1 What Data Should I Include in a Summary Table?

Summary tables are flexible and can be customized to best suit the aspects of your proposal and ultimately to best highlight the research gap (Table 4.1). The standard items included as column headings in a summary table are **Author/Year, Study Design**, and **Study Population**. The Study Design column for epidemiologic studies is typically limited to cohort (prospective or retrospective), cross sectional, case–control, and ecologic/correlational or subvariations of these studies. The Study Population column typically includes the sample size and the study location. In addition, if you are considering proposing a study limited to a certain study population (e.g., Hispanics or children), list the percentage of people in these subgroups within the "Study Population" column for each study.

An **Exposure Assessment** column concisely describes the tool used to measure your exposure. For example, using our prior example, this column would state how postmenopausal hormone use was assessed (e.g., self-reported questionnaire, medical record abstraction). It might also be useful to state how this variable was parameterized (e.g., as a dichotomous variable, a categorical variable, or a continuous variable). Some summary tables list these categories in a **Contrast** column (see the example summary table at the end of this chapter).

Similarly, an **Outcome Assessment** column concisely describes the tool used to measure your outcome as well as how it was parameterized. For example, using our

TABLE 4.1 Example summary table for organizing the epidemiologic literature

AUTHOR, YEAR	STUDY DESIGN	STUDY POPULATION	EXPOSURE TYPE OF PHYSICAL ACTIVITY	EXPOSURE WHEN ASSESSED	OUTCOME BIRTH WEIGHT	CONTRAST	EFFECT ESTIMATE
Jones, 2012	Prospective cohort	500 prenatal patients; NYC	Occupational	Once at 20 weeks gestation	Medical record abstraction	Active job vs. sedentary	⇐ 1.60 (95% CI 1.10–1.90)
Smith, 2010	Prospective cohort	3000 prenatal patients; Utah	Total	Once at 23–26 weeks gestation	Birth certificates	High work/exercise vs. low work/exercise	⇒ 0.75 (95% CI 0.45–0.92)
Tyler, 2008	Prospective cohort	250 prenatal patients; Australia	Occupational, household	Each trimester at 17, 28, and 36 weeks gestation	Medical record abstraction	Kcal/min nominal categories	⇕ Nonsignificant mean differences
Frank, 2007	Prospective cohort	800 prenatal patients; Sweden	Recreational	Each trimester	Medical record abstraction	Heavy exercise vs. no exercise	⇒ 0.61 (95% CI 0.48–0.85)

prior example, this column would state how Alzheimer's disease was assessed (e.g., proxy questionnaire, medical record abstraction). Both of the Exposure and Outcome Assessment columns can also state key factors such as the timing of assessment (e.g., at 6-month postintervention or at baseline) and whether the assessment tools were validated.

Another key column is **Results**. The Results column should concisely provide findings on your association of interest. Provide the actual magnitude of association (e.g., RRs, odds ratios, correlation coefficients) between the exposure and outcome as opposed to simply listing p-values.

A pitfall to avoid Be as specific and concise as possible in the Results column. Present the actual numerical findings here, as opposed to quoting a narrative of the text of the findings. For example, "OR = 3.2, 95% CI 2.1–4.5" is more concise than a statement like *The authors found a positive association between postmenopausal hormone use and risk of Alzheimer's disease.* The latter sentence is not only cumbersome to read, but it does not provide key information on the magnitude of association. Based on this sentence alone, the reader would not know if the authors found only a 10% increased risk or a fourfold increased risk. Even more simply, you may consider creating a version of your summary table that only displays arrows in the Results column, that is, up arrows for positive associations, down arrows for inverse associations, and cross arrows for null associations. In this manner, you can quickly scan across this column to assess the overall thrust of prior study findings.

Other potential columns to consider include a **Covariates** column that lists all the adjustment factors and an **Exclusions** Column.

If you have several outcome variables, it may be preferable to use separate tables for each outcome type. On the other hand, if you have one outcome variable but several exposure variables, you may want to create separate tables for each exposure type. In both of these situations, the same papers may be included in both tables; however, key measurement columns as well as Results columns will differ, and you will find it useful to have the entire details of these studies in both tables.

4.5.2 Reviewing the Table to Identify Research Gaps

As mentioned earlier, your goal in creating the table is to not only summarize the prior literature but to make the research gaps clearly evident. In reviewing the table, make note of trends (weaknesses) across studies. For example, looking down the *Study Design* column, ask yourself questions such as "Are all the studies cross sectional?" "Are all the studies based on small sample sizes?" Look at the characteristics of the participants and note if any groups at high risk of your outcome are not included. These are *research gaps*. If your study will be filling these research gaps, then you'll want to highlight these facts when writing the literature review (as described in Chapter 7, *Background and Significance Section*).

Continue to examine the table and note whether study findings in the **Results** column differ according to the study designs or measurement techniques used. For example, ask yourself, "Do all studies that support a certain conclusion use one method of measurement, while those that support a different conclusion use a different method?" "Do all studies that support a certain conclusion control for key confounding factors?"

Now that you have examined the summary table with this goal in mind, you may want to make modifications to the table. This may involve including or expanding your column headings, or column content, to make the research gaps most apparent. For example, if you will be the first to use a new measurement technique, you'll want to be sure that your **Exposure Assessment** column lists the measurement technique used by each study. In this way, a scan of that column will make it evident that no prior study used your proposed measurement technique. If your study is the first study to adjust for body mass index (BMI), you'll want to include a **Covariates** column that lists all the adjustment factors. In this way, a scan of that column will make it clear that no prior study evaluated BMI. For example, in a proposed study of physical activity and preterm birth, I included a column titled, **Validated Exposure Assessment**. The response under this column for each study was *no* making it clear that no prior study had used a measure of physical activity validated in pregnant women—a key research gap.

Remember that the goal of the literature review is to identify gaps in the literature. The crux of the proposal is filling, at least in part, these research gaps and thereby extending prior research. Having this summary table in hand when you start the writing process (see Chapter 7, *Background and Significance Section*) will make this process go much more smoothly. It is also reasonable at this point to consider altering your hypotheses in light of your findings. Remember if it is not clear to you that you will be extending the prior literature, then it certainly will not be to your reviewers.

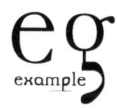

eg *example* Imagine that you are proposing to evaluate the association between physical activity during pregnancy and birth weight. After reviewing the summary table (Table 4.1), you note two themes: (1) few studies measured physical activity at more than one time point in pregnancy, and (2) only one study measured total activity (e.g., occupational + household + recreational). Therefore, you revise your proposal to measure *total physical activity at all three trimesters* of pregnancy—becoming the first study to date to do so.

4.5.3 Should I Include the Summary Table in My Proposal?

It is likely that a dissertation proposal will have adequate space to include a summary table, and inclusion of the table will clearly demonstrate your knowledge and grasp of the state of the literature to the dissertation committee. However, due to space limitations, it may not be possible to fit your table into a grant proposal. Regardless, the table will still be critical in your writing process. Your acquired grasp of the prior published literature in your area—the number of studies and their trends as to methods, findings, and gaps—will readily come across in the literature review write up (as discussed in Chapter 7, *Background and Significance Section*). The summary table will allow you to more readily convince yourself and your reviewers that you have identified the research gaps. Also note that, as side benefit, the table may be useful for a subsequent review article publication.

4.6 EXAMPLES

4.6.1 Example #1

Stress and Hypertensive Disorders of Pregnancy in Black Women

Literature Review Outline

    a. Introduction: Public Health Impact of Hypertensive Disorders of Pregnancy
        i. Impact of hypertensive disorders of pregnancy on maternal and fetal health
        ii. Rates of hypertensive disorders of pregnancy in US women
        iii. Rates of hypertensive disorders of pregnancy in black women
        iv. Established risk factors for hypertensive disorders of pregnancy
    b. Physiology of Stress—Hypertensive Disorders of Pregnancy
        i. Neuroendocrinological mechanism
        ii. Inflammatory mechanism
    c. Epidemiology of Stress—Hypertensive Disorders of Pregnancy
        i. Epidemiologic studies observing a positive association
        ii. Epidemiologic studies observing an inverse association
        iii. Epidemiologic studies observing null findings
    d. Summary of Significance and Innovation

4.6.2 Example #2

Physical Activity and Duration of Second Stage of Labor in Hispanic Women

Literature Review Outline

    a. Introduction: Public Health Impact of Second Stage of Labor
        i. Mean duration of second stage of labor
            1. Among all women
            2. Among Hispanic women
        ii. Impact of duration of second stage of labor on maternal and fetal health
        iii. Known risk factors affecting duration of second stage of labor
            1. Risk factors prolonging duration of second stage of labor
            2. Risk factors reducing duration of second stage of labor
    b. Physiologic Evidence for the Effect of Physical Activity on Duration of Second Stage of Labor
        i. Pelvic floor muscle training leading to a better perineal muscle tone and reduction in second-stage duration
        ii. Increased activity leading to lower BMI. Increased maternal BMI known to cause dystocia and need for augmentation
        iii. Physical activity leading to changes in oxytocin, adrenaline, and endorphins levels in blood responsible for regulating the process of birth

c. Epidemiologic Evidence for the Effect of Physical Activity during Early and Midpregnancy on Duration of Second Stage of Labor
      i. Epidemiologic studies on effect of physical activity during early or midpregnancy or entire pregnancy on duration of second stage of labor
      ii. Epidemiologic studies among Hispanic women regarding physical activity and second stage of labor
   d. Summary of Significance and Innovation

4.6.3 Example #3

Use of NSAIDS and Risk of Endometrial Cancer in Postmenopausal Women

Literature Review Outline and Summary Table (Table 4.2)

   a. Introduction: Public Health Impact of Endometrial Cancer
      i. Significance of endometrial cancer
      ii. Rates of endometrial cancer in the United States and in postmenopausal women
      iii. Established risk factors for endometrial cancer
      iv. Modifiable risk factors for endometrial cancer
         1. Risk factors known to increase the risk of endometrial cancer
         2. Risk factors known to decrease the risk of endometrial cancer
   b. Physiology of NSAIDS and Endometrial Cancer Relationship
      i. Hormone-mediated mechanism
      ii. Insulin-mediated mechanism
      iii. Inflammatory mechanism
   c. Epidemiology of NSAIDS and Endometrial Cancer Relationship
      i. Epidemiologic studies observing a positive association
      ii. Epidemiologic studies observing an inverse association
      iii. Epidemiologic studies observing null findings
   d. Summary of Significance and Innovation

TABLE 4.2 Example summary table for a proposal to evaluate the use of NSAIDS and risk of endometrial cancer in postmenopausal women

AUTHOR, YEAR	STUDY DESIGN	STUDY POPULATION	EXPOSURE: NSAIDS TYPE	EXPOSURE: WHEN/HOW	STRATIFIED BY	OUTCOME: WHAT	OUTCOME: HOW	CONTRAST	EFFECT ESTIMATE	ADJUSTMENT FACTORS
Smith et al., 2013	Case-control study	400 matched pairs, age 35–50, received medical services at Georgia Hospital, 2010–2012	A: Aspirin	Self-administered questionnaire	BMI	Cases: endometrial cancer; controls: nonneoplastic conditions	Cases and controls identified from tumor registry	(a) A: Regular users vs. nonusers; (b) A: Obese users vs. normal weight users	(a) ↔OR: 0.96 (95% CI: 0.71–1.31); (b) ↓OR: 0.45 (95% CI: 0.22–0.87)	Age, education, BMI, parity, age at menarche and menopause
Jones et al., 2013	Prospective cohort study	50,000 female teachers, age 30–55 years in US	A: Aspirin, NA: Non-aspirin NSAIDS	Self-administered questionnaire at baseline	BMI	Self-reported cases of endometrial cancer	Cases confirmed by physicians reviewing medical records	(a) A: Past vs. never users; (b) A: Current vs. never users; (c) A: Obese current users vs. obese never users	(a) ↔RR: 1.17 (95% CI: 0.94–1.47); (b) ↔RR: 1.08 (95% CI: 0.88–1.32); (c) ↔RR: 0.61 (95% CI: 0.41–0.91)	Age, BMI, smoking, OCP use, PMH use, age at menarche and menopause, hypertension, diabetes
Frances et al., 2012	Case-control study	200 cases, 205 controls, age 50–70, New York	Any: Any NSAIDS, A: Aspirin, NA: Non-aspirin NSAIDS	Interview	BMI	Cases of endometrial cancer diagnosis	Cases: Dept. of Health and State Cancer Registry; controls of <65 years of age by random dig. dialing; controls of >65 years by CMS	(a) Any: Users vs. nonusers; (b) A users vs. nonusers; (c) NA: Users vs. nonusers; (d) NA: Lower vs. higher BMI	(a) Slight ↓OR: 0.6 (95% CI: 0.4–0.98); (b) slight ↓OR: 0.6 (95% CI: 0.3–1.0); (c) slight ↓OR: 0.7 (95% CI: 0.4–1.3) (d) slight ↓OR: 0.7 (95% CI: 0.4–1.4)	Age, BMI, education race, menarche, hormone therapy, OCP use, age at menopause, parity, family history of endometrial cancer

Dodge et al., 2011	Prospective cohort study	65,000 women in Taipei Diet and Health Study, age 50–71 years, 2010–2013	*Any:* Any NSAIDS, *A:* Aspirin, *NA:* Non-aspirin NSAIDS	Mailed questionnaire	BMI	Cases of endometrial cancer	North American Association of Central Cancer Registries	(a) *Any:* Users vs. nonusers; (b) *A:* Users vs. nonusers; (c) *NA:* Users vs. nonusers; (d) *A:* Obese users vs. obese nonusers	(a) ↔RR: 0.7 (95% CI: 0.5–0.97) (b) ↔RR: 0.7 (95% CI: 0.4–1.0) (c) ↔RR: 0.8 (95% CI: 0.5–1.3) (d) RR: 0.7 (95% CI: 0.4–1.4)	Age at menarche and menopause, race, PMH use, parity, OCP, smoking, BMI, physical activity, diabetes, hypertension, heart disease, family history of breast cancer
Grainger et al., 2011	Case–control study	250 cases and 405 controls, age 50–74 years (2007–2010)	*Any:* Any NSAIDS, *A:* Aspirin	In-person interview	BMI	Cases of endometrial cancer; controls: cases of ovarian cancer	Cases: cancer surveillance system affiliated with SEER; controls: random dig. dialing	(a) *Any:* Users vs. nonusers; (b) *A:* Users vs. nonusers; (c) *Any:* Obese users vs. nonusers	(a) ↔OR: 1.01 (95% CI: 0.8–1.5); (b) ↔OR: 1.02 (95% CI: 0.6–1.77); (c) ↔OR: 0.91 (95% CI: 0.61–1.42)	Age, residence, calendar year, BMI, hormone therapy use
Roth et al., 2010	Prospective cohort study	12,000 females, age 55–69 years, Western Health Study 2000–2010	*A:* Aspirin, *NA:* Non-aspirin NSAIDS	Mailed questionnaire at baseline	BMI (data not shown)	Cases of endometrial cancer	Identified from State Health Registry	*A:* Users vs. nonusers; *NA:* Users vs. nonusers	(a) ↔HR: 0.77 (95% CI: 0.59–1.01); (b) ↔HR: 0.87 (95% CI: 0.67–1.10)	Age, BMI, age at menarche and menopause, history of OCP use, history of diabetes and hypertension

Scientific Writing 5

In Chapter 4, I described a step-by-step process for conducting the literature search for your proposal, starting with how to create a literature review outline, techniques and tips for conducting a targeted search, and ending with how to assimilate those search findings into a summary table. After identifying the research gap with the help of your summary table and confirming and/or refining your topic, you are now ready for the process of actually writing the literature review!

Therefore, this chapter focuses on writing style and how to write for a scientific audience. Specifically, the chapter goes over tips as well as specific stylistic guidelines for writing with a scientific audience in mind. As with any writing, you will want to factor in time for (1) writing a first draft, (2) editing (i.e., checking the draft for completeness, cohesion, and correctness), and (3) rewriting and revising the draft.

5.1 TIP #1: CONSIDER YOUR AUDIENCE

Your target audience is the scientific community regardless of whether you are writing a dissertation proposal, submitting a grant proposal, or writing a journal article. As noted in Chapter 1, *Ten Top Tips for Successful Proposal Writing*, grant reviewers do not always have expertise in your proposed area. That is, while one reviewer may have a specific background in your area, others are assigned based on their expertise with the proposed methodology (e.g., epidemiology), and others are assigned to review the statistical analysis section. For example, a grant designed to identify risk factors for uterine cancer may be assigned to the following three reviewers: (1) an oncologist, (2) an epidemiologist who has conducted case–control studies among cancer patients, and (3) a statistician. It is even possible that the physician or the epidemiologist will not have direct experience with uterine cancer specifically but are instead more generalist reproductive cancer researchers.

However, it is reassuring to note that, if your proposal is well written, even a generalist reviewer will be able to assess (1) whether your goals are clearly stated, (2) whether your proposal clearly justifies how it extends prior work in the field, (3) what is innovative about your proposal, as well as (4) the impact of your potential findings on public health and clinical practice.

5.2 TIP #2: AVOID USING THE FIRST-PERSON SINGULAR

Using the first-person singular (e.g., *I* or *myself*) is appropriate for writing an editorial but not for writing a scientific proposal. Most simply stated, the first-person singular voice puts you at risk of sounding subjective and expressing simply a personal opinion.

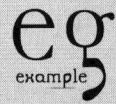

> *e.g.* example
>
> **Original Version**
> In this review, I will establish what I believe to be a major weakness in the literature on weight loss programs. Namely, my observation is that most of the evidence on the impact of the programs on cardiovascular disease risk factors is purely descriptive and anecdotal. While reading the following literature review, you should keep in mind...
>
> **Improved Version**
> The popularity of weight loss programs has resulted in numerous articles reporting claims about the impact of such programs.[1-7] The articles tend to provide (a) purely descriptive, anecdotal accounts of the programs' impact on cardiovascular disease risk factors[1-3] or (b) descriptions of design and guidelines for developing a weight loss program.[5-7]

The *improved version* has a number of advantages: First, the improved version avoids the use of the first-person singular by not referring to the writer(s) at all. As an alternative, the improved version also could have considered the use of the first-person plural (i.e., *we*) if the review was written by a group of investigators or a convened panel. Note that, in the improved version, the background section appears more scientifically sound as it does not appear that the proposal writer is stating their own personal opinions.

Secondly, the *improved version* cites scientific publications to support the points raised. This further reinforces the objectivity of the assertions made. Thirdly, the use of a numbered list provides structure and organization to the paragraph and gives the impression that the writer has conducted a thorough review and knows how to organize and present results. Overall, the entire impression is one of rigor and fact as opposed to conjecture and personal conversation.

5.3 TIP #3: USE THE ACTIVE VOICE

Use of the active voice as opposed to the passive voice is always preferable in scientific writing. Unfortunately, students often feel tempted to use the passive voice in an attempt, albeit misguided, to sound more sophisticated. However, it may be somewhat surprising to learn that, instead, the use of active voice comes off sounding more impressive. The active voice has other advantages: it avoids indirect sentence constructions, which, in addition to being harder to read, also takes up more space. And, as you know, space is vital when writing a grant proposal.

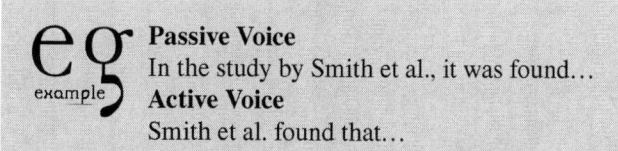

> **Passive Voice**
> In the study by Smith et al., it was found...
> **Active Voice**
> Smith et al. found that...

As you can see, the improved version is more concise and easier to read.

If you read scientific journals (always recommended to improve your writing!), you will see that these journals provide further evidence that the active voice is preferable. For example, one of the highest-ranked and rigorous journals, *The New England Journal of Medicine*, uses active voice. A quick glance through a typical article in *The New England Journal* will yield such sentences as the following:

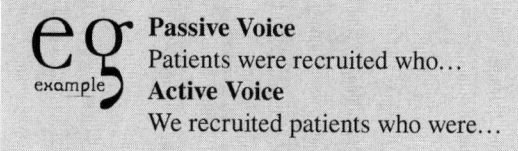

> **Passive Voice**
> Patients were recruited who...
> **Active Voice**
> We recruited patients who were...

5.4 TIP #4: USE TRANSITIONS TO HELP TRACE YOUR ARGUMENT

This tip fits under the rubric of being kind to your reader (as described in Chapter 1, *Ten Top Tips for Successful Proposal Writing*). For example, let's say that you would like to introduce three related points. In this case, it is helpful to the reader to begin sentences or paragraphs describing these points with such terms as *first, second,* and *third*. These terms provide guideposts for your reader, keeping them up to date on your plan and helping them to identify relationships among sections of your proposal. These transitions also have the secondary effect of ensuring that you are internally consistent—ensuring that you do not inadvertently drop one of your arguments. Similarly, the list format also helps to ensure that all your points are relevant to your overall argument as opposed to being extraneous. Other transition phases, aside from a numbered list, include *the next example, in a related study,* and *a counterexample*. In summary, these phrases serve the purpose of alerting the reader to the purpose of each paragraph and therefore are *kind* to the reader/reviewer.

5.5 TIP #5: AVOID DIRECT QUOTATIONS BOTH AT THE BEGINNING AND WITHIN THE LITERATURE REVIEW

Graduate students and early-career faculty are often tempted to start a proposal with a direct quotation or, more often, to use a direct quotation when summarizing the conclusions of authors of prior literature in the field. The greatest temptation to use a direct quotation seems to occur when summarizing the results of a review article written by a leader in the field. While the use of direct quotations may be fairly typical of a creative writing piece such as a novel, they are less useful, and I would suggest actually detrimental, in the context of a proposal. I describe several reasons for this below.

In the context of a scientific proposal, direct quotations are by definition presented out of context and as such may not convey the original author's intent. Addressing this concern by going on to explain the context of the quotation uses even more space, can serve to detract from your main purpose, and is likely to confuse the reader with nonessential details.

Instead, paraphrasing prior literature in your own words, even when you feel that another author's thoughts are vital to your proposal, is always preferable. This technique eliminates disruptions in the flow due to the different writing styles and avoids extraneous details.

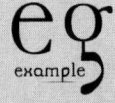

> *e.g. example* Imagine a proposal to evaluate the association between socioeconomic status and some aspect of health that starts out with the following quote:
>
>> The place and roles that individuals take up in the socioeconomic structure of the society shapes and defines the life conditions that characterize the different social classes and are the source of the differences in the quality of life and the differential exposure to conditions (e.g., different types of behaviour and lifestyle characteristics of different social groups) that on the one hand protect and benefit health and on the other hand deteriorate and limit health, resulting in the appearance of disease and death. (Smith et al. 2012)

First, and most importantly, the proposal would need to take some time *translating* this quote into what it actually means in the context of the proposal. The quote is very dense, the wording is cumbersome, and it is unlikely that the writing style and terminology used in the rest of the proposal will be consistent with this quote. Secondly, note the potential for differences in style and spelling conventions between the quote (i.e., the use of the British spelling for *behaviour*) and what is likely to be in the body of the proposal. Thirdly, to be kind to your reviewer, you want to use consistent terms to refer to your exposure of interest. The quote does not follow this guideline and instead uses a variety of terms for socioeconomic status (e.g., *socioeconomic structure, social class, social groups*). If socioeconomic status will be your exposure of interest in the proposal, then you might even be introducing yet another synonym. Even though various authors have chosen their own variant on this term, the proposal should have one voice—your own. Therefore, in paraphrasing the key thoughts behind this quote, it is important to replace all these synonyms for socioeconomic status with your term of choice.

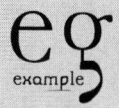

> **Improved Version**
> Socioeconomic status constitutes a variety of factors (e.g., lifestyle and behavioral factors) and, in turn, has been found to impact morbidity and mortality.[1-3]

5.6 TIP #6: AVOID SAYING *THE AUTHORS CONCLUDED*...

This tip is very closely related to the prior tip. While it is tempting to use quotations, it is almost more common for students to say *the authors concluded* when describing the findings of prior studies in the field. This is often motivated by a lack of confidence in stating one's own conclusions. Students may believe that they are gaining credibility by directly quoting the author, when instead they are actually inadvertently undermining the reviewer's confidence in their own abilities as an independent researcher.

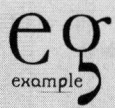

> **Original Version**
> The authors concluded that their findings were unlikely to be due to selection bias.
>
> **Improved Version**
> Because women who participated in the study did not differ significantly from women who did not participate in the study in terms of sociodemographic factors, it is unlikely that the findings could have been due to selection bias.

Remember that authors are not always correct in their conclusions. Some authors might minimize the impact of potential biases on their study findings. Other authors may either incorrectly describe their study design or use a vague term when describing their study design (e.g., retrospective study vs. *case–control study*). Even when the authors are correct, it is still preferable to state their conclusions in your own words. Note that the improved version has the additional advantage of avoiding the use of epidemiologic jargon by defining *selection bias* in lay person's terms.

5.7 TIP #7: OMIT NEEDLESS WORDS

A common aphorism is that, in most writing, every third word can be eliminated.

Of course, this cannot be taken literally, but at its heart, this phrase means that all writing has a *flab* factor, particularly in early drafts. I cannot think of any proposal that I have reviewed in the past that would not be strengthened by this approach.

Vigorous writing is concise. As described in the classic guide to writing, *Strunk and White*, "A sentence should contain no unnecessary words, a paragraph no unnecessary sentences, for the same reason that a drawing should have no unnecessary lines and a machine no unnecessary parts. This requires not that the writer make all his sentences short, or that he avoid all detail and treat his subjects only in outline, but that every word tell."

George Orwell was an early-twentieth-century English novelist and journalist who had a profound impact on language and writing. His writing reflects clarity, intelligence, and wit. Orwell was unhappy with vague writing and professional jargon and felt that poor writing was an indication of sloppy thinking. He excused neither the scientist nor the novelist from his strict requirement for good, vigorous writing.

Orwell's Writing Rules
1. Never use a long word where a short one will do.
2. If it is possible to cut a word out, always cut it out.
3. Never use the passive where you can use the active.
4. Never use a foreign phrase, a scientific word, or a jargon word if you can think of an everyday English equivalent.
5. Break any of these rules sooner than say anything outright barbarous.

Therefore, in rereading your proposal for a second and third time, your main focus will be removing extraneous words that detract the reader from quickly and directly getting to your main point. Extra prepositional phrases will detract from your points.
Many expressions in common use violate this principle:

- *The question as to whether...* can be written as *Whether....*
- *There is no doubt but that* can be written as *no doubt* (*doubtless*).
- *This is a subject that...* can be written as *This subject....*
- *The reason why is that...* can be written as *Because....*

The use of definite, specific, concrete language is the surest way to arouse and hold the attention of the reviewer:

- *Since* actually refers to a span of time and should not be used in place of *Because*.
- *Though* can be written as *Although*.
- *In order to...* can be written as *To....*

The improved example below omits needless words from a sentence found in the background section of a proposal.

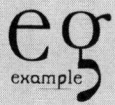

> **Original Version**
> Using accelerometers, light-intensity physical activity has been found to be positively associated with kidney function.
>
> **Improved Version**
> Using accelerometers, light-intensity physical activity has been positively associated with kidney function.

5.8 TIP #8: AVOID PROFESSIONAL JARGON

In the spirit of writing clearly and concisely, one of the keys is to avoid the use of professional jargon. (Or, if you must include the jargon, at the least you will want to accompany it with a brief explanation.) *Professional jargon* refers to use of the terms such as *selection bias*, *information bias*, and *confounding* as stand-alone terms without a lay person description. This tip may appear counterintuitive at first, because you may feel that such jargon is brief and self-explanatory. However, even for an audience of experts, simply using these terms without describing the bias scenario that you are concerned about puts the burden on the reviewer to imagine how the study under discussion may be facing, for example, recall bias. Therefore, clarifying your jargon in a direct manner using simple terms will show the reviewers that you have a clear grasp of the potential limitations that your study faces. Secondarily, by doing this work for the reviewer, you will be following the principle of being *kind* to the reviewer.

For example, imagine you are conducting a study of oral contraceptives and risk of diabetes.

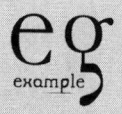

> **Original Version**
> Study findings of an increased risk of diabetes among oral contraceptive users may have been due to detection bias.
>
> **Improved Version**
> Detection bias is possible because women who take oral contraceptives are monitored more closely for diabetes than nonusers of oral contraceptives.

The improved example retains the term *detection bias* but also includes a clear explanation of what detection bias means in this scenario.

5.9 TIP #9: AVOID USING SYNONYMS FOR RECURRING WORDS

The avoidance of synonyms is a key principle to follow as their use is one of the largest sources of reader/reviewer confusion and ultimately frustration. We are taught in creative writing courses to find synonyms for terms in order to keep reader interest and to keep from being repetitive. In contrast, this approach is discouraged in scientific writing. Given the complexity of the terms and methods used in proposals, the more clear and simple you can be stylistically, the easier it will be for the reviewer to understand your proposal and thereby to evaluate its merits.

> **Original Version**
> The Athena cohort was taught to correctly identify heart-healthy food groups and was brought back to be studied by three researchers twice, once after 6 months and again at the end of the year. The other group of youngsters was asked to answer the set of questions only once, after 6 months, but they had been taught to label the food groups by name rather than by health effects. The performance of Group 1 was superior to the performance of Group II. The superior performance of the experimental group was attributed to...
>
> **Improved Version**
> The experimental group was taught to identify heart-healthy food groups and was retested twice at 6 month intervals. The control group was taught to identify the food groups by name and was retested only once after 6 months. The performance of the experimental group was superior to the performance of the control group. The superior performance of the experimental group was attributed to...

You probably found yourself reading the original example several times to make sense of it. Imagine your frustration as a grant reviewer facing a stack of proposals to read with an impending deadline.

You can see in the original example that several synonyms are used: *Athena cohort*, *Group 1*, and *experimental group*. Additionally, it is unclear who constitutes the *other group of youngsters*. Confusion grows because we don't know if Group 1 refers to (1) the Phoenix cohort or (2) the *other group of youngsters* or (3) represents a third group that has yet to be defined.

In the improved example, it is now clear that there are only two groups and, even more importantly, which one is the experimental group and which one is the control group.

5.10 TIP #10: USE THE POSITIVE FORM

This tip is closely related to tip #3 suggesting the use of active voice. The use of positive form is always recommended for proposals. Simply, in place of stating what you chose *not* to do, instead state what you chose to do.

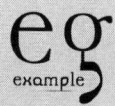

> **Original Version**
> We did not think that a case–control design was appropriate for our proposed study.
> **Improved Version**
> We thought a prospective cohort study was the appropriate design for our proposed study.
> **Original Version**
> We chose not to recruit women who were less than age 16 years.
> **Improved Version**
> We chose to recruit women who were aged 16 years and older.

The one caveat to note as regards this point is that the discussion of alternatives (e.g., what you chose *not* to do) does actually have an appropriate home in the proposal (see Chapter 13, *How to Present Limitations and Alternatives*). The main emphasis here is to first use the positive form—for example, put your best foot forward. Then, save the discussion of alternatives to the "alternatives" section dedicated to that purpose.

5.11 TIP #11: PLACE LATIN ABBREVIATIONS IN PARENTHESES; ELSEWHERE USE ENGLISH TRANSLATIONS

The following table lists the correct usage of some standard Latin abbreviations. Note that English translations of these terms are used outside of parentheses. Caution should be taken with the punctuation used in the Latin abbreviations, although modern software spell-checkers should correct any errors you make in use of these terms:

- i.e., = *that is,*

    We propose to evaluate diabetes risk factors (i.e., glucose, insulin, adiponectin).

    We will evaluate diabetes risk factors, that is, glucose, insulin, adiponectin.

Note that the Latin abbreviation is in parentheses, while the English translations are outside parentheses:

- e.g., = for example,
    We propose to evaluate sociodemographic factors (e.g., age, income, education).
    We propose to evaluate sociodemographic factors, for example, age, income, and education.
- vs. = versus
- etc. = and so forth
- et al. = and others (this is the only exception where the Latin abbreviation goes outside of parentheses)

5.12 TIP #12: SPELL OUT ACRONYMS WHEN FIRST USED; KEEP THEIR USE TO A MINIMUM

Proposal writers often resort to acronyms as a way to save space. While this is acceptable for commonly accepted acronyms (e.g., MI for myocardial infarction), this practice is discouraged for acronyms that are either not commonly used or, even worse, that are created solely for the purposes of your proposal.

Imagine that you are writing a proposal to evaluate the impact of high-impact physical activity and you find yourself using that term repeatedly. It is still not acceptable to create a new acronym to save space (e.g., HIPA for high-impact physical activity). Using such nontraditional or customized acronyms will make your proposal much more difficult for a reviewer to follow—leading to reader frustration. Some proposal writers, intent on saving space, have tried to get around this tip by including an acronym glossary as a table near the beginning of their proposal. However, such a glossary either requires the reader to constantly flip pages back and forth to refer to the glossary or page up and down, thereby impeding the flow of their reading. Anything to make the review process easier for the reviewer, even at the expense of a slight increase in word count, will pay off in terms of a happier reviewer who can clearly see the impact of your application.

5.13 TIP #13: AVOID THE USE OF CONTRACTIONS

Another technique that proposal writers sometimes use to save space is the use of contractions. Contractions are common in casual usage (and in this textbook!) but are not appropriate for scientific writing. Common contractions include such words as *don't*, *didn't*, and *can't*. Just as with Stylistic Tip #12, the use of contractions runs the risk of diminishing the quality of your proposal by prioritizing space saving over scientific writing quality.

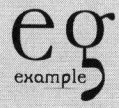

> **Original Version**
> Given the differences in barriers to physical activity according to ethnicity, it's critical to evaluate whether the findings differ by ethnicity.
>
> **Improved Version**
> Given the differences in barriers to physical activity according to ethnicity, it is critical to evaluate whether the findings differ by ethnicity.

5.14 TIP #14: SPELL OUT NUMBERS AT THE BEGINNING OF A SENTENCE

All numbers, no matter how large, must be written out when they appear at the beginning of a sentence. We are certainly used to seeing numbers less than 10 written out, and this is actually required by many scientific journals. Even for numbers between 10 and 100, seeing these terms written out in proposals is not unusual. However, dedicating space to writing out numbers larger than 100 when they appear at the beginning of a sentence is not wise. Therefore, instead, it is preferable to rearrange your sentence.

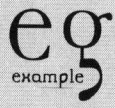

> **Original Version**
> 1876 women were enrolled in the study.
>
> **First Improved Version**
> A total of 1876 women were enrolled in the study.
>
> **Second Improved Version**
> We enrolled a total of 1876 women in the study.

The second improved version is even further improved by using active voice *and* avoiding starting the sentence with a large number. In contrast, you can see that it would be cumbersome to start a sentence with *One thousand eight hundred seventy six women were enrolled*.

5.15 TIP #15: PLACEMENT OF REFERENCES

In writing a proposal, you will cite published articles in the body of your proposal (in-text citations), and the references in full will appear at the end of your proposal in a bibliography. Journals often require their own specific reference style, and certain granting agencies have reference requirements as well. For a dissertation proposal, the reference style is typically defined by the graduate school guidelines. Overall, reference styles and requirements vary widely so it is important to make sure you are using the correct formatting, not only for in-text citations, but also for the body of the bibliography/reference list.

However, there are certain basic rules that you can typically rely upon. When the proposal guidelines require superscripted in-text citations, they are placed after punctuation like this.[1] In contrast, when proposal guidelines require in-text citations to be in parentheses, they are placed before the punctuation like this (1). Other in-text citation types range from first author's name and publication date in parentheses (e.g., Smith et al. 2012) to all authors' names and publication date (Smith A, Jones B, Brown C, 2006).

If you are writing an NIH grant or are in a situation where the reference style is up to you, there will be several issues to consider. First, given that space is typically at a premium in a grant proposal, the choice of superscript is preferable. This style has the second advantage of allowing the text to flow in a relatively unimpeded fashion. On the other hand, if it is important to your argument that you are citing the key authors in the field, you may want to select the reference style that includes author name and date. This may be particularly relevant in an area where there is a small body of research. Either way, it is important to note that the reviewer will have access to the full citation in the bibliography—the question is whether or not you feel it is critical that they see the authors' names in real time as they read your study rationale.

5.16 STRIVE FOR A USER-FRIENDLY DRAFT

To ensure a happy reviewer, it is vital to meticulously read your draft. The avoidance of sloppy errors and consistency in style and terminology reflects well upon you as not only a writer but also as a researcher. It is certainly true that some of the brightest researchers have not been strong writers, and vice versa. However, from a reviewer's standpoint, the proposal writing style is the first impression that you will make upon your reviewer. It is rare that a meticulously written proposal does not represent a conscientious researcher. Therefore, your writing style not only provides evidence of your care in preparation but also avoids errors that will detract from your proposal and reflect poorly on the quality of your scholarship.

Classic errors to avoid are lack of callouts to figures and tables in the text, missing or misnumbered figures or tables, and other editorial mistakes. While these mistakes seem small, they can lead to a very frustrated reviewer who is trying to hunt down the appropriate figure/table.

Other reviewer-friendly stylistic practices include the use of standard margins, avoidance of *cute* touches such as clip art, use of different size fonts, or any other special touches that may distract the reader by calling attention to the format of your paper instead of its content. While some online grant submission interfaces allow the use of color highlighting, it is important to note that many reviewers print out their assigned proposals on their own black and white printers. Unless they have paged through your proposal prior to printing, they will not be aware that they will be losing the color highlighting and any point that you were trying to make via this highlighting will be lost. Instead, consider the use of bolding or underlining, being sure to follow proposal guidelines at all times. You could also consider italics, but some reviewers find italics difficult to read.

In this vein, it is important to spell-check, proofread, and edit your proposal. Other suggestions particularly important for dissertation proposals include numbering all pages and double-spacing the draft. Numbering the draft enables the reader/reviewer to more readily provide written comments for you—as they may want to refer to a particular page or ask you to move a section from page x to page y. Also, for dissertation proposals, the use of double spacing, if allowed, is preferable, as single-spaced documents make it difficult for the reader to write in specific comments or suggest alternate phrasing.

5.17 TAKE ADVANTAGE OF WRITING ASSISTANCE PROGRAMS

For the graduate student and early-career faculty member, writing assistance is available. Most universities have graduate writing programs. Similarly, university faculty development offices often offer grant-writing retreats or other writing assistance. As noted in Chapter 1, *Ten Top Tips for Successful Proposal Writing*, some departments will fund early-career faculty to attend local and national grant-writing workshops and will compensate outside scientists, with expertise on the proposed topic, to review and critique your grant proposals. Lastly, many departments will support their early-career faculty by making the services of a grant writer available. This person will likely not be an expert in your field but will be well able to review your application and ensure that you are clearly and concisely conveying your aims and methods. By encouraging the faculty member to be as clear as possible, the best grant writers help the faculty member to further refine their specific aims and convey the potential impact of their findings.

5.18 SOLICIT EARLY *INFORMAL* FEEDBACK ON YOUR PROPOSAL

I would encourage you to ask your colleagues and mentors for early feedback on your proposal—even if they are not experts on your topic. Remember, as noted in Chapter 1, *Ten Top Tips for Successful Proposal Writing*, it is likely that some of your assigned grant reviewers will also not have expertise in your area of interest.

After writing a first draft, ask your readers to point out elements that are not clear. The process of verbally responding to their concerns and points of confusion in your proposal will be invaluable in helping you to better articulate your thoughts in writing. First, such an interchange will enable you to identify areas that you have not clearly conveyed to the reader. Secondly, through orally explaining any confusing concepts to the reader, you will learn how to better explain these concepts when you return to the writing. This practice of peer reviewing and receiving verbal comments back in real time has been an invaluable practice that I use in my course on scientific writing. It is always better to receive comments from a colleague early in the process, when there is still time to make changes, as opposed to delaying and waiting for the formal reviewers' feedback after proposal submission—when it may be too late to make any changes. We call this early feedback *low stakes*. The more feedback you can receive from your colleagues and mentors, the less likely that you will hear concerns from reviewers that you have not already addressed.

Solicit feedback on content, not just style It is important to get feedback on the *content* early in the redrafting process. If your first draft contained stylistic and organizational errors, such as misspellings or misplaced headings, your reviewer may feel compelled to focus on these stylistic errors and defer comments on content until the manuscript is easier to read. If this occurs, be prepared to ask for comments on content. Did you cover the literature adequately? Are your conclusions about the topic justified? Are there gaps in your review? How can the proposal be improved?

5.19 WHO MUST READ YOUR PROPOSAL

For graduate students, there is often little choice as to who should read the proposal; this is dictated by rules regarding constitution of the dissertation committee (see Chapter 2, *Starting a Dissertation Proposal*). For those writing a grant, the coinvestigators should all be allowed the opportunity to review the complete proposal. It is considered customary to provide your coinvestigators with a complete copy of the draft of your proposal at least 1 month before it is due. In this way, they will have 2 weeks to read the proposal, and then you have 2 weeks to incorporate their comments. There is nothing more inconsiderate of a colleague's time than to ask for their feedback but not to include it in the final draft—due to lack of time. This is not to say that you cannot disagree with this preliminary feedback, but if so, there should always be a time for a discussion of any substantive suggestions that you chose not to incorporate. Allow plenty of time for the feedback and redrafting process.

5.20 INCORPORATING FEEDBACK

In this process of review, it is essential to remember that the reader is always right. If one person misunderstands your points, or finds them hazy, then it is highly likely that a large portion of the future readers will also misunderstand these same points.

If the reader has not understood one of your points, the communication process has not worked and the draft should be changed to make it clearer for the reader. Do not try to defend the draft manuscript. Instead, try to determine why the reader did not understand it: Did you provide insufficient background information? Would the addition of more explicit transition terms between sections make it clearer? These questions should guide your discussion with the reader.

Early in one's career, it is instinctive to blame the reader. *They just don't understand my points* or even worse *They are not smart enough to understand my points* is a common knee jerk reaction. Further complicating this is the tendency of students and early-career faculty to mistakenly believe that they have to write using jargon in order to impress. Instead, the most impressive writing is the most simple writing. It takes much longer to write something short and concise, than to write a long thought laden with jargon, that when closely scrutinized may not really have substance.

One way to get an *ear* for how to write in a scientific manner is to read numerous reviews of literature, paying attention to how they are organized and how the authors make transitions from one topic to another.

5.21 HOW TO RECONCILE CONTRADICTORY FEEDBACK

It is inevitable that you will encounter differences of opinion among those that read your draft. The likelihood for contradictory feedback increases in direct proportion to the number of people that you solicit as reviewers. This is not to say to limit the number simply to make the process easier but instead to choose carefully such that each investigator/committee member is playing a key role. This will ultimately be appreciated by grant review agencies and can lead to a higher review score.

Reconcile contradictory feedback by seeking clarification from the readers. An example of contradictory feedback is when one reviewer/committee member asks for additional details about a prior study, while another may ask you not to include the prior study at all. It is likely that there is truth in each reviewer's suggestion.

First, make sure that the different opinions were not due to one person's failure to comprehend your argument. This would be the easiest misunderstanding to clear up. Second, it is your responsibility to seek further clarification from both sources and to negotiate a resolution.

Once you identify the source of confusion, the text of the proposal must be revised to make this point clear and avoid such misunderstanding by future readers. I am always surprised when a proposal writer believes it is simply sufficient to clarify the issue verbally with the reviewer and leave the text unchanged. As mentioned earlier, if one reviewer is confused by your writing, then it can be expected that future reviewers will also be confused by the same point.

In our example above, each reviewer had a difference of opinion on whether a prior article should be cited. After such a discussion, the manuscript should be revised to clarify the relevance of that citation. For example, *while Smith et al. studied the relationship between x and y, this does not directly relate to our work which used a different technique to study the relationship between x and y.* This approach shows that you have a mastery of the literature and did not accidently leave out the study by Smith et al. due to ignorance of his body of work and instead shows enough familiarity with the study to say why this work was not relevant. Remember that it is possible that Smith may be one of your proposal reviewers!

5.22 ANNOTATED EXAMPLE

A proposal to evaluate the association between race and heat illnesses among a military population.

Paragraph #1
A hot topic among environmentalists today is global warming and the corresponding public health need to study risk factors for heat-related illnesses. Current findings suggest an increase in the number of heat waves resulting in the unforeseen deaths of hundreds of US children and adults alike.

Comment: In general, the tone in paragraph #1 is too casual and the paragraph sounds more like an editorial or a commentary for the lay press. Citations are lacking throughout. There are other more relevant ways to justify the public health need to study heat illnesses such as (1) specifying changes in the incidence rates of heat illnesses over time as well as (2) the impact of heat illnesses on other diseases or disabilities or work lost days.

Paragraph #2
Dozens of heat illness studies have shown that the primary populations at risk are the young and the elderly. Of these, some have also pointed to trends suggesting that men and blacks may also be more susceptible. To our knowledge, there has not been a single study focusing on race and risk of heat illnesses. The one prior study of ethnicity and heat illness found no association (RR = 1.1, 95% CI 0.9–1.2) between Hispanic ethnicity and heat illnesses (2). However, as the authors noted, possible recall and selection biases were weaknesses of the study. Therefore, this proposal will focus on the hypothesis that among soldiers, black men are at higher risk of heat stroke and exhaustion than white men.

Comment: Overall, paragraph #2 is too vague. Citations should be inserted throughout. While it is often a strength to be conducting the first study in an area, the lack of any studies could be due to the fact that the hypothesis is not adequately grounded in either the physiologic or epidemiologic literature. Therefore, a brief justification for the proposed hypothesis should be added. The paragraph uses professional jargon (e.g., recall bias and selection bias) without clarifying the study limitations in simple terms. The phrase *as the authors noted* should be removed, and instead the proposal writer should state their own view. Most importantly, the study population (i.e., soldiers) comes as a surprise to the reader. Much earlier in the document, the writer should highlight that soldiers are at particular risk of heat illnesses, giving incidence rates and citations.

PART TWO

The Proposal: Section by Section

Specific Aims

6

Welcome to Part Two of this textbook, *The Proposal: Section by Section*. In this part of the textbook, I will walk you through each section of a proposal step by step, with a particular focus on strategically meeting NIH guidelines specific to each section. I use NIH guidelines as the primary example of writing a grant proposal as it is the most typical funding source for epidemiology and preventive medicine, particularly for larger awards—the ultimate career goal. Depending upon your institution's guidelines, a dissertation proposal can also be formatted in the same fashion as an NIH grant proposal. Using the NIH format will give you, as a graduate student, great practice in writing an actual grant proposal under the dedicated mentorship of a faculty committee. If the proposal format at your institution is not in the model of an NIH grant proposal, it may be useful to ask if you could modify the format to make it more relevant.

Your choice of specific aims will dictate the content of the remainder of your proposal—the Background and Approach sections. For example, following this chapter, Chapter 7, *Background and Significance Section*, continues where this chapter leaves off, with guidelines for summarizing the prior epidemiologic literature as well as the physiologic or behavioral mechanism supporting your exposure–outcome relationship.

6.1 PURPOSE OF THE SPECIFIC AIMS PAGE

Writing the Specific Aims page of your grant proposal really kicks off the meat of the proposal. This section can arguably be considered the most critical component of the body of the proposal. After the Abstract (described in Chapter 15, *Abstracts and Titles*), the Specific Aims page is the first section to be read by the review (or dissertation) committee and therefore is of paramount importance. A well-written Specific Aims page serves not only to *grab* the reader's attention but also immediately brings to the forefront the scientific importance and impact of the proposal.

As noted in Chapter 1, *Ten Top Tips for Successful Proposal Writing*, most funding agencies, including NIH, consider the scientific impact and importance of the proposed topic as one of the top criteria in funding decisions. For example, the NIH directs reviewers to "provide an **overall impact** score to reflect their assessment of the likelihood for the project to exert a sustained, powerful influence on the research field(s) involved. An application does not need to be strong in all categories (e.g., Significance, Investigators, Innovation, Approach, Environment) to be judged likely to have major scientific impact."

Also remember that, as noted in Chapter 1, the majority of the NIH review committee, with the exception of the two to four assigned to your application, may only ever read the Specific Aims page of your proposal. Yet they will all be voting on your proposal! Even, more importantly, the majority of the NIH review committee may only be reading this page in the immediate moments before your review. Therefore, the Specific Aims page has to grab their attention with the importance of your study, be clear and easy to read, and give a quick snapshot of the study methods, the aims, as well as the implication of the study findings. The *so what* factor has to be quickly addressed. Give the reader a reason to read on!

6.2 A WORD OF CAUTION

If you have skipped directly to this chapter in an attempt to move more quickly through the proposal-writing process or to expedite the process, you will actually find the opposite. A key part of your proposal's potential to have a strong overall impact is your ability to clarify how the proposed work will extend prior research in the field. Through your work in organizing the prior literature and identifying the research gap (as described in Chapter 4, *Conducting the Literature Search*), and by following the stylistic guidelines for scientific writing (as described in Chapter 5, *Scientific Writing*), you have set the stage for this step.

Indeed, writing the Specific Aims page will be much more challenging and, at worst, potentially misdirected, without following those tasks set forth in Chapters 4 and 5. It is only now that you have done your *homework*, that is, identification and refining of the research gap that your proposal will fill, that the writing process will now flow easily.

Now you are ready to write!

6.3 OUTLINE FOR THE SPECIFIC AIMS PAGE

The NIH grant application starts with a **one-page** description of your specific aims. The goal on this page is to not only list your specific aims in their entirety but also to provide a brief context for your aims, a synopsis of the study design, as well as a brief summary of your significance and innovation. You will have room to expand upon your proposal's significance and innovation on the following pages (as described below), but a brief one- to two-sentence summary is useful on this page.

Goals of the Specific Aims page
Your first goal for the Specific Aims page is to give an overview of the problem—What is known? What is the remaining question? Your second goal is to explain—How are you going to answer the question? What is the long-term goal of this line of research?

During my time as a standing and ad hoc member of several NIH study sections, I have found the following outline to be the most successful approach for the Specific Aims page:

Detailed Outline: Specific Aims Page

1. *Paragraph #1*: Study Background and Research Gap
   a. Brief summary of Public Health Impact of Outcome.
   b. Brief summary of the Physiology of Exposure–Outcome Relationship.
   c. Brief summary of the Epidemiology of the Exposure–Outcome Relationship.
      i. Describe the prior studies of this topic and how the previous research is limited (e.g., the **research gap**).
   d. The overall goal of your proposal and how it will fill this research gap.
2. *Paragraph #2*: Synopsis of the Study Methods
   a. Specify the proposed (1) study design, (2) sample size, (3) measurement tools, and (4) length of follow-up (if relevant).
   b. Mention any related preliminary studies.
3. *Paragraph #3*: Your Aims and Corresponding Hypotheses
4. *Paragraph #4*: Summary of Innovation and Significance

6.3.1 Paragraph #1: Study Background and Research Gap

This paragraph should briefly summarize the public health importance of the topic—typically your outcome of interest—using citations. The paragraph would then segue into your exposure of interest and the potential physiological or behavioral relationship between your exposure and your outcome. Subsequent sentences should comment on the prior epidemiologic literature in the area and highlight the research gap. Often, a well-written paragraph #1, *study background and research gap*, in combination with paragraph #2, *synopsis of study methods*, can serve as the basis of your abstract (see Chapter 15, *Abstracts and Titles*).

It is important to note here that a fully developed section on the epidemiology and physiology of your exposure–outcome relationship will be part of the Background section following the Specific Aims page (see Chapter 7, *Background and Significance Section*). Instead, here in the Specific Aims page, your goal is to **briefly** summarize the physiological or behavioral mechanisms that link your exposure to your outcome. The ability to be brief in conveying this link also provides evidence that you have a firm grasp on this mechanism and can summarize the key points concisely. It is always more difficult to write a short explanation than a long one!

The importance of the research gap Failure to identify a research gap is one of the most common flaws of an application. In other words, it is essential that this paragraph clarifies, through the gap, how it will extend prior research in this area. Simply proposing to repeat prior studies is typically not sufficient to receive funding. Instead, there must be an identified gap such as a methodological weakness or a study population in which this topic has not been evaluated that this study will fill. Luckily, you will have already identified this research gap by creating and reviewing the summary table as described in Chapter 4, *Conducting the Literature Search*. To maintain a semblance of objectivity, I find that it is most effective to wait until the next paragraph before describing your proposed study. Instead, this first paragraph is meant to be an objective description of the state of the science to date. And it is not until the next paragraph that you will indicate how your proposal will fill this gap.

A friendly reminder This is a good point to remind you that it is common to become discouraged to find that a study has already been published evaluating your exposure–outcome relationship of interest. As mentioned earlier in this book, many studies of varying designs and methodologies are required before causality can be determined. In addition, often these previously published studies may have conflicting findings. That is, some studies may have observed associations that were not statistically significant, while others observed an increased risk of the health outcome for those who were exposed.

In this case, the proposal can highlight in this paragraph that *few studies have evaluated the relationship between x and y, and among these studies, findings have been conflicting*. The paragraph can then go on to discuss potential reasons for these conflicts—such as different measurement tools and limitations in methodology. In other words, even in the situation of previously published studies on your exposure–outcome relationship, you are able to clearly identify a worthy research gap. One definitely doesn't have to be proposing the first study in an area in order for the proposal to be of high scientific importance.

Lastly, the final sentence of this paragraph can present your overall study goal.

Example Paragraph #1

Women diagnosed with gestational diabetes mellitus (GDM) are at substantially increased risk of developing type 2 diabetes and obesity, currently at epidemic rates in the United States. **GDM, therefore, identifies a population of women at high risk of developing type 2 diabetes and thus provides an excellent opportunity to intervene years before the development of this disorder.** Recent epidemiologic studies have suggested that women with higher levels of physical activity have reduced risk of GDM.[8-10] However, to date, primary prevention studies have not intervened to test whether making a change in physical activity reduces risk of developing GDM among women at high risk of this disorder. **Therefore, we propose to test the hypothesis that an exercise intervention is an effective tool for preventing GDM among women with a history of GDM.**

6.3.2 Paragraph #2: Synopsis of the Study Methods

This second paragraph of your Specific Aims page should provide a brief summary of your study methods. It is critical in this paragraph to provide the sample size, the measurement tools that will be used (e.g., food frequency questionnaires, activity monitors, and biomarkers), and the study design. Leaving these key pieces of information out is a common pitfall even among experienced investigators. Their omission will leave the reviewer wondering how you will be conducting the study.

It may be helpful here to imagine that your primary assigned NIH reviewer will be describing your study to the rest of the review panel—who have not yet read your proposal. A well-written synopsis of the proposed study methods can serve double duty as their script in presenting your proposal. By having written this *script* for them, you not only ensure that their *pitch* to the committee will be accurate, but you are also being kind to the reviewer in creating this script for them. In addition, if there is space, this paragraph can reappear later in the proposal at the beginning of your Approach/Methods section as a synopsis of your protocol (see Chapter 9, *Study Design and Methods*).

Lastly, this paragraph would be the place to mention your prior experience with the proposed topic and/or methods. You can do this concisely by citing the grant number and funding source in parentheses for any highlighted preliminary studies. This parenthetical information should also state your role (e.g., Dr. Smith PI).

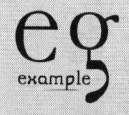

> **e.g. example** A total of 320 multiparous women who had GDM in a prior pregnancy (58% will be from minority groups) will be recruited in early pregnancy (10 weeks gestation) and randomized to either an exercise intervention (n = 160) or a comparison health and wellness intervention (n = 160). The overall goal of the intervention is to encourage pregnant women to achieve the American College of Obstetricians and Gynecologists Guidelines for physical activity during pregnancy. The intervention consists of a 12-week program ending at routine GDM screen (24–28 weeks gestation) with approximately 14 weeks of follow-up (ending at birth). The intervention draws from the theory of stages of motivational readiness for change and social cognitive theory constructs for physical activity behavior and will take into account the specific social, cultural, economic, and environmental challenges faced by women of diverse socioeconomic and ethnic backgrounds. It addresses the rapidly changing context of pregnancy, which brings opportunities for adoption and maintenance of new behaviors. GDM will be assessed via American Diabetes Association criteria, and biochemical factors associated with insulin resistance will be collected at baseline and 24–28 weeks gestation. Physical activity will be assessed via

> 7 days of accelerometer monitoring and the Pregnancy Physical Activity Questionnaire at baseline, at 22–24 weeks gestation, and at 32–34 weeks gestation. The intervention protocol builds upon our pilot work (American Diabetes Association Career Award #xxxx; PI: Yourself) and can readily be translated into clinical practice in underserved and minority populations.

6.3.3 Paragraph #3: Your Aims and Corresponding Hypotheses

This paragraph will be a numbered list of your specific aims and hypotheses using the techniques outlined in Chapter 3, *How to Develop and Write Hypotheses*.

A typical grant proposal to NIH—be it small or large—typically has three to five related aims. The trick is to avoid being too ambitious while at the same time not being too narrow. Mentors, outside readers, and coinvestigators can help you identify the appropriateness of your aims. Feedback should very quickly be obtained from them before proceeding further.

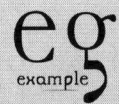

> *eg example*
>
> I. Specific Aims
> Specific Aim #1: Evaluate the impact of a 12-week individually targeted exercise intervention on risk of recurrent GDM among prenatal care patients with a history of GDM.
> > Hypothesis #1: Compared to subjects in the comparison health and wellness intervention, women in the individually targeted exercise intervention will have a lower risk of recurrent GDM.
>
> Specific Aim #2: Evaluate the impact of a 12-week individually targeted exercise intervention on biochemical factors associated with insulin resistance among prenatal care patients with a history of GDM.
> > Hypothesis #2: Compared to subjects in the comparison health and wellness intervention, women in the individually targeted exercise intervention will have lower fasting concentrations of glucose, insulin, leptin, TNF-α, CRP, and higher concentrations of adiponectin.
>
> Specific Aim #3: Evaluate the impact of a 12-week individually targeted exercise intervention on the adoption and maintenance of physical activity during pregnancy among prenatal care patients with a history of GDM.
> > Hypothesis #3: Compared to subjects in the comparison health and wellness intervention, women in the individually targeted exercise intervention will participate in more physical activity in mid- and late pregnancy.

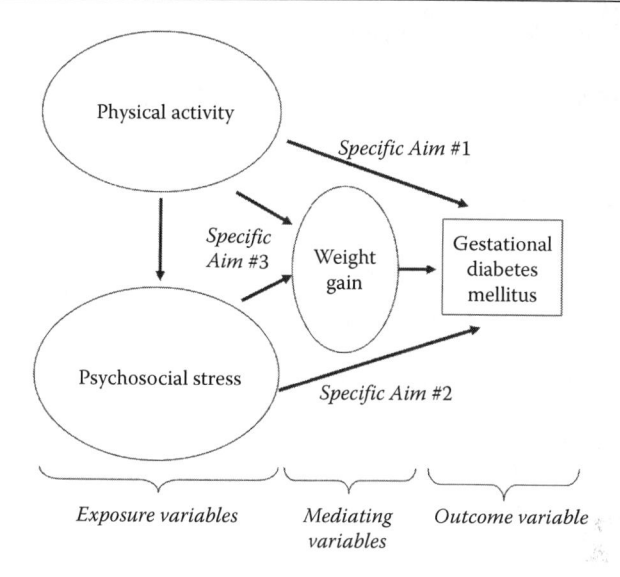

FIGURE 6.1 Specific aims figure from a proposal to evaluate the association between physical activity, stress, and risk of GDM.

If there is adequate space, a figure of your specific aims is highly recommended. If space is not adequate, this figure can be placed in the Background section (see Chapter 7, *Background and Significance Section*). Figure 6.1 is from a proposal to conduct an observational cohort study to evaluate how physical activity (exposure #1) and stress (exposure #2) impact risk of GDM (outcome) via certain physiological and behavioral mediating variables.

6.3.4 Paragraph #4: Summary of Significance and Innovation

Significance The Specific Aims page should include a brief synopsis of the significance of your proposal. Later, in the Background section, you can expand further upon significance, but it is essential to point it out on this first page as well.

The NIH defines **significance** as addressing the following questions:

- Does the project address an important problem or a critical barrier to progress in the field?
- If the aims of the project are achieved, how will scientific knowledge, technical capability, and/or clinical practice be improved?
- How will successful completion of the aims change the concepts, methods, technologies, treatments, services, or preventative interventions that drive this field?

As you can see from these questions, *significance* in this context does not **only** mean that you plan to study a very important public health issue. *Significance* is also assessed by reviewers in terms of how data from your study will **inform the field**. Be clear as to how currently available data need to be refined and extended. For example, obesity is a significant public health problem in the United States. But how will your study drive the field forward: Will it identify susceptibility genes or maybe point the way to better preventive interventions?

A perfectly designed study about an unimportant question is not considered significant. But a study that considers a topic of extremely high significance in terms of public health but has flaws in the study design that can affect validity of the findings is not significant either.

Objectively assess these multiple aspects of significance and summarize these in two to three sentences on the Specific Aims page.

Innovation Similarly, the Specific Aims page should include a brief synopsis of the innovation of your proposal. Later, in the Background section, you can expand further upon innovation, but it is essential to point it out on this first page as well.

The NIH defines **innovation** as addressing the following questions:

- Does the application challenge and seek to shift current research or clinical practice paradigms by utilizing novel theoretical concepts, approaches or methodologies, instrumentation, or interventions?
- Are the concepts, approaches or methodologies, instrumentation, or interventions novel to one field of research or novel in a broad sense?
- Is a refinement, improvement, or new application of theoretical concepts, approaches or methodologies, instrumentation, or interventions proposed?

> *example*
>
> Strengths of the study include our prior experience with recruitment and follow-up of the study population, a validated intervention program, the racial/ethnic diversity of the population, the use of multidimensional (subjective and objective) measures of physical activity, multiple and fasting measures of biochemical factors associated with insulin resistance, and collaboration among a team of scientists representing multiple disciplines. The proposal is innovative in being the first, to our knowledge, to test a physical activity intervention designed to prevent GDM among high-risk women. The significance of the study lies in the fact that changes in modifiable risk factors may reduce the morbidity associated with GDM and risk of subsequent type 2 diabetes, obesity, and cardiovascular disease in women.

An important caveat Often in epidemiology and preventive medicine, you will be proposing to use standard population-based methods to achieve your specific aims. In this case, your aims will be innovative through addressing **novel hypotheses** even though your methods may not be innovative. It is important to note that a project that employs standard methodologies can nevertheless result in essential information that will advance the field. Do not feel that you have to propose the development of a new methodology to achieve the *innovation* guidelines.

6.4 TIP #1: HOW TO DEAL WITH THE ONE-PAGE LIMITATION FOR THE SPECIFIC AIMS PAGE

Specific Aims are designed to be concise and to the point. How, therefore, does one decide what merits mentioning in the aims and hypotheses aside from the independent and dependent variables and the proposed direction of effect? One of the key determinants is whether the additional details will make a critical difference to reviewers in determining whether to fund your study—again with the thought in mind that some reviewers will only read your abstract and aims. Therefore, priority should be given to mentioning study attributes that reflect key advances in the field. It may be helpful to consider that if a reviewer were **only** to read your hypotheses, what are the key factors (i.e., advances) of your proposal that you would want them to know? In summary, the specific aims and hypotheses should be clear and succinct while encapsulating both the key features of your project's methods and your anticipated findings.

6.5 TIP #2: AVOID INTERDEPENDENT AIMS

Years ago, when NIH funding paylines were higher, it was often considered acceptable to include pilot feasibility or validation studies as the first specific aim of a large R01-type grant application. That is, your first Specific Aim #1 would be to develop the tools/intervention/methods that would then be used in your Specific Aims #2–#5. These days, such study development aims need to be conducted prior to applying for an R01—for example, as part of a smaller R21, R03, K award, or foundation grant. The other advantage of starting small in this fashion (see Chapter 1, "Tip #1: Start Early") is that it is easier to grow in a stepwise fashion from smaller to larger grants. First, such smaller grants like a K award or career foundation grant will be more likely to be funded due to their critical role in supporting your subsequent career plans—this is often the main funding criteria used by reviewers of these small grants. Second, having successfully applied for, received, and conducted any type of smaller grant will demonstrate to the reviewers that you have the ability to successfully carry out larger projects. Third, the generation of publications from these smaller grants will further indicate that you can translate findings into publications—another key factor in reviewers' eyes.

6.6 TIP #3: AIMS INVOLVING THE USE OF AN EXISTING DATASET—PROS AND CONS

As the majority of diseases are relatively rare, epidemiologic studies typically require large numbers of participants and many years of follow-up. In addition, the IRB approval process for human subjects' protection can be quite lengthy. Therefore, graduate students don't typically have enough time in their degree programs to propose to launch a new study from scratch and then recruit and follow enough people to have sufficient statistical power to test their hypotheses. In other words, by the time the student writes the proposal, submits the proposal to a funding agency, resubmits the proposal after a likely first rejection, obtains an IRB approval, develops forms, follows subjects, enters data, and cleans data, many years will have passed by.

In contrast, proposing to evaluate your specific aims within the context of an existing dataset capitalizes on work already conducted by investigators and is an excellent first step in your proposal-writing career. This approach can also be viewed by funding agencies as a cost-efficient way to answer an important research question. Such existing datasets could be local (e.g., collected by a mentor or colleague) or national (e.g., collected as part of a national surveillance system). It is important to note that this approach would still require that your aims and hypotheses address important research questions. In addition, you would want to be sure that your proposed aims are not already included as part of the aims of the original grant that funded the existing dataset.

In summary, there are several **advantages** to utilizing an existing dataset:

- In a climate of low NIH funding paylines, this approach can be seen as cost efficient.
- It provides an efficient way to *mine* existing data for other important questions.
- By nature of the fact that you would be working on an existing project, you will have the accompanying benefit of an established research team. These investigators can be an invaluable resource for you, and listing them on your proposal will be seen as a strength.
- You will not be subject to the vagaries of not meeting your stated recruitment and follow-up rates. The reviewers can be assured that you already have the data in hand, and it is less risky for them to have confidence that you will be able to achieve the stated aims of the application.

There are also several **disadvantages** to utilizing an existing dataset:

- Because the overall study was not designed with your research topic in mind, you may be missing data on important covariates.
- In addition, exclusions may have been made to the original sample that are not relevant to your research question.
- Detailed data on your exposure and outcome variables of interest may not be available.

However, these concerns are usually somewhat addressable. For example, one of my doctoral students proposed to examine smoking and risk of preterm birth within the context of our existing larger dataset designed to examine the association between physical activity and gestational diabetes. As part of our original grant, we had already collected information on smoking as well as preterm birth as important covariates of our focus on gestational diabetes. For the doctoral student, a key potential confounding factor in her analysis was history of preterm birth. The dataset, however, did not have complete information on that variable as preterm birth was not our focus. As a way to address this, the student proposed to conduct a sensitivity analysis, repeating her primary analysis among women who were nulliparous. In other words, by proposing to repeat her analysis within a strata of women that had no history of preterm birth, she assured the reviewers that she would be able to evaluate potential concerns regarding confounding by this variable.

6.7 TIP #4: SHOULD YOU AIM TO CONDUCT ANALYTIC OR DESCRIPTIVE STUDIES?

Specific aims, at the level of a dissertation or grant proposal, typically propose to assess measures of association between an exposure of interest and an outcome of interest. These types of aims are termed *analytic*. However, for pilot or feasibility studies, it is reasonable to propose specific aims designed simply to measure the distribution of an outcome, regardless of its association with an exposure. Or, alternatively, specific aims may be designed simply to measure the distribution of an exposure, independent of its association with an outcome. These types of aims are termed *descriptive* or univariate. The main point to keep in mind is that these descriptive-type analyses are typically only appropriate for feasibility or pilot studies or as a Specific Aim #1 in a proposal, which also contains analytic aims as Specific Aim #2, #3, and/or #4.

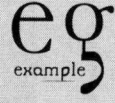

> **Descriptive Aim**
> Specific Aim #1: To estimate seasonal trends in the prevalence of tick-borne diseases during 2007–2011 in the Northeastern United States.
> **Analytic Aim**
> Specific Aim #1: To evaluate the association between seasonal trends in the prevalence of tick-borne diseases and corresponding trends in Lyme disease incidence.

In this example above, the descriptive aim simply describes the prevalence of an exposure (i.e., tick-borne diseases). In contrast, the analytic aim evaluates the association between tick-borne diseases (the exposure) with Lyme disease incidence (an outcome).

6.8 TIP #5: HOW TO DECIDE WHETHER TO INCLUDE EXPLORATORY OR SECONDARY AIMS

It is common practice for proposal writers to include exploratory or secondary aims when they lack the statistical power to achieve these aims. By labeling these aims as *exploratory*, for example, they reduce the risk of being held accountable for such a lack of power. The advantage of including such aims is that you can show off the potential of your project to achieve numerous other aims—thereby increasing its potential value. However, the theme to keep in mind throughout the proposal-writing process is that the proposal is a cohesive whole. What this means is that each section of the proposal influences the other. In other words, each aim should be supported in the Background and Significance section as well as in the Data Analysis section. By including these extra aims, you run the risk of an overly ambitious proposal and also must add more text to support these aims. Without them, the proposal is more likely to fit into the restrictive page requirements that your university or granting mechanism promulgates. One compromise may be to simply add a sentence about the future potential uses of your collected data.

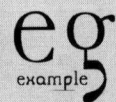

> **eg** *example*
> The collection and storage of cord blood as part of this proposal will also facilitate future applications designed to evaluate the association between the *in utero* environment and risk of childhood diseases.

6.9 TIP #6: DON'T BE TOO AMBITIOUS

As a general rule of thumb, for a large NIH grant, avoid having more than four to five aims. For a smaller grant, three aims are likely sufficient, and it is particularly dangerous to include more without being viewed as overly ambitious. Because this is a common pitfall of new investigators, review panels are particularly wary of multiple aims in small grant proposals.

Let's imagine that you are writing a large R01-type NIH grant and you find yourself in love with eight aims; consider the following options:

Ask yourself if the aims form natural groupings. For example, is there a natural split where four aims fit under one overall goal while the other four fit under another overall goal? If so, consider two separate grant proposals. However, there is an important caveat to this approach. That is, this option should only be considered for a large

R01-type grant mechanism if you already have preliminary studies to support each aim. If you have more preliminary data for one set of aims than another, then by all means, focus on the set that has the most preliminary data!

Ask yourself if your aims are too specific. Consider how broadly or narrowly you are writing your aims.

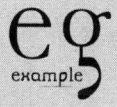

> **eg example**
>
> **Original Version**
> Specific Aim #1: We propose to evaluate the association between light-intensity physical activity and risk of preterm birth.
> Specific Aim #2: We propose to evaluate the association between moderate-intensity physical activity and risk of preterm birth.
> Specific Aim #3: We propose to evaluate the association between vigorous-intensity physical activity and risk of preterm birth.
>
> **Improved Example**
> Specific Aim #1: We propose to evaluate the association between light-, moderate-, and vigorous-intensity physical activity and risk of preterm birth.

The improved example recognizes the fact that the three subtypes of physical activity all fall within one overall domain of physical activity and therefore can be combined into one aim. Note, however, that the improved example still mentions these three subtypes by name within the aim to indicate the output that will be achieved by conducting this aim as well as to reassure the reviewer that you are aware of the intricacies of the field.

6.10 TIP #7: REMEMBER THAT ALL AIMS SHOULD BE ACCOMPANIED BY HYPOTHESES

The importance of hypothesis writing was described in Chapter 3, *How to Develop and Write Hypotheses*. The ideal hypothesis should make testable predictions. As an NIH review panel member, I've seen grants triaged, or considered fatally flawed, for failing to include hypotheses.

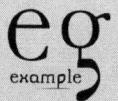

> **eg example**
>
> Specific Aim #1: Identify activities in each trimester that are major contributors to total energy expenditure.
> Specific Aim #2: Directly measure the metabolic cost (intensity) of physical activity.

Looking at the example, such an application that only included specific aims would just be a simple to-do list, often termed a *laundry list*. The act of writing hypotheses requires the investigator to assimilate the prior literature and state of evidence in a particular area and to take the next step of proposing what direction of effect they expect to see in their proposed study.

The need for hypotheses is vital **even** if your aims are simply designed to be *hypothesis generating*. Hypotheses are also critical regardless of your study methods—that is, they are necessary for both qualitative and quantitative studies. For example, Specific Aim #1 above could be an aim for a qualitative study using focus groups to generate hypotheses for major contributors to total energy expenditure. Alternatively, Specific Aim #1 could be an aim for a quantitative analysis of an existing dataset. Regardless, it requires a hypothesis. For example, Hypothesis #1a could be as follows: *Sports and exercise will be the major contributors to total energy expenditure, while occupational and household activities will be minor contributors.*

Including hypotheses does not mean that the investigator will be correct. It instead means that it is your best educated guess based on your expert knowledge of the state of the literature. Later in the proposal, you will include *alternatives and limitations*, which discuss approaches that will be taken if the hypothesis is not found to be correct (see Chapter 13, *How to Present Limitations and Alternatives*).

I've heard from some early-career investigators that they have been advised that simply proposing to collect data, without proposing hypotheses, will be viewed as sufficient. This may be true for a small internal seed grant offered by your institution or another small foundation grant. However, in the current economic culture and in view of the low NIH paylines, this cannot be viewed as a strategic approach to take.

Similarly, proposals to simply continue follow-up of existing prospective cohort studies or existing data registries also tend to not do well—even if these data sources are unique. This has become a problem especially in the last couple of years, where NIH institutes have decreased funds available to fund such resources through a request for applications (RFA, grants and cooperative agreements) or request for proposals (RFP, contracts). Instead, you need to include hypotheses that justify the continued follow-up of this cohort.

6.11 TIP #8: IF YOU PLAN TO EVALUATE EFFECT MODIFICATION IN YOUR METHODS, THEN INCLUDE THIS AS A SPECIFIC AIM

If you plan to consider any of your covariates as possible effect modifiers of the relationship between your exposure and disease, it will be important to include this *a priori* as a study aim(s) and hypothesis. This will help to assure your reviewers that you will not be *data dredging* for statistically significant findings if you fail to observe an overall association between your exposure and outcome of interest. In other words, when writing the proposal, you will want to carefully consider which covariates might be possible effect modifiers based upon feasible physiological mechanisms and/or findings from the prior literature. For a definition of effect modification (i.e., interaction) and how it differs from confounding, see Chapter 12, *Review of Bias and Confounding*.

6.12 WHEN TO CONSIDER DISCARDING YOUR ORIGINAL AIMS AND HYPOTHESES

If, after reading the above guidelines, you find you cannot clearly articulate the significance and innovation of your specific aims, it may be reasonable to consider discarding your original aims and starting over. As discussed in Chapter 19, *Review Process*, the overall impact of your specific aims is the driver of the final score of an NIH grant.

Reasons to consider discarding or revising your original aims are as follows

- If you cannot identify the public health or clinical significance of your potential findings
- If you cannot identify a means by which your aims will extend the prior published literature (e.g., even via a new study population, study design, or measurement tool)
- When, after conducting power calculations, you discover that you have insufficient statistical power even after considering such techniques described in Chapter 11, *Power and Sample Size*.

6.13 ANNOTATED EXAMPLES

6.13.1 Example #1: Needs Improvement

Exercise Intervention to Reduce Gestational Weight Gain (GWG)

Specific Aims Page

Paragraph #1: Excessive GWG is associated with increased complications of pregnancy, labor, and delivery[1] and is also a major risk factor for obesity later in life.[2] Latinas have higher rates of overweight and obesity when they become pregnant, experience higher rates of excessive GWG, and experience more maternal and neonatal complications compared to non-Latinas. Lifestyle interventions with pregnant non-Latinas have been found effective, especially among normal weight women.[3] To date, no randomized controlled trials have been conducted to test interventions targeting excessive GWG among pregnant Latinas. The primary objective of this study is to evaluate a comprehensive behavioral intervention to reduce excessive GWG among Latinas. Interventions developed for non-Latinas need to be culturally adapted for Latinas to address cultural differences in beliefs and values that may influence the effectiveness of gestational weight management.[4] Further, interventions addressing dietary intake among Latinas should involve the family, particularly the partner.[5] Findings from our previous couple-based randomized trial aiming to promote smoking cessation among expectant Latino fathers and promote physical activity and improved nutrition among pregnant Latinas suggest that counseling alone did not significantly improve fruit and vegetable consumption or physical activity, but we did find that women in the intervention arm consumed less fat in pregnancy than those in the control arm. Our findings suggest that a more intensive intervention is required to affect key drivers of GWG.

Comment: This paragraph is too long. It is important to quickly convince the reader of the importance of your topic and then shift to a new paragraph on study methods. It is also difficult for reviewers to wade through long paragraphs. Bolding or otherwise highlighting a key sentence will make it clear to the reviewer what you feel is the most important point. Having preliminary data is a real strength and should be highlighted by including the funding source, grant number, and investigator's role on this prior project to this paragraph. Avoid first stating the null findings of the preliminary data (i.e., no impact on fruit and vegetables); instead, first state the significant findings (i.e., a decrease in fat). Indeed, the fat findings are likely more relevant to the proposal than the fruit and vegetable findings.

Paragraph #2: In the proposed study, we are partnering with local community organizations that already address obesity in the Latino community. We propose a two-arm trial in which we compare (1) intervention arm, an intervention that includes activities to promote physical activity and improved nutrition (n = 200), versus (2) standard care arm (n = 200). The primary outcome is the proportion of women who gain weight within the IOM recommendations. Secondary outcomes include perinatal outcomes such as GDM and preterm birth and changes in physical activity and nutrition.

Comment: The term *partnering* is vague. Instead clarify if this group is a collaborator on the proposal. The paragraph should also clarify how weight, physical activity, and diet will be measured.

Paragraph #3

Primary Aim

Aim 1. To assess whether a culturally adapted, comprehensive lifestyle intervention reduces excessive GWG.

Hypothesis 1. At 32 weeks gestation, women in the intervention arm will be more likely to gain weight within IOM recommendations than women in the control arm.

Secondary Aims

Aim 2. To assess the effect of a lifestyle intervention on maternal physical activity and dietary intake at the end of pregnancy (32 weeks gestation), 6 weeks, and 6 months postpartum.

Aim 3. To assess whether the effect of the intervention on weight, physical activity, and dietary intake at the end of pregnancy, 6 weeks postpartum, and at 6 months postpartum is mediated by psychosocial factors (motivation, self-efficacy, perceived risk, outcome expectations, pregnancy-related weight beliefs, and social support).

Aim 4. To assess the effect of a lifestyle intervention on perinatal and infant outcomes.

Comment: Typically, there should be more primary aims than secondary aims (e.g., three primary aims and one secondary aim would be preferable). As written, reviewers may immediately become concerned that there is inadequate statistical power to achieve aims #2, #3, and #4 and that is why they are listed as *secondary*. In addition, none of the secondary aims are accompanied by hypotheses. Due to the large number of possible perinatal and infant outcomes, this aim comes off at best as overly ambitious and, at worst, as indicating a lack of knowledge about the area. Lastly, this example is also missing a statement summarizing the significance and innovation of the proposal.

6.13.2 Example #2: Does Not Need Improvement

Exercise Intervention to Reduce Postpartum Diabetes

Specific Aims Page

Diabetes and obesity have reached epidemic proportions in the United States with rates consistently higher among Hispanic as compared to non-Hispanic whites. Among Hispanic women diagnosed with GDM, 50% will go on to develop type 2 diabetes within 5 years of the index pregnancy. Although randomized controlled trials among adults with impaired glucose tolerance have shown that diet and physical activity reduce the risk of type 2 diabetes, such programs have not been tested in high-risk postpartum women. **The overall goal of this randomized controlled trial is to test the efficacy of a culturally and linguistically modified, individually tailored lifestyle intervention to reduce risk factors for type 2 diabetes and cardiovascular disease among postpartum Hispanic women with a history of abnormal glucose tolerance during pregnancy.**

Eligible Hispanic women will be recruited after routine GDM screening and randomly assigned to a lifestyle intervention (n = 150) or a comparison health and wellness (control) intervention (n = 150). Multimodal contacts (i.e., in-person, telephone counseling, and mailed print-based materials) will be used to deliver the intervention from randomization (~29 weeks gestation) to 12 months postpartum. Targets of the intervention are to achieve and maintain (1) postpartum weight reduction to prepregnancy weight, (2) at least 150 min per week of moderate-intensity physical activity, and (3) reduction in postpartum total caloric intake via reduced consumption of popular calorie-dense foods and reduced portion size as recommended by the American Diabetes Association. The intervention draws from social cognitive theory and addresses the specific social, cultural, economic, and environmental challenges faced by underserved Hispanic women. Measurements of adherence will include accelerometers and dietary recalls. The intervention will be based on our efficacious exercise and dietary interventions for Hispanics (R01XX000000).

> **Specific Aim #1**: Evaluate the impact of a lifestyle intervention on **postpartum weight loss** among Hispanic women with a history of abnormal glucose tolerance in pregnancy.
>> **Hypothesis #1**: Participants randomized to the lifestyle intervention will have greater adherence with IOM postpartum weight-loss guidelines at 6 and 12 months postpartum as compared to participants randomized to the comparison health and wellness intervention.
>
> **Specific Aim #2**: Evaluate the impact of a lifestyle intervention on **postpartum biomarkers of insulin resistance** among Hispanic women with a history of abnormal glucose tolerance in pregnancy.
>> **Hypothesis #2**: Participants randomized to the lifestyle intervention will have lower fasting concentrations of glucose, insulin, HbA_{1c}, leptin, and TNF-α and higher concentrations of adiponectin as compared to participants randomized to the comparison health and wellness intervention.
>
> **Specific Aim #3**: Evaluate the impact of a lifestyle intervention on other **postpartum biomarkers of cardiovascular risk** among Hispanic women with a history of abnormal glucose tolerance in pregnancy.

> **Hypothesis #3**: Participants randomized to the lifestyle intervention will have lower total cholesterol, LDL cholesterol, triglyceride concentrations, systolic and diastolic blood pressure, CRP, fetuin-A, and albumin-to-creatinine ratio (ACR) and higher HDL cholesterol as compared to participants randomized to the comparison health and wellness intervention.
>
> This proposal is innovative in capitalizing on the postpartum window of opportunity and by utilizing objective measures of adherence with exercise (i.e., accelerometers). The intervention can readily be translated into clinical practice in underserved and minority populations. The public health impact of such lifestyle modifications is likely to be greatest in ethnic groups, such as Hispanics, with consistently high rates of obesity, diabetes, and the highest rates of sedentary behavior.

Background and Significance Section 7

The goal of the Background and Significance section of the proposal is to convince your reader that you have a solid command of the current research in the field and that you can be objective and thoughtful in your evaluation of this prior literature. In fact, a well-written Background and Significance section will lead the reader to ask the same research questions that you are asking in your specific aims. Through the tips below, I will show how this section will ultimately provide the rationale for your aims and hypotheses.

One quick point about terminology Depending on your dissertation or grant proposal guidelines, this Background and Significance section may simply be titled Background or Significance.

7.1 REFER BACK TO YOUR LITERATURE REVIEW OUTLINE

Your Background and Significance section will draw directly from your specific aims and hypotheses and the corresponding literature review outline that you developed in Chapter 4, *Conducting the Literature Search*. Let's use the same example used in Chapter 4.

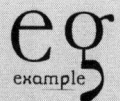

> **example**
>
> **Specific Aims**
> Specific Aim #1: We propose to assess the relationship between postmenopausal hormone use, antioxidants, and Alzheimer's disease in a cohort of women participating in the Phoenix Health Study.
> Hypothesis #1a: Postmenopausal hormone use will be inversely associated with Alzheimer's disease.
> Hypothesis #1b: Antioxidant use will be inversely associated with Alzheimer's disease.

Literature Review Outline:

Background and Significance

    a. Introduction: Public Health Impact of Outcome (Disease)
        i. Number and percent affected by Alzheimer's disease
        ii. Sequelae of Alzheimer's disease
        iii. Established risk factors for Alzheimer's disease
    b. Physiology of Exposure–Outcome Relationship
        i. The physiologic relationship between postmenopausal hormone use and Alzheimer's disease (Hypothesis #1a)
        ii. The physiologic relationship between antioxidants and Alzheimer's disease (Hypothesis #1b)
    c. Epidemiology of Exposure–Outcome Relationship
        i. The prior epidemiologic studies on the relationship between postmenopausal hormone use and Alzheimer's disease (Hypothesis #1a)
        ii. The prior epidemiologic studies on the relationship between antioxidants and Alzheimer's disease (Hypothesis #1b)
    d. Summary of Significance and Innovation

7.2 BACKGROUND AND SIGNIFICANCE SHOULD BE MADE UP OF SUBSECTIONS CORRESPONDING TO EACH HYPOTHESIS

As you can see in the example above, the literature review outline is divided into subsections, which directly correspond to each hypothesis. In creating and titling your subsections, you will want to use similar wording as used in the hypotheses to make it clear to your reviewers that you have summarized the state of the research in each area of your hypotheses. This technique of cross-checking these two sections (i.e., the Specific Aims/Hypotheses with the subsections of the Background and Significance section) will ensure that there are no omissions. That is, that there are no hypotheses that you have failed to support via the prior literature nor vice versa: extra Background and Significance sections that do not correspond to a hypothesis. The latter is of particular concern in grant proposal given the strict space limitations.

7.3 SECTION a: SUMMARIZE THE PUBLIC HEALTH IMPACT OF THE OUTCOME (DISEASE)

The public health impact of your study can be supported by specifying the prevalence and/or incidence rates of your outcome (disease) of interest. For example, depending upon your study outcome, this data can be found on such websites as the

Center for Disease Control and Prevention (CDC) and Surveillance, Epidemiology, and End Results (SEER) Program or in published findings from large surveillance studies such as the *National Health and Nutrition Examination Survey*. Another efficient way to locate such incidence/prevalence data can be found by carefully reading the introductions of journal articles that you included in your summary table (see Chapter 4, *Conducting the Literature Search*). A well-written introduction to a journal article will cite current rates and provide a corresponding citation. By obtaining these cited articles, you can get a head start on identifying sources of such data.

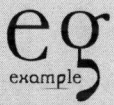

> **eg** **Imagine a proposal to conduct a randomized lifestyle intervention:**
> *example*
> Epidemiological evidence suggests that an estimated 5.2 million Americans of all ages have Alzheimer's disease.[1] More women than men have Alzheimer's disease; almost two thirds of Americans with Alzheimer's are women.[2]

The public health impact of your study can also be supported by specifying the sequelae of your outcome (disease) of interest (e.g., increased mortality and cardiovascular disease). In addition, in this section, it is also useful to summarize the established risk factors for your outcome of interest.

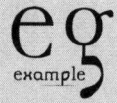

> **eg** Alzheimer's disease leads to increased rates of infection, organ failure, and eventually disability and mortality.[1] Established risk factors for Alzheimer's disease include age, family history, and genetic factors.[2]

7.4 SECTION b: SUMMARIZE THE PHYSIOLOGY OF EXPOSURE–OUTCOME RELATIONSHIP

Your goal in this section is to briefly summarize the physiologic or behavioral mechanisms that link your exposure to your outcome. The need for brevity is driven by the limited-space requirements in the typical grant application. However, the ability to be brief in conveying this physiologic link also provides evidence that you have a firm grasp on this mechanism and can summarize the key points concisely. It is always more difficult to write a short explanation than a long one!

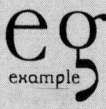

> **e.g. example** Numerous animal and laboratory studies have shown that antioxidant nutrients can protect the brain from oxidative and inflammatory damage, but there are limited data available from epidemiological studies.[14–17]

As noted in the literature review outline instructions (see Chapter 4, *Conducting the Literature Search*) in this section, it is important to avoid focusing on simply the physiology of your outcome or your exposure in isolation. One can assume that the scientific reader is familiar, for example, with the basic mechanisms behind Alzheimer's disease. Instead, one wants to focus on the mechanism for how your exposure, antioxidants, could *impact* Alzheimer's disease.

If your specific aims involve the examination of several exposures or outcomes, including a figure in the Background section is highly recommended. This figure would display your exposure(s) of interest and how they relate to each other and to your outcome(s) of interest. This figure can also help to demonstrate the proposed physiologic pathways between these variables.

Figure 7.1 is from a proposal to conduct an observational cohort study to evaluate how physical activity (exposure #1) and stress (exposure #2) impact risk of GDM (outcome) via certain physiologic and behavioral mediating variables.

Figures displaying your *theoretical model* can also be helpful.

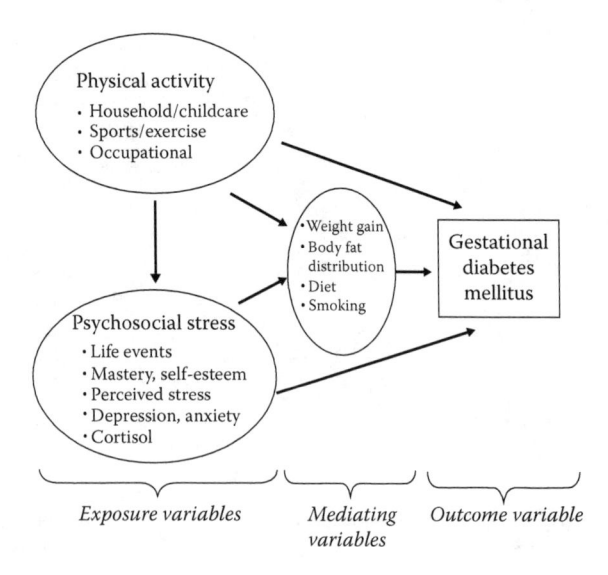

FIGURE 7.1 Mechanisms from a proposal to evaluate the association between physical activity, stress, and risk of GDM.

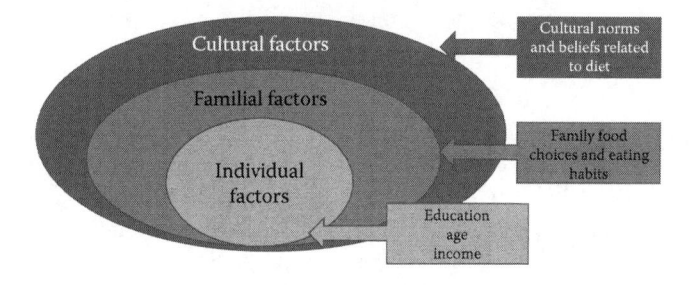

FIGURE 7.2 Underlying theoretical model behind a dietary intervention.

Figure 7.2 shows the underlying theoretical model behind a dietary intervention.

7.5 SECTION c: SUMMARIZE THE EPIDEMIOLOGY OF EXPOSURE–OUTCOME RELATIONSHIP (DESCRIBE STUDIES IN GROUPS)

Following the outline, the goal of Section c is to summarize the prior epidemiologic literature. Therefore, this epidemiologic literature review section should open with a paragraph that gives the reader an overview of the number and designs of the prior epidemiologic studies which have evaluated your exposure–outcome association of interest.

Remember that the goal is to quickly give the reader a synopsis of the state of the research in this area. For example, is this a well-studied area? Or are prior studies sparse? What is the research gap? This type of overview can be achieved by describing the prior studies in groups. You will be well positioned to do this after creating the summary table of the prior literature as part of Chapter 4, *Conducting the Literature Search*.

In contrast to a simple listing (e.g., laundry list) of all the prior studies, organizing the body of prior literature in meaningful categories provides a service for the reviewer. It shows your understanding of the body of work in the field and forms the basis on which you can build the argument for your research gap. In contrast, describing each prior study on this topic, one by one, fails to organize the material for the reviewer nor show your mastery of the area. In addition, due to space requirements in a grant proposal, this approach is really not feasible.

Which groupings to choose? The choice of categories to use in the opening paragraph is dictated by the research gap that you want to highlight. For example, if one of your study strengths is your prospective cohort design, and few prior studies used this design, you will want to group the studies in categories by study design. In this way, you make clear to the reader that the number of prior prospective studies is sparse and therefore efficiently demonstrate that your study will be extending this prior literature by adding to the small body of prior studies of this design.

In addition, or alternatively depending on the point you would like to make, you could also choose other categories by which to *group* (i.e., organize) the prior epidemiologic studies (e.g., by study design or by study methods; see examples below).

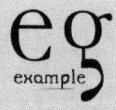

> **eg example** Prior studies of antioxidant use and Alzheimer's disease have been contradictory.[1-21] Fifteen of the 21 published studies observed decreased risk of Alzheimer's disease for women who regularly used antioxidants compared with nonusers.[1-15] No overall association between antioxidant use and Alzheimer's disease was found in four studies.[16-19] Higher levels of antioxidant use were associated with an increased risk of Alzheimer's disease in the Framingham cohort study[20] and the Turkish case–control study.[21]

In the above example, the writer chose to group the studies according to their findings.

In this example, the first sentence informs the reader of the total number of publications in the field that have evaluated antioxidant use (one of the exposures of interest) and Alzheimer's disease (the outcome of interest). The following sentences group the prior studies according to the direction of their findings (i.e., decreased risk, null, and increased risk).

In contrast, in the example below, the writer chose to group the studies according to their methods.

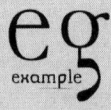

> **eg example** A total of 15 epidemiologic studies have evaluated the relationship between antioxidant use and Alzheimer's disease.[1-15] These studies, however, have assessed women's dietary supplement use only[1-5] or dietary (nonsupplement) sources only.[6-13] Only two studies have measured both supplement and dietary sources of antioxidant use.[14,15]

7.5.1 In Summarizing the Epidemiologic Literature, Note the Relationships between Study Methods and Their Corresponding Findings

Use your summary table to identify possible explanations for the differences in study findings such as different methodologies or different populations.

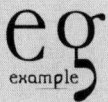

> **eg example** While the two studies that used mailed questionnaires support the finding that inhalant use among adolescents increased risk of autism, the three studies that used face-to-face interviews did not observe an increased risk.

This example identifies differences in study methods (i.e., questionnaires vs. face-to-face interviews) as a possible explanation for the differences in study findings.

7.5.2 Finding the Research Gap in the Prior Epidemiologic Literature

The **key principle** here in Section c is to report sparingly on the details of these studies and to instead describe them in groupings—carefully selected to implicitly highlight the research gap that your proposal will be filling.

The items in Table 7.1 can all serve as excellent examples of a research gap. In other words, they can serve to answer the question, what is the demonstrated need for this new study? The more research gaps that you can point out to the reviewer that you will be filling with your proposal, the better. In other words, at least one is necessary but more are value added.

7.5.3 How Big a Research Gap Do I Need to Fill?

The research gap does not need to be large—but it needs to be clearly elucidated and be of scientific importance in direct proportion to the size of the grant. This is a point that I can't emphasize enough. I've found that graduate students and early-career faculty are sometimes dissuaded by the presence of even one prior study in the literature that evaluated their exposure–outcome relationship. They fear that the presence of this study removes the need for their study. However, in epidemiology and preventive medicine, it is important to remember that causality can only be determined by a multiplicity of studies of varying designs in varying study populations.

As you can see by the example above of the proposal to study antioxidants and Alzheimer's disease, a total of 21 prior epidemiologic studies in your area can be considered insufficient if, for example, their findings have been conflicting, or if few of them used your proposed study methods, or even if few of these studies utilized your study design or study population.

TABLE 7.1 Example research gaps

PRIOR LITERATURE IS...
Limited to particular study designs
Limited to particular methodology
Limited sample size
Conflicting findings
Limited control for confounding factors
Limited to particular study populations
Limited number of prior studies

7.5.4 Highlight the Limitations of Prior Studies That Your Proposal Will Be Able to Address

Below are two example excerpts of an identified research gap.

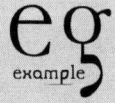

> **eg** *example* Prior studies were limited by self-reported assessment of antioxidant use. In contrast, we propose to assess biomarkers of oxidative stress.

> **eg** *example* Prior studies of antioxidant use and risk of Alzheimer's disease have been limited by cross-sectional study designs; therefore, we propose to conduct a prospective cohort study of the association between antioxidant use and Alzheimer's disease.

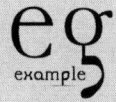

For the second example above, if your study will **also** be cross sectional, it will not be useful to include this phrase, because this is a limitation that your proposed study shares with the prior literature. Instead, you will want to highlight a different research gap that your study will be filling. In other words, the goal of the Background and Significance section is to show how you will extend prior research, and this can only be done by filling gaps. It is not that you will hide the problems that you share with the prior literature (e.g., a cross-sectional design). Instead, you will discuss these limitations in your Limitations and Alternatives section—a subsection of the Approach section (Chapter 13, *How to Present Limitations and Alternatives*).

Sometimes graduate students and early-career faculty are hesitant to point out the limitations of prior studies for fear of offending the authors of these works, whom, they fear, might be serving as potential reviewers of their proposal. However, remember that all authors are aware of the limitations of their studies and even have presented these openly in the Discussion sections of their published work. It is fine to point out these concerns simply and directly. In addition, if, in your opinion, these authors have not identified all their limitations, it is also fine to factually state what you view are additional study limitations. For example, an author of a previous cross-sectional study will know that their study design has limitations, by definition, over and above a prospective cohort study.

Below is an example of simply and directly summing up the limitations of the prior literature in the area of antioxidant use and risk of Alzheimer's disease. Note that all the limitations mentioned are those limitations that the proposal writers feel that they will be improving upon in their own proposal.

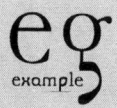

> **e.g.** *example* — In summary, the prior epidemiologic studies of antioxidant use and Alzheimer's disease have several limitations: (1) the majority involved small numbers of nonminority women and men limiting the generalizability of results, (2) few assessed the validity of their measure of self-reported antioxidant use, and (3) many failed to account for confounding variables that can lead to misleading results.

7.5.5 What Should You Do if the Prior Literature Is Conflicting?

7.5.5.1 Let reviewers know that you are aware of controversies

The first and foremost approach to dealing with controversies or conflicting findings in the prior literature is not to hide or dodge them. Instead, you will want to objectively present each opposing finding or theory. Indeed, remember that your reviewers may have published in the same field and may be the authors of the very works that you are discussing. Imagine their perception of your scholarship if your proposal leaves out their findings.

The worst-case scenario The worst-case scenario (always healthy to imagine) is that you have left out the reviewer's study because it is not consistent with your hypothesis. In other words, you decide to only present studies that found a positive association between your exposure and outcome to further justify your hypothesis of a positive association. Therefore, you omit the reviewer's study that found an inverse association. The reviewer would conclude that not only do you not have an adequate grasp of the literature but you are purposefully spinning prior findings. In fact, it is always a useful exercise to envision that one of the reviewers is indeed an author of one of the prior studies in the field.

7.5.5.2 Give clear reasons for taking a side

In the context of prior conflicting findings, it is important to make the decision process underlying your final hypothesis transparent to the reviewer. You will want to (1) present the conflicting findings, then (2) describe the strengths and limitations of these prior studies, and (3) describe how you weighted these strengths and limitations to come up with your final hypothesis. In this section, do not be shy in presenting prior study limitations. Remember that you are simply proposing to test a particular hypothesis. You are not proposing to determine causality. Therefore, your goal is to convince the reviewer that you are open minded enough to reject your hypothesis if your experimental results indicate.

7.5.6 Highlight Key Studies

After the summary paragraph, if space allows, it is ideal if you can highlight several of the key studies that were included in your groupings. This is usually more feasible in a graduate proposal than in the tight space limitations of a grant proposal. As a reminder, these would be studies that appeared in your summary table of the epidemiologic association between your exposure and your outcome.

Which studies to highlight? In choosing which prior epidemiologic studies to highlight, you have several options. For example, you may choose to highlight the most recent studies to give a sense of the current state of the field. Often proposal writers will highlight what they feel, as a result of their comprehensive literature review, are the strongest prior studies in the area. Details on these studies will give your reviewer a sense of the state of the art in the field and will also provide further support for your methods—if they are similar to those in these highlighted studies. Other studies that you may want to highlight are the studies most similar to your own—which can provide support for your hypotheses and/or methods. Caution should be taken, however, to still clarify how your study will improve or differ from these highlighted studies. That is, you don't want to obviate the need for your study.

Make explicit the reasons for highlighting noncurrent articles. Such reasons could include the fact that the study is a landmark study, or perhaps the study is the only evidence available on a given topic; or perhaps by including this older study, it helps the reader to understand the evolution of a research technique that you are proposing.

How to highlight a particular study? When highlighting studies, first, state why you think the highlighted study is important. For example, *In the most recent study to date, Smith et al. enrolled...* or *In the first prospective study of risk factors for Alzheimer's disease, Smith et al. enrolled....*

Then, be sure to concisely delineate the following **key attributes** about the highlighted study—ideally within several sentences:

- Author
- Study design
- Size
- Brief methods
- Measure of association
- Brief limitations

Below is an example of a highlighted study from the same proposal designed to assess the association between antioxidants and Alzheimer's disease.

> *example* — In the only prospective study to assess frequency and dose of lifetime supplement use, Jones et al. administered the Antioxidant Questionnaire to 2000 women at the onset of menopause.[39] Heavy antioxidant users had a decreased risk of Alzheimer's

> disease (OR = 0.78, 95% CI 0.56–0.94) as compared to light users. These findings, however, may be due to self-selection; women who regularly take antioxidants could be healthier in some overall way that improves cognitive function.

Note that, as demonstrated in the example above, when describing the measure of association, the key is to provide the absolute magnitude of the results, not just whether the results are statistically significant. It is important to remember that statistical significance only indicates whether the observed findings might be due to chance. Statistical significance does *not* mean that the findings are clinically significant nor that the difference is not due to bias or confounding. In other words, the highlighted study may have found statistically significant findings, but these may have been small, clinically insignificant, or due to bias. Therefore, it is always preferable to state the actual magnitude of findings (as well as the corresponding measure of variation) that the study observed. Examples include relative risks (RRs) (and corresponding confidence intervals [CIs]) or mean differences (and corresponding standard errors).

Also, note that in the above example, you are not expected to dissect and discuss every flaw of each highlighted study. In contrast, graduate school courses involving journal article critiques typically require students to evaluate studies for each possible bias and limitation. Instead, in a grant proposal, you are expected to only comment on the most important/major limitations of the prior epidemiologic studies with a focus on those limitations that your proposal will improve upon.

The other strength of the example is that the authors avoided using professional jargon when briefly summarizing the study limitations. By clearly defining what they meant by *self-selection*, they demonstrated their understanding of this limitation and made it easier on the reviewer who would have been left with the task of trying to deduce their point.

7.6 SECTION d: SUMMARIZE THE SIGNIFICANCE AND INNOVATION

Corresponding to your literature review outline, Section d of the Background and Significance section should summarize the **significance** and **innovation** of your proposal.

The NIH defines **significance** as addressing the following questions:

- Does the project address an important problem or a critical barrier to progress in the field?
- If the aims of the project are achieved, how will scientific knowledge, technical capability, and/or clinical practice be improved?
- How will successful completion of the aims change the concepts, methods, technologies, treatments, services, or preventative interventions that drive this field?

As you can see from the questions above, *significance* in this context does not **only** mean that you plan to study a very important public health issue. *Significance* is also assessed by reviewers in terms of how data from your study will **inform the field**. Be clear as to how currently available data really need to be refined and extended. For example, obesity is a significant public health problem in the United States. But, how will your study drive the field forward: Will it identify susceptibility genes or maybe point the way to better preventive interventions?

A perfectly designed study about an unimportant question is not considered significant. But a study that considers a topic of extremely high significance in terms of public health but has flaws in the study design that can affect the validity of the findings is not significant either.

The NIH defines **innovation** as addressing the following questions:

- Does the application challenge and seek to shift current research or clinical practice paradigms by utilizing novel theoretical concepts, approaches or methodologies, instrumentation, or interventions?
- Are the concepts, approaches or methodologies, instrumentation, or interventions novel to one field of research or novel in a broad sense?
- Is a refinement, improvement, or new application of theoretical concepts, approaches or methodologies, instrumentation, or interventions proposed?

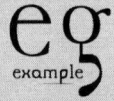

> *example* **Imagine a proposal to conduct a randomized lifestyle intervention:**
>
> This proposal is innovative in being the first, to our knowledge, to test a physical activity intervention designed to prevent Alzheimer's disease among high-risk women. The significance of the study lies in the fact that changes in modifiable risk factors may reduce the morbidity associated with Alzheimer's disease. Findings of this low-cost, high-reach intervention can readily be translated to clinical practice in high-risk populations.

7.7 TIP #1: SHOULD YOU HAVE ONE CONSOLIDATED BACKGROUND AND SIGNIFICANCE SECTION?

If you have multiple specific aims, NIH allows you to address background/significance (and approach as described in Chapter 9, *Study Design and Methods*) for each specific aim individually. In this case, you would repeat each aim prior to its individual Background and Significance section. This decision as to whether to have one collective Background and Significance section that addresses all your aims (albeit still has subparagraphs) versus repeating each aim above its own Background and Significance section largely depends upon how interrelated your specific aims and study methodology are, the collective approach being best suited to interrelated aims and the separate approach being more suited to disparate aims.

7.8 TIP #2: BE SURE TO EXPRESS YOUR OWN OPINIONS ABOUT A PRIOR STUDY'S LIMITATIONS

It is important to show evidence of independence in your ability to critique the prior literature when writing a grant proposal. In other words, be sure to summarize the study limitations in your own words. Avoid quoting directly from the author's description of their own study limitations (e.g., from the Discussion section of the published article). In addition, avoid deferring to the authors of the study by saying, for example, *The authors stated that their findings might be due to confounding*. This approach is problematic for several reasons. First, the authors may be incorrect. Second, the authors are certainly not as unbiased as you theoretically are. Third, your opinion of the primary limitation of their study (which you selected to highlight the need for your own study) may differ from their opinion.

The only exception to this advice is when citing a review article as noted in Tip #3 below.

7.9 TIP #3: YOU MAY REFER TO COMMENTS FROM A REVIEW ARTICLE

A review article can provide useful authority on a topic, and its conclusions can sometimes provide further support for the rationale for your study. In this situation, citing a review article is like calling in the *big guns*. For example, many review articles will comment upon the limitations of prior studies and point out the need for and type of future studies that should be conducted in the area. If these conclusions are consistent with the thrust of your proposed study, then it would be helpful to cite the review article.

> *e.g.* example
> Prior studies were limited by lack of control for key confounding factors. In fact, in a recent review article of risk factors for bladder cancer, Taylor et al. concluded that prior studies faced uncontrolled confounding.
> In a review of risk factors for preterm delivery, Berkowitz et al.[29] concluded that there is insufficient data to assess the effect of recreational activity on prematurity.

7.10 TIP #4: OCCASIONALLY YOU MAY PROVIDE THE HISTORICAL CONTEXT

Providing a historical context is especially desirable for dissertation proposals with the goal of demonstrating the graduate student's comprehensive knowledge of the literature.

> **e.g. example**: As early as 1892, Osler described the coronary-prone person as a 'keen ambitious man, whose engines are set at full speed ahead.'

On the other hand, for grant proposals, you may be unlikely to have space to dedicate to the historical evolution of a concept unless it is somehow key to your proposed methodology. For example, you would want to comment that your proposal is innovative if it is the first to advance the methods used since a prior date.

7.11 TIP #5: SUMMARIZE AT THE END OF EACH SECTION IN THE BACKGROUND AND SIGNIFICANCE SECTION

It is important to summarize at least once in the Background and Significance section. If space permits, a brief summary at the end of the epidemiology section and at the end of the physiology section is even more preferable. These summaries can take the form of a single summation sentence of the take-home message of that particular paragraph, typically reemphasizing the research gap.

One approach is to highlight this summary sentence in bold. Indeed, I suggest bolding or otherwise highlighting one key sentence in each paragraph of the Background and Significance section. This tip fits under the concept of being kind to your reviewer. That is, this bolding does the work for the reviewer of locating the key sentence in each paragraph and identifying it for them. Indeed, the act of searching for this key sentence provides you with the added benefit of ensuring that each paragraph has a key point. With space at a premium in grant proposals (e.g., current limits for the research strategy for smaller NIH grants can be as low as six pages), each paragraph needs to count. This point is particularly relevant for the Background and Significance section as this section is usually densely packed with text, and reviewers may have difficulty picking out the key points.

7.12 TIP #6: AVOID BROAD AND GLOBAL STATEMENTS IN THE BACKGROUND AND SIGNIFICANCE SECTION

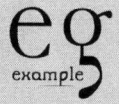

> **Original Version**
> Obesity reduction is important to both the economy of the United States and to the rest of the world. Without obesity prevention, we will face a catastrophic public health crisis in the next millennium...
>
> **Improved Version**
> Tailored exercise and dietary interventions have been credited as the most effective form of weight-reduction programs.[1,2] Over the past 5 years, randomized trials of such interventions have found...

The improved example clarifies the specific topic that will be evaluated, and it is now clear what will be measured and studied. Other improvements include the addition of citations. In addition, the time frame of interest is now clarified.

7.13 TIP #7: BE COMPREHENSIVE AND COMPLETE IN CITATIONS

One important detail is to be sure that your citations are internally complete. That is, the opening sentence of the summary paragraph of the prior epidemiologic literature must cite all the studies highlighted in this section.

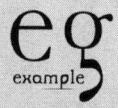

> A total of 15 epidemiologic studies have evaluated the relationship between physical activity and birth weight.[1-15] These studies, however, have assessed women's occupational activities only,[1-5] recreational activities only,[6-11] or a combination of occupational and household activities.[12,13] Only two studies have measured total activity (recreational, occupational, and household).[14,15]

Note that in this example above, the first sentence cites references 1–15, and the subsequent sentences divide this total into subcategories (i.e., 1–5, 6–11, 12, 13, 14, 15).

These subcategory citations add up to the total number of 15 cited at the beginning of the sentence. In addition, given that this first sentence is developed based on your summary table of the literature created in Chapter 4, *Conducting the Literature Search*, this total number should be the same as the total number of studies that you included in that summary table. In this way, the reader can easily see the specific number of studies in each subcategory and what percent they are of the whole body of literature on your topic.

Lastly, if you then choose to go on and highlight particular studies, they should also have been included in the citations from this opening sentence. In other words, in the example above, any subsequent epidemiologic study that you highlight should be a citation between 1 and 15 inclusive.

7.14 TIP #8: REFERENCES SHOULD DIRECTLY FOLLOW THE STUDIES THAT THEY RELATE TO

A common practice among proposal writers is to group citations at the end of the sentence in spite of the fact that the sentence may describe several data points derived from several different citations.

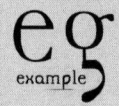

> **Original Version**
> Previous studies have found that 35%–50% of college students report participating in an online alcohol abuse prevention program.[1-3]
>
> **Improved Version**
> Previous studies have found that 35%[1-2] of college students to 50%[3] of college students report participating in an online alcohol abuse prevention program.

In the original example, the reviewer will not know which of the three cited studies reported which percentage. If the reviewer is questioning one of your presented rates (e.g., if they feel that 50% seems high), the burden will be upon the reviewer to look through each of the three citations to see which one observed this high rate. In the improved example, the citations immediately follow the corresponding percentages.

7.15 TIP #9: IF YOU ARE COMMENTING ON A TIME FRAME, BE SPECIFIC

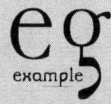

Original Version
In recent years, there has been an increase in child abuse.
Improved Version
Child abuse incident reports increased by 50% between 2008 and 2013, totaling more than 5 million reports in 2013.[1]

The improved version provides a time frame for the increase, making the statement less general and more specific, which is always preferable.

7.16 ANNOTATED EXAMPLES

7.16.1 Example #1: Needs Improvement

NSAIDS and Risk of Endometrial Cancer

Background and Significance

Paragraph #1: Endometrial cancer is one of the most common invasive gynecological malignancies affecting postmenopausal women.[1] It is the fourth most common cancer, accounting for 6% of female cancers, following breast, lung, and colorectal cancer.[2] The American Cancer Society estimates that there will be 46,470 new cases and 8,120 deaths attributable to endometrial cancer in 2011 in the United States.[3] Endometrial cancer develops in the body or corpus of the uterus. The most common histological type of endometrial cancer is endometrioid adenocarcinoma, which typically presents with postmenopausal vaginal bleeding or spotting. Within the United States, incidence rates are higher in non-Hispanic white women as compared to black or Asian women.[4] However, the mortality rates are higher in black women with endometrial cancer than in white women. The possible reasons for disparity in mortality rates could be inequalities in treatment, access to health care, and a higher prevalence of more aggressive types of endometrial cancer.

Comment: This paragraph addresses Section a, of the outline (public health impact of the outcome of interest). The sentences on disparities in rates between white and black women should only have been included if the proposal included an aim designed to evaluate effect modification by race/ethnicity. Instead, because the proposal will be evaluating effect modification by obesity, this section should present rates of endometrial cancer in obese women as compared to normal weight women.

Paragraph #2: Several studies have suggested that women with a family history of endometrial cancer are at increased risk of endometrial cancer.[5] Women with a mutation in one of the HNPCC genes usually develop endometrial cancer before 50 years of age.[6] High levels of endogenous or exogenous estrogen are one of the underlying causes of endometrial cancer.[7] Risk factors such as early menarche,[8] late menopause,[9] and anovulation[10] are associated with increased levels of endogenous estrogen. Other risk factors known to increase the risk endometrial cancer are nulliparity,[11] obesity,[12] diabetes, and hyperinsulinemia.[13] Conversely, increased parity[14] and cigarette smoking[15] have been suggested to reduce the risk of endometrial cancer.

Comment: This paragraph appears to continue to address Section a, of the outline (public health impact of the outcome of interest). However, the paragraph is disjointed and unorganized. The paragraph should be reorganized to start out by stating, *Established risk factors for endometrial cancer include....* Sentences referring to endometrial cancer among premenopausal women can be deleted because the proposal is focusing on postmenopausal women.

Paragraph #3: Unopposed estrogen theory implicates long-term estrogen exposure unopposed by progesterone as one mechanism for increased risk of endometrial cancer. Estrogen causes the endometrium to undergo mitotic division during the follicular phase of the menstrual cycle.[16] Inflammatory mechanisms are also hypothesized to play a role in the development of endometrial cancer.[17] This mechanism is supported by the fact that inflammatory cells induce rapid cell division and high levels of free radicals that may subsequently damage DNA.[18] Insulin-mediated mechanisms have also been suggested to play a role in the etiology of endometrial cancer.

> Comment: This paragraph can be deleted because it only focuses on the general etiology of endometrial cancer. Instead, this section should focus on describing the physiologic mechanism **linking** NSAIDS to risk of endometrial cancer as the writer does in the next paragraph.

Paragraph #4: In recent years, there has been some *in vitro* evidence suggesting that the use of NSAIDS may impact risk of endometrial cancer by affecting inflammatory pathways.[20] However, epidemiological evidence for the protective role of NSAIDS is conflicting and inconsistent. Furthermore, the effect of dose, duration, frequency, and type of NSAIDS has not been evaluated together in a single study.[21-26] Additionally, some of these studies were not able to evaluate the modifying effect of BMI and postmenopausal hormone use on the association between NSAIDS and endometrial cancer.[28-30]

> Comment: This paragraph describes the physiologic mechanism between NSAIDS and endometrial cancer as well as the prior epidemiologic studies (Sections b and c of the outline). No changes necessary.

Paragraph #5: Given the uncertainties in the association between NSAIDS and endometrial cancer, it is crucial to evaluate the importance of the protective role of dose, duration, and type of NSAIDS on endometrial cancer. Therefore, we propose to investigate the relationship between use of NSAIDS and risk of endometrial cancer using data from Pyramid Health Study. This study is innovative in that it will be the first to have detailed on NSAIDS use and on suspected and established risk factors for endometrial cancer. This will provide us a unique opportunity to carefully examine the relation between NSAIDS use and endometrial cancer in a large prospective study.

> Comment: This paragraph summarizes the significance and innovation of the proposal (Section d of the outline). No changes necessary.

7.16.2 Example #2a: Grant Proposal Version *Not* in Need of Improvement

Stress and Risk of Hypertensive Disorders of Pregnancy

Background and Significance

Hypertensive disorders of pregnancy affect up to 8% of pregnancies and can result in poor outcomes for both mother and child.[1] Additionally, there are sparse data on the Latina population, a group at a twofold increased risk of preeclampsia relative to non-Latina white women.[2] Additionally, this group is a growing segment of the US population[3] and has a higher birthrate than non-Latina white women.[4] There are few modifiable risk factors for hypertensive disorders of pregnancy, and research suggests that stress may play a role in a woman's risk of developing these conditions.

Stress may increase risk of hypertensive disorders of pregnancy through a number of pathways, including neuroendocrinological mechanisms and through an inflammatory response to stress. Previous research has shown a link between adrenocorticotropic hormone and cortisol and both stress and hypertension.[5] CRP[6] and TNF-α,[7] markers of inflammation, are also elevated among women with high stress levels and are associated with increased blood pressure[8] and preeclampsia.[9]

Previous epidemiologic data suggest an association between psychosocial stress and hypertensive disorders. While limited in some respects, previous data suggest that high levels of job stressors, as well as depression, may result in a twofold increased risk of preeclampsia.[10–12] However, prior research has yielded conflicting results with one study showing no association between job stress and preeclampsia.[13]

Given the serious nature of hypertensive disorders of pregnancy and their sequelae, the proposed study will be significant by evaluating the association between general stress and this disease in a Latina population, an understudied high-risk group with high rates of stress. The proposal is innovative by using a validated measure of psychosocial stress in the underrepresented Latina population.

7.16.3 Example #2b: Dissertation Proposal Version *Not* in Need of Improvement

Stress and Risk of Hypertensive Disorders of Pregnancy

Background and Significance

Gestational hypertension and preeclampsia comprise the hypertensive disorders of pregnancy, disorders which affect some 8% of pregnancies (1) and can result in serious complications for both mother and child (2). Gestational hypertension is characterized by *de novo* hypertension after 20 weeks gestation; preeclampsia is defined as gestational hypertension with proteinuria occurring in the latter half of pregnancy. Hypertension in pregnancy is the second leading cause of maternal death, accounting for 20% of maternal deaths, and presents an increased risk of complications for the fetus, including increased NICU involvement, preterm delivery, low birth weight, and even fetal death (3). In addition to the risk they present to the pregnancy, hypertensive disorders of pregnancy have been linked to future high blood pressure and cardiovascular disease in women (4).

Psychosocial stress may contribute to risk of hypertensive disorders via neuroendocrinological mechanisms, including adrenocorticotropic hormone and cortisol, and the inflammatory response associated with stress (5). Although there is little research on the physiologic impact of stress on hypertensive disorders of pregnancy, the data that do exist suggest a positive association (6).

Epidemiologic research in the area of psychosocial stress and hypertensive disorders of pregnancy is sparse. To our knowledge, no previous studies have addressed the relationship between general perceived stress and hypertensive disorders of pregnancy. The three previous studies in this area have examined the relationship between work-related stress and hypertensive disorders of pregnancy, without regard to stress experienced outside of the workplace (7–9). Other studies have focused on the role of depression and anxiety in pregnancy and the association between these conditions and hypertensive disorders of pregnancy (10).

One further study evaluating the relationship between a psychiatric diagnosis, including depression, anxiety disorder, panic disorder, social phobia, and bulimia nervosa, and pregnancy outcome found a slightly elevated risk, though not statistically significant, of hypertensive disorders of pregnancy for women with a psychiatric diagnosis (11). Additionally, stress-reduction programs have been shown to significantly decrease systolic and diastolic blood pressure measurements in a cohort of minority men over age 55 (12).

Jones and colleagues (7) published the most recent and largest study examining the association between psychosocial stress and hypertensive disorders of pregnancy. The authors evaluated this relationship among 3000 nulliparous members of a larger prospective cohort study of 8000 pregnant women in Amsterdam who completed a questionnaire describing their stress levels prior to 24 weeks gestation and continued the pregnancy to at least 24 weeks gestation. This study found no association between work-related stress and hypertensive disorders of pregnancy (RR = 1.10, 95% CI 0.95–1.20). While this is the largest study conducted evaluating the association between stress and hypertension in pregnancy, it is limited in that it was conducted in a predominantly white population in nulliparous women and may, therefore, have limited generalizability.

Smith and colleagues (8) were the first to evaluate the relationship between psychosocial work stressors and hypertension in pregnancy in a prospective cohort study of 600 women, including 16 cases of gestational hypertension and 11 cases of preeclampsia. Women were interviewed in the first trimester, and responses were categorized into low, medium, and high levels of complexity and decision latitude, with high levels considered the lowest stress. A second variable combined job pressures and level of control, with low pressure/high control considered the least stressful. Compared to women with high job complexity, women with low job complexity (n = 8) had a twofold, although not statistically significantly, increased risk of gestational hypertension (OR: 2.2, 95% CI: 0.7–10.5). Women with low decision latitude at work had a similarly increased risk of gestational hypertension, as did women in the medium job pressure/control group and the high job pressure/low control group, although none of these results were statistically significant. Among women with low occupational status (score below the median on the Occupational Status Scale), each standard deviation decrease in decision latitude was associated with a twofold increased risk of hypertensive disorders of pregnancy (preeclampsia and gestational hypertension combined) (OR: 1.9, 95% CI: 0.7–3.8). This study among predominantly white women had limited power to detect an association between stress and hypertensive disorders of pregnancy due to small sample size and has limited generalizability due to the exclusive focus on job-related stressors.

In the final of only three studies evaluating the relationship between stress and hypertension in pregnancy, Taylor et al. (9) performed a case–control study among 300 cases (200 with gestational hypertension and 100 with preeclampsia) and 400 controls to evaluate the association between job-related stressors and hypertensive disorders of pregnancy. Job titles were ascertained from subjects after delivery, and the degree of job-related stress was derived by assigning a psychological demand (high/low) and decision latitude data (high/low) using data from Population Health Survey (PHS), a national survey among Canadians. No individual data on work-related stressors were collected; rather women were assigned to one of the four job classifications with data from the PHS. Women in high-demand and low-decision-latitude jobs (considered high-stress jobs) for at least 1 week in pregnancy prior to 20 weeks gestation had a twofold increased risk of preeclampsia relative to women in low-demand and high-decision-making jobs, considered lower stress (OR: 2.0, 95% CI: 1.0–4.0). The increased risk was similar for women who stayed at the high-demand and low-decision-latitude job for 20 weeks of pregnancy. Similarly, women who worked more than 35 h per week in high-demand and low-decision-latitude jobs had an increased risk of preeclampsia (OR: 2.1, 95% CI: 1.2–4.2) relative to women who spent no time per week in such a job. There were no significant effects for gestational hypertension in this study. This study is limited through its failure to collect an individual stress measure. Additionally, the sample was made up of predominantly white, nulliparous women, and the results may have limited generalizability.

In summary, no previous studies have evaluated the effect of general psychosocial stress on risk of hypertensive disorders of pregnancy. The few prior studies on the relationship between job-related psychosocial stress and hypertensive disorders of pregnancy have mixed results, with one suggesting no association and two suggesting a positive association between high stress levels and risk of hypertension in pregnancy. This previous research has been limited to predominantly white populations, with little racial or ethnic minority representation including few Latinas. Additional limitations include inadequate measures of exposure (9) and small sample sizes (8).

Therefore, we propose to investigate the relationship between psychosocial stress and hypertensive disorders of pregnancy using data from Estudio GDM, a prospective cohort study of 1231 Latina prenatal care patients, and Estudio GDM II, an ongoing prospective cohort study of approximately 900 Latina prenatal care patients. We will use Cohen's Perceived Stress Scale to measure stress in early pregnancy. Given the serious nature of hypertensive disorders of pregnancy and their sequelae, the proposed study will be significant by evaluating the association between general stress and this disease in a Latina population, an understudied high-risk group with high rates of stress. The proposal is innovative by using a validated measure of psychosocial stress in the underrepresented Latina population.

Summarizing Preliminary Studies 8

Preliminary data can be defined as data that relate, in some manner, to your proposed specific aims. The purpose of the **preliminary data section** of a grant proposal is to show evidence of your expertise—both in regard to the proposed subject area and in terms of the feasibility of your proposed methods. Preliminary results, when available, are critical to a grant application as they not only provide evidence supporting your proposed hypotheses but also can serve to support your ability to *pull it off.*

This chapter provides you with strategies for selecting which preliminary data might be relevant and strategies for how to find or collect preliminary data if you believe that you currently do not have any. Just as importantly, this chapter provides you with tips for describing and summarizing preliminary results in a manner that best positions your proposal for successful review.

A caveat Preliminary data are not typically required for a dissertation proposal. However, the tips presented below are relevant for describing your own data once your proposal is approved. Therefore, graduate students should view this chapter as useful for how to write up their **results section** once they have completed their data analysis.

8.1 WHAT ARE PRELIMINARY STUDIES?

Preliminary studies can take many forms:

- **Pilot studies** that address the same aims, or very similar aims, to those that you are proposing in your current proposal
- **Feasibility studies** of your proposed methods

Most typically, **pilot studies** address the same aims, or very similar aims, to those that you are proposing in your current proposal **within a small sample**. This small sample does not typically have adequate power to decisively answer your proposed hypotheses but ideally suggests an association, therefore motivating the rationale for the larger proposed study. Pilot studies may also be conducted in an existing dataset (i.e., secondary data analysis). However, this dataset will likely differ from your proposed study in important ways—via characteristics of the study population (e.g., age and race/ethnicity) or via study design (e.g., cross sectional) or via study methods utilized (e.g., less precise measurement tools). All of these reasons would, again, help to motivate the rationale for your proposed study. Regardless of the type of pilot study, the goal of the pilot is to provide findings that in some way support your proposed aims and justify the need for your proposed study (e.g., improved measurement device, stronger study design, different study population).

In terms of the second example above, **feasibility studies** demonstrate to reviewers that you can logistically pull off your proposed study. Feasibility studies can provide key data on a number of factors. They can provide evidence that you, as a PI, are able to recruit subjects and collect data and that the proposed study is feasible in the planned study population. Such preliminary data have the added benefit of providing key figures necessary for calculating power and sample size calculations for your current proposal. Participant satisfaction surveys administered in a feasibility study can also provide data on the acceptability of your methods. Validation studies of your proposed methods (as described in Chapter 14, *Reproducibility and Validity Studies*) can provide assurance that a study based upon these methods will work. In summary, ideally, the goal is to show proof of principal and demonstrate to the reviewers that you can *pull it off*. So, for example, if you are in the midst of conducting a pilot study of your proposed aims, but results are not yet ready, this study may still yield useful feasibility data.

Data Generated from Preliminary Studies

- Pilot studies
    - Measures of association and variation (e.g., mean differences and SD)
- Feasibility studies
    - Eligibility rates
    - Recruitment rates
    - Retention rates
    - Participant satisfaction survey results
    - Validation studies of your proposed methods

8.2 DO PRELIMINARY DATA NEED TO BE PREVIOUSLY PUBLISHED?

Pilot studies can be published or unpublished. However, if they are published, then it is important to include the citation in the proposal as it will further increase your chances of success. A track record of relevant publications will (1) provide evidence that peer reviewers considered your findings of scientific merit and (2) provide evidence that you, as an investigator, have the ability to translate your findings into publications. This latter ability is an important concern among reviewers who want assurance that the findings of your current proposal will also be translated to the scientific community via publications. Therefore, citing the preliminary study findings, when published, is important.

Include preliminary studies by your coinvestigators

It is also important to note that preliminary studies can not only include prior work that you have conducted but also work by any of your coinvestigators on the proposal. In a sense, your coinvestigators on a proposal become part of your *research team*. As long as you clarify the source of the preliminary data, their preliminary data are relevant. In addition, it is likely that they will have relevant preliminary data—as that is probably one of the main reasons that you invited them to serve as coinvestigators!

8.3 HOW TO DESCRIBE PRELIMINARY DATA

A concise one-paragraph description of the preliminary data will typically suffice.

e.g. example Behaviors Affecting Adolescents (BAA) Study (ASPH/CDC 1234, PI: yourself). This pilot study was conducted at the proposed study site in conjunction with Drs. Taylor, Smith, and Jones (coinvestigators). The primary goals were to investigate the effect of an individually tailored 12-week exercise intervention on serum biomarkers associated with insulin resistance. Adolescents (n = 25) were predominantly overweight/obese (98%), young (48% < 24 years), and low income (43% < $15,000/year). After the 12-week intervention, during a time when exercise typically decreases, the exercise arm experienced a higher increase in sports/exercise (0.9 MET-hours/week) versus the control arm (−0.01 MET-hours/week; p=0.02) (Figure 8.1).[1] Intervention participants reported being satisfied with the amount of information received (95%), and 86% reported finding the study materials interesting and useful. **These data support the feasibility and efficacy of the exercise component of the proposed lifestyle intervention.**

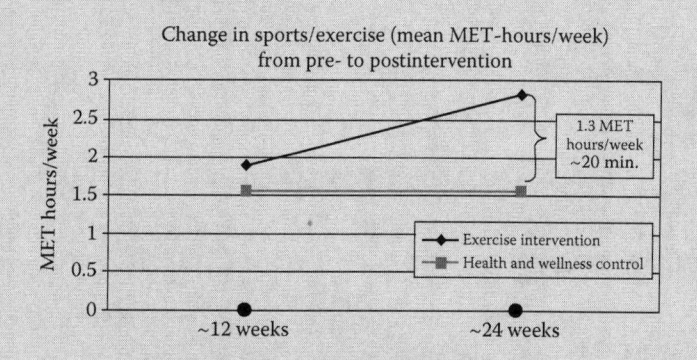

FIGURE 8.1 Preliminary data from a pilot exercise intervention.

Note that this paragraph includes the following key items:

- Pilot grant name, number, and Principal Investigator (PI) (if funded)
- Citation (if published)
- A table/figure of the findings relevant to the current proposal
- Brief text summary of findings including magnitude of results
- Relation of preliminary data to current proposed aims

If your preliminary data were based on a grant-funded pilot study, then state the grant number and PI's name early in the paragraph. If you were not the PI, then clarify in parentheses the role of that PI on your proposal (e.g., S1234 ASPH/CDC PI: Jones, coinvestigator on the proposed study). The body of the paragraph should contain a brief description of the methods and findings. Findings ideally should be shown in a table/figure if there is space with a one- to three-sentence description of the take-home message. Ideally, references in this section should be included citing the publication of these preliminary data by you or your coinvestigators on the proposal.

The final sentence of each preliminary study paragraph should end with a sentence specifying the rationale for why it is relevant to the current proposal. This summary sentence removes the burden on the reviewer. It is your job to connect the dots between your preliminary work and how it relates to or supports your proposed aims. The act of creating these sentences also serves a dual purpose of ensuring that you are not including extraneous preliminary findings not directly relevant to your aims. In other words, if you can't make the connection, then the reviewer will certainly not be able to.

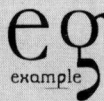

> **e.g.**
> *example*
>
> **Examples of Last Sentences of Preliminary Study Descriptions:**
>
> - This study adds further evidence of our experience conducting randomized trials among low-income, low-literate Hispanics and intervening for dietary change.
> - This study supports our ability to recruit, retain, and intervene on weight loss, physical activity, and diet with the postpartum population.
> - These data support the feasibility, acceptability, and efficacy of a high-reach, low-cost, individually tailored mailed intervention among high-risk adolescents.

8.4 USE THE PRELIMINARY STUDIES SECTION TO DEMONSTRATE ESTABLISHED RELATIONSHIPS WITH YOUR COINVESTIGATORS

Another way that you can assure your reviewers that you can *pull it off* is by demonstrating in the preliminary studies section that you have established relationships with the coinvestigators on your proposal. Relationships with more senior colleagues are critical if you are a graduate student or early-career faculty. Their involvement on your proposal will be a key factor supporting your ability to logistically conduct the project—particularly if these senior investigators have a track record of conducting similar projects in similar populations.

It is important to reassure the reviewers that these coinvestigators do not appear in name only. There are several ways in which you can prove established working relationships:

- Coauthored publications
- Submitted publications under review
- Copresentations
- An established mentoring relationship (e.g., as part of a training grant)
- Coinvestigators on an already funded grant

Of course, much of this information will appear in your biosketch and that of your coinvestigators. But you cannot rely upon the reviewers to connect the dots between you and your coinvestigators. Instead, you want to make it easy for the reviewers by clearly delineating this prior collaboration in your Preliminary Studies section.

8.5 WHAT IF YOU DO NOT HAVE PRELIMINARY DATA?

There are several approaches that you can take if you do not have preliminary data as defined above:

- *Does your research team have preliminary data?* Remember that when you are writing a grant, your coinvestigators and/or mentors in the case of a K award become your research team. If they have preliminary data, then your team, by definition, has preliminary data. This is likely as it is likely that part of the reason that you chose these coinvestigators/mentors was their expertise in the area of your grant proposal. The preliminary studies paragraph can state *Our research team has also conducted…* and then include a brief description of their preliminary studies as described above.
- *Consider a different funding mechanism.* Certain funding mechanisms are themselves designed to generate pilot data (e.g., preliminary data) such as particular R21s, or R03s, or seed grants that do not require preliminary data. In contrast, an R01 requires substantial preliminary data—ideally led by the PI themselves but at a minimum by the research team. Remember that if you yourself have not been the PI of significant grant-funded research, then applying for an R01 is premature. Even if your *research team* has significant grant-funded research, the reviewers will still want assurance that you, as a

PI, can logistically pull off a large R01 size from a feasibility point of view. A strong prior publication and grant record, as well as project management experience, can also work to minimize these concerns in the absence of your own personally led preliminary data (with the caveat that your team does indeed have preliminary data). This may be the time to take one of your ultimate R01 aims and use it to motivate a seed grant/R21 and obtain preliminary data for that R01 aim. In fact, ideally, a career mentor has sat down with you as a junior faculty member and mapped out your progress from small seed grants to smaller NIH mechanisms and/or foundation grants to the R01 with each subsequent step providing preliminary data for the ultimate R01.

- Cast a wide net and consider *tangential* preliminary studies. For example, if you are proposing to recruit a sample of participants, any previous experience with recruitment—even in a different setting and with different methods—may still be helpful in terms of demonstrating your experience in recruiting and retaining a study population. In this case, including a table of characteristics of your previous study population will show concrete evidence of how many participants you recruited and that you know how to collect and present data. Similarly, any management experience of grant-funded projects can also be helpful.

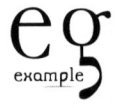

example: Let's imagine that you are proposing to conduct a randomized trial of a lifestyle intervention (which consists of diet and exercise advice) to treat diabetes in older African-American men. Your prior studies that only included dietary interventions, or only exercise interventions, would be relevant even though your proposed intervention is broader. Your prior studies of lifestyle interventions in non-Hispanic white populations would also be relevant to support your logistical experience in conducting such an intervention study. Prior studies conducted by your research team validating the exercise and diet compliance measures that you will be using will also be relevant.

8.6 WHAT IF YOUR PRELIMINARY DATA CONTRADICT YOUR PROPOSED HYPOTHESES?

If your preliminary data contradict your proposed hypotheses (e.g., show the opposite direction of effect from your proposed hypotheses), this is often considered a *fatal flaw* by reviewers. First, step back and be sure to consider the statistical significance of your pilot data. Any pilot findings are usually accompanied by wide variability (e.g., a wide CI), so be sure that you believe that these findings are indeed contradictory.

However, if you do determine that your pilot findings contradict your hypotheses, then unless you have an excellent reason to explain this opposite finding and also a clear rationale for why you expect to see the opposite in your proposal—do not proceed with your hypotheses as written. Instead, reconsider your hypotheses. This may also entail reconsidering the topic of the entire grant.

Avoid trying to explain away your contradictory findings by saying that they are not supported by the prior literature. If the reviewers see such opposite results from your own lab, this will call into question not only the rationale for your proposed hypothesis but also the validity of your methods.

8.7 DOUBLE-CHECK THAT ALL YOUR PRELIMINARY FINDINGS RELATE TO ONE OR MORE OF YOUR PROPOSED HYPOTHESES

It is not considered appropriate to *pad* the preliminary studies section simply to look like a more established researcher. Instead, as noted above, you will want to show that each preliminary study presented relates specifically to one of your proposed hypotheses or, at the least, a subcomponent of a hypothesis. The only exception to this rule is to show evidence of your study management skills as noted above. But even in this case, you will need to explicitly state this point to the reviewer in your brief justification at the end of that preliminary study paragraph.

Also, in summarizing the findings of preliminary studies, remember that the top priority is the relevance of these findings to your proposed research hypotheses and not their statistically significance. Once you describe findings that are relevant to your hypotheses, then you may go on and mention other unexpected or unusual significant findings (if space permits), but the hypotheses of the proposal need to be supported first.

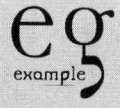

> **example**
>
> **Hypothesis #1a: Frequency of television viewing will be negatively associated with the school readiness of preschoolers.**
> In the preliminary results section
> **[Address hypothesis #1a first]**
> Correlational analysis between television viewing time and IQ demonstrated that television time was negatively related to school readiness ($r = -0.70$, $p = 0.02$).
> **[Include other findings second]**
> We also found that children's television viewing time was significantly and negatively related to parental instruction ($r^2 = -0.35$, $p = 0.01$).

8.8 PITFALLS OF PRELIMINARY DATA

While your preliminary data should directly relate to one or more of your hypotheses, it should not fully answer that hypothesis. If it did, then you have removed the motivation for including that hypothesis in your current proposal.

Often, your preliminary data will be based on a smaller sample than the proposed study. This small size may lead to findings that are suggestive but not statistically significant, therefore requiring a larger study (i.e., the proposed study) with adequate statistical power to address the promising result that you observed in your preliminary studies.

Or your proposed study could be improving in a substantive way on this preliminary data—for example, via an improved measurement device, stronger study design, and different study population.

Therefore, in these cases, it will be critical to justify the advantage of the proposed study, over and above the preliminary study, to the reviewer in the last line of the preliminary study paragraph.

8.9 WHERE TO PLACE PRELIMINARY STUDIES IN AN NIH GRANT PROPOSAL?

For new applications, NIH allows the inclusion of preliminary studies in the Approach section. This issue is discussed in more detail in Chapter 18, *Submission of the Grant Proposal*.

8.10 SHOULD I INCLUDE PRELIMINARY RESULTS EVEN IF THE GRANT DOES NOT REQUIRE THEM?

Some foundation grants and certain NIH grants do not require the inclusion of preliminary studies. These include exploratory/developmental research grants (R21/R33), small research grants (R03), and academic research enhancement award (AREA) grants (R15). For R01 applications, reviewers are instructed to place less emphasis on the preliminary data from early-stage investigators (ESIs) than from more established investigators. However, almost without exception, including the results from preliminary studies can serve to increase your chances of a favorable review. As noted above, even if you have conducted a pilot study that has not yet yielded results, preliminary recruitment rates can help to establish the feasibility and therefore the likelihood of the success of the proposed project.

8.11 PRELIMINARY STUDIES WITHIN PROPOSALS BASED UPON EXISTING DATASETS

It is fairly common for grant proposals, particularly by graduate students and early-career faculty, to propose to use data from an existing dataset. Such studies involve proposing to conduct a secondary data analysis using data from a study that has already been conducted. Such a dataset could have been collected by your mentor or colleagues, or this could be a national dataset to which you have access. Examples could include the Health Professionals Follow-Up Study (HPFS), the Nurses' Health Study (NHS), the Women's Health Initiative (WHI), the Behavioral Risk Factor Surveillance System (BRFSS), the National Health Interview Survey (NHIS), and the National Health and Nutrition Examination Survey (NHANES).

Indeed, the practice of using preexisting data is **efficient and economical**, aspects that are particularly attractive given the current funding environment. In recognition of this, some NIH requests for proposals and program announcements are limited to secondary analyses of existing datasets only—as in the example below.

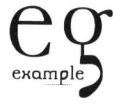

> **Secondary Dataset Analyses in Heart, Lung, and Blood Diseases and Sleep Disorders (R21)**
>
> The National Heart, Lung, and Blood Institute (NHLBI) invites 3R21 applications for well-focused secondary analyses of existing human datasets to test innovative hypotheses concerning the epidemiology, pathophysiology, prevention, or treatment of diseases/conditions highly relevant to the NHLBI mission. Applicants may use data from a variety of sources, including, but not limited to, investigator-initiated research activities, contracts from public or private sources, administrative databases, and the NHLBI BioLINCC resource.

In these situations, your preliminary studies will involve a complete description of this existing dataset, that is, information on how the dataset was derived, characteristics of the study population, and any relevant preliminary findings. Describe the recruitment, eligibility, and follow-up rates. A table may be an efficient way to present these data. It will also be critical to describe any loss to follow-up. You will also want to clarify your previous experience with this dataset, if any, as well as your access to this dataset. That is, do you already have the data in hand?

Basing a proposal on an existing dataset can be a two-edged sword in that reviewers may expect you to show more preliminary data than if you were proposing a study de novo. In this vein, you might be expected to show the distribution of your exposure of interest among the participants. Such a table will assure the reviewers that your study population has sufficient variability in exposure distribution such that it will be feasible to see an association with your outcome of interest (see Chapter 11, *Power and Sample Size*). For example, if you propose to use an existing dataset to study alcohol consumption and risk of bladder cancer, but almost all your participants are nondrinkers, this will raise a concern among reviewers. Because reviewers know you have these data, they may think that you are hiding something by not showing it.

8.12 TIP #1: INCLUDE TABLES AND FIGURES IN THE PRELIMINARY STUDIES SECTION

As mentioned in Chapter 1, *Ten Top Tips for Successful Proposal Writing*, the more figures and tables in a grant application, the better. Not only does the process of creating these figures and tables help you to crystallize your preliminary findings, but they are also kinder to the reviewers. As compared to dense text, tables and figures are easier for the reviewer to digest and help them grasp your findings more quickly. They save space—reducing the text—critical for the page limitations of most proposals.

e.g. example **A Proposal to Evaluate Coffee Drinking and Melanoma Risk**

- Option #1: Text Version

    We investigated the association between coffee drinking (cups/day) and risk of melanoma in our pilot study. There was no increase in risk with increasing coffee consumption ($p_{trend} = 0.20$). As compared to those with no coffee consumption, the RR for melanoma among those with 1 cup/day of consumption was 0.79 (95% CI = 0.18–1.30); for 2 cups/day of consumption, the RR was 1.47 (95% CI = 0.55–1.56); for 3 cups/day of consumption, the RR was 3.03 (95% CI = 0.95–8.55); and for 4 or more cups/day, the RR was 1.30 (95% CI = 0.54–1.35). Lack of statistically significant findings may have been due, in part, to the small sample size, particularly among those with the highest level of coffee consumption.

- Option #2: Table Version (Table 8.1)
- Option #3: Figure Version (See Figure 8.2)

TABLE 8.1 Preliminary data for a proposal to evaluate coffee drinking and melanoma

COFFEE CONSUMPTION	CASES	RR	95% CI
None	15	1.0	Referent
1 cup/day	10	0.79	0.18–1.30
2 cups/day	9	1.47	0.55–1.56
3 cups/day	2	3.03	0.95–8.55
4+ cups/day	2	1.30	0.54–1.35

FIGURE 8.2 Preliminary data for *A Proposal to Evaluate Coffee Drinking and Melanoma Risk*.

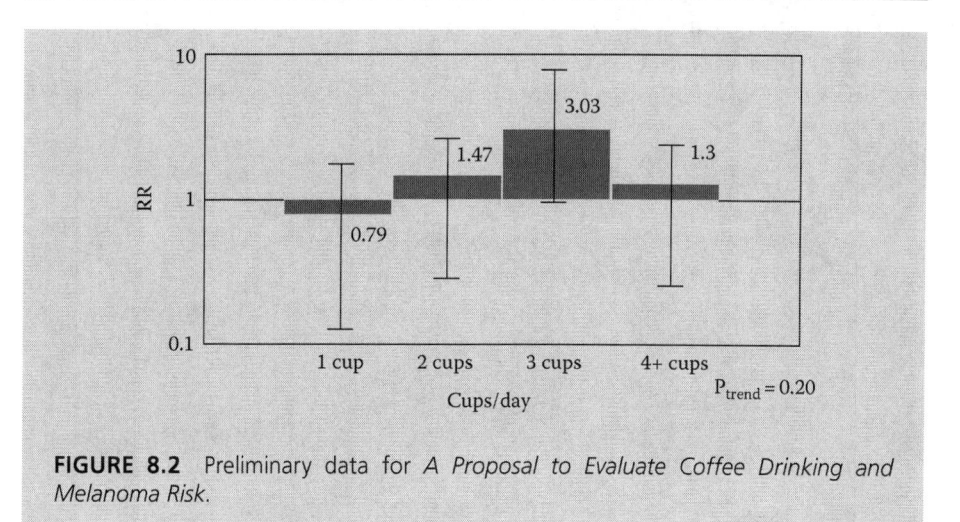

As you can see, the figure version is the clearest way to show a potential trend to the reviewers. It saves the work for the reviewer of translating dense text or numerical findings to a visual image. It is important to note that the use of a table or figure is not meant to completely replace the text. Instead, it reduces the amount of text necessary as discussed in Tip #2 below.

8.13 TIP #2: WHEN DESCRIBING RESULTS IN A TABLE OR FIGURE, POINT OUT THE HIGHLIGHTS FOR THE REVIEWER

While pictures say a thousand words, it is not sufficient to only include preliminary results tables and figures in the proposal without accompanying text. You will also need to include some brief text that walks the reader through the table/figure and points out the important points. In this way, you are guiding the reviewer to what you feel is the **take-home message**.

Therefore, the first approach in writing text to accompany a set of preliminary results tables is to look through the tables and circle what you believe are the most important findings in each table. These would be findings that directly show support for your primary hypotheses or some aspect of your hypotheses.

In the text, avoid repeating each value that appears in the tables/figures. Remember that the reader can see all of these data. Instead, limit yourself to **highlighting two to three data points per table**. This is a critical exercise and much more challenging than it originally appears. However, it is an integral exercise not only for describing preliminary results in a proposal but also subsequently when you are writing up a journal article submission of your findings.

In your text description, be sure to point out the **magnitude of your findings** (e.g., mean differences and RRs) with their accompanying measures of variation (e.g., SD and CIs) and not just their statistical significance. Indeed, because preliminary data are usually underpowered to detect a statistically significant effect, it would be even less effective to only present the statistical significance in this section.

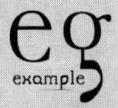

> **example**
>
> **Original Version**
> We did not observe a statistically significant association between coffee drinking and risk of melanoma in our pilot study.
>
> **Improved Version**
> As compared to those with no coffee consumption, the RR was 3.03 (95% CI = 0.95–8.55) for those who drank 3 cups/day and 1.30 (95% CI = 0.54–1.35) for those who drank 4 or more cups/day. Lack of a statistically significant trend of increasing risk with increasing coffee consumption (p_{trend} = 0.20) may have been due, in part, to the small sample size, particularly among those with the highest levels of coffee consumption (n = 2 cases).

Note that this example above follows the principles of presenting the magnitude of study findings (i.e., selected RRs and 95% CIs) and highlights two to three main points for the reviewers to have as a take-home message.

Finally, results can also contain one-liners of data that do not justify presentation in a table or figure.

> **example**
>
> Although we controlled for diabetes in the prior analysis, we repeated the analysis excluding those with diabetes. Results were virtually unchanged.

8.14 TIP #3: INCLUDE DESCRIPTIVE TABLES OF THE STUDY POPULATION

When proposing to use an existing dataset, it is common practice to show a table of descriptive characteristics of the study population. In this way, you help the reviewer to *see* or envision your study population. In addition, inclusion of this table provides implicit evidence that you have access to the data and know how to quantify it.

If space permits, it is beneficial to not only present characteristics of the overall study population but also to include additional columns stratifying the study population by categories of your exposure. For example, if you are proposing to conduct a study of alcohol consumption and risk of bladder cancer, your study population table would not only show characteristics of the total population but also stratify participants according to categories of alcohol consumption (e.g., nondrinker, drinker) (Table 8.2).

TABLE 8.2 Characteristics of the study sample according to alcohol consumption

CHARACTERISTIC	TOTAL SAMPLE	DRINKER	NONDRINKER
Total in 2009 (n)	450	250	200
Obesity (%)	25.2	24.3	26.5
History of hypertension (%)	10	11	9
History of high cholesterol (%)	20	15	25
History of diabetes (%)	5	3	7
Cigarette smoking (%)	10	12	8
Regular physical activity (%)	30	40	20

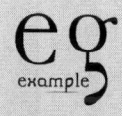

> *example*
>
> **Original Version**
> Drinkers and nondrinkers were similar.
> **Improved Version of Example**
> Among the participants, 200 (44.4%) reported that they almost never consumed alcoholic beverages, while 250 (55.6%) drank 5 g or more per day. History of hypertension appeared to be similar among drinkers and nondrinkers. Obesity and a history of high cholesterol and diabetes were less common among drinkers, while smoking and regular physical activity were more common.

In describing how these groups differ, you again want to avoid listing general summaries and at the same time want to avoid listing every value.

The improved example does some work for the reviewer and does not simply regurgitate all the findings in the table. That is, it **describes the findings in groups:** listing those characteristics that were (1) similar among both exposure groups, (2) less common among the exposed than the unexposed, and (3) more common among the exposed than unexposed. The reviewer's eye would naturally be trying to do this as they look at your table, so instead you have saved them precious time in their review.

8.15 TIP #4: DESCRIBE PRELIMINARY FINDINGS IN LAYPERSON'S TERMS

The key principal in describing your preliminary findings is to avoid epidemiologic jargon. Describing results concisely and in layperson's terms is important as not all your reviewers will be epidemiologists. In addition, describing your results in layperson's terms will also serve you well in your career when you are ultimately communicating your important findings with the press.

8.15.1 How to Describe a Relative Risk in Layperson's Terms

Let's say you conducted an analysis of history of severe sunburns (exposure variable) and melanoma (outcome variable). Melanoma is a dichotomous outcome variable (yes, no), so you chose multivariable logistic regression. Your model yielded an OR of 1.2.

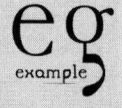

> **example**
>
> **Original Version**
> The multivariate RR of melanoma was 1.9 (95% CI 1.1–2.5) (Table 1).
>
> **Improved Version**
> After controlling for age, race, and BMI, men who had ever had a severe sunburn had almost two times the risk of melanoma compared to men who had never had a severe sunburn (95% C.I. 1.1–2.5) (Table 1).

The original example has several limitations. It does not articulate what the comparison was—that is, who were the exposed and who were the unexposed. Therefore, the sentence does not clarify that the RR is a comparison of the risk of melanoma for those who had ever had a severe sunburn (exposed) as compared to those with no history of severe sunburn (unexposed).

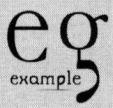

> **example**
>
> **Original Version**
> The RR of liver cancer was 1.2 (Table 2).
>
> **Improved Version**
> Men who had consumed 5 or more g of alcohol per day had a 20% increased risk of liver cancer as compared with never drinkers (95% CI 1.12–1.36) (Table 2).

8.15.2 How to Describe a Beta Coefficient in Layperson's Terms

Students often struggle with how to interpret a beta coefficient in layperson's terms. A beta represents the mean change in the outcome variable for a unit change in the exposure of interest. For example, let's say you conducted an analysis of television watching (exposure variable) and weight (outcome variable). Weight is a continuous outcome variable (pounds [lb]), so you chose multivariable linear regression. Your model yielded a beta coefficient of 0.2.

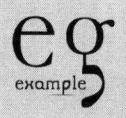

> **eg** *example*
> **Original Version**
> The beta coefficient was 0.2 (SE = 0.45) (Table 3).
> **Improved Version**
> Every 1 h increase in television watching was associated with, on average, a 0.2 lb increase in weight (SE = 0.45) (Table 3).

8.15.3 How to Describe Effect Modification in Layperson's Terms

Effect modification can be challenging to write up in layperson's terms. Let's say that you included a hypothesis to evaluate the possibility of effect modification in your proposal. Your exposure of interest is hemorrhage size and your outcome of interest is 3-month mortality. You have preliminary data that support the presence of effect modification by gender.

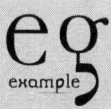

> **eg** *example*
> **Specific Aim #2. The association between hemorrhage size and 3-month mortality will differ according to gender.**
> **In the results section:**
> We found that gender modified the association between hemorrhage size and mortality. The association between hemorrhage size and risk of mortality was stronger in women than in men (Table 4).

8.16 STYLISTIC TIP #1: DESCRIBE TABLES IN NUMERIC ORDER

The text should describe the tables in numeric order. Avoid going back and forth between consecutive tables. In other words, after you describe Table 2, do not return again to Table 1. If you are having trouble doing this, this may mean that you have to restructure your tables so that the narrative can flow in sequence. At all costs, try to avoid having your reviewer bounce forward and then backward between study tables. This can annoy a tired reviewer and is not good scientific practice.

8.17 STYLISTIC TIP #2: TRY TO DESCRIBE TABLES FROM TOP TO BOTTOM

Within a table, try to describe it from top to bottom. This is not always possible, and it is often better to break this rule than to have to reorder the table. However, as mentioned above, it is often useful to group findings for the reviewer according to similarity in findings. For example, in the alcohol table (Table 8.2), it would not be appropriate to reorder the table rows according to the post hoc observance of study findings, because tables are meant to be structured *a priori* (e.g., before findings are known). However, all other things being equal, try to describe the key results in order from top to bottom as they appear in the table.

8.18 STYLISTIC TIP #3: SPELL OUT NUMBERS THAT START SENTENCES

Sentences should never start with a number in digit form. Instead, numbers should be spelled out if they start a sentence.

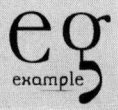

> **Original Version**
> 25 adolescents agreed to participate in our pilot study.
> **Improved Version**
> Twenty-five adolescents agreed to participate in our pilot study.

However, in the case of large numbers, it is best to restructure the sentence so that you avoid spelling out the number (which is cumbersome to the reader and takes up valuable space). Instead, write the sentence so that the number is not the first word.

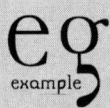

> **Original Version**
> Seven thousand six hundred thirty-four women are included in the National Health Survey dataset.
> **Improved Version**
> A total of 7634 women are included in the National Health Survey dataset.

8.19 STYLISTIC TIP #4: AVOID PRESENTING CONFIDENCE INTERVALS AND p-VALUES

Like a p-value, a CI also provides information about the statistical significance of a finding. However, the CI has the additional advantage of providing the range that will include with a 95% probability of the true measure of association. Therefore, presenting CIs as well as p-values is repetitive.

How can we tell if a finding is statistically significant by looking at the CI? If the CI includes the null value for the association being calculated, then the observed association is not statistically significant.

For example, if a CI for an RR spans the value of 1.0 (the null value), then it is not statistically significant.

- If the CI spans 1, then the RR is not statistically significant. The p-value is ≥0.05.
- If the CI does not include 1, the RR is statistically significant. The p-value is <0.05.
    - RR = 1.75, 95% CI = (1.12–2.75) = statistically significant
    - RR = 1.43, 95% CI = (0.92–2.25) = *not* statistically significant
    - RR = 0.35, 95% CI = (0.14–0.89) = statistically significant

8.20 STYLISTIC TIP #5: AVOID REFERRING TO YOUR TABLES AS ACTIVE BEINGS

Tables should not be the subject of sentences and instead should simply be referred to in parentheses within sentences describing the table contents. This approach is also more space efficient.

> **Original Version**
> Table 1 shows that cases are older than controls.
> **Improved Version**
> Cases are older than controls (Table 1).

Similarly, another space-saving technique is to avoid the practice of writing a sentence that tells the reviewer what type of data you will be presenting in the table **and** then writing a second sentence that tells the reviewer what results the table actually shows. Instead, jump straight to describing the table contents.

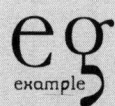

> **Original Version**
> Table 1 shows characteristics of cases and controls in our dataset. Cases are on average older than controls (mean 35 years vs. 30 years, respectively).
> **Improved Version**
> Cases are on average older than controls (mean 35 years vs. 30 years, respectively) (Table 1).

8.21 STYLISTIC TIP #6: TIPS FOR TABLE TITLES

- Table titles should be as concise, yet informative, as possible.
- Table titles should name the statistics presented in the tables (e.g., means and SDs or RRs and 95% CIs).
- The table title should refer to the variables that were measured.
- Table titles should be freestanding such that the title and table could stand alone from the remainder of the proposal.

In addition, a table should list your exposure and outcome variables. If there are too many exposure and outcome variables to fit concisely in the title, then the corresponding umbrella terms should be used. For example, if your outcome variables included markers of cardiovascular disease such as HDL, LDL, and triglycerides, it would be more efficient to simply use the umbrella term *cardiovascular disease risk factors*. Similarly, if your exposures involved lifestyle behaviors such as diet, exercise, and weight management, instead using the term *lifestyle behaviors* would be preferable.

When writing a table title, it is a useful exercise to imagine that the table has become separated from the rest of the document. In other words, it should be written so that it is **freestanding**—understandable separate from the rest of a proposal. Therefore, well-written table titles should state the study name and dates of conduct:

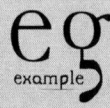

> *eg example*
> - Table 1. Number of Participants by Gender and Grade Level; the Idaho Women's Health Study, 2000–2004.
> - Table 2. Means and Standard Deviations of Reading and Mathematics; the Idaho Women's Health Study, 2000–2004.
> - Table 3. Analysis of Variance for Reading Scores; the Idaho Women's Health Study, 2000–2004.

Note that all three examples follow the titling guidelines. That is, they all name the variables, statistics, and study name and dates.

8.22 PRELIMINARY STUDY EXAMPLES

Below are two preliminary studies to support *A Proposal to Conduct a Lifestyle Intervention in Hispanic Women*. Note that the first preliminary study focuses more on supporting the proposed hypotheses that the intervention will be efficacious. The second preliminary study focuses more on supporting the feasibility and acceptability of the intervention.

8.22.1 Preliminary Study #1

Estudio Salud (*Grant # xxxx*, PI: Smith). A randomized controlled trial was used to test the intervention among overweight/obese Hispanics with low income and acculturation.[1] Participants (n = 93) reported that having materials that addressed culture-specific barriers was helpful in terms of setting realistic goals (87%), endorsed reading most/all of the physical activity information (85%), gaining knowledge about exercise via reading the materials (97%), finding it enjoyable (95%), and wearing pedometers (90%). Moderate-intensity (or greater) activity increased from an average of 16.6 min/week (SD = 25.8) at baseline to 147.3 (SD = 241.6) at 6 months in the intervention arm and from 11.9 min/week (SD = 22.0) to 96.8 (SD = 118.5) in the wellness contact control arm. In addition, there was a significant association between baseline BMI and change in social support (family) from baseline to 6 months (b = −0.89, SE = 0.33, p < 0.01). Retention rates were high (87%) for a hard-to-reach Hispanic group, and there were no differences in follow-up according to participant characteristics or study arm. **These data support the feasibility, acceptability, and efficacy of a high-reach, low-cost, individually tailored mailed intervention among high-risk Hispanic women.**

8.22.2 Preliminary Study #2

Estudio Vida: A Pilot Lifestyle Intervention for Gestational Diabetes among Overweight/Obese Hispanic Women (*Grant # xxxx*; PI: Yourself). The goal of this pilot was to develop and evaluate the feasibility of the proposed lifestyle intervention as a complete unit among pregnant and postpartum overweight/obese Hispanic women.[2] Participants (n = 68) endorsed the interest and utility of the study materials (86%), amount of information (*appropriate* 100%), ability to access a telephone for telephone interviews (100%), and the amount of time spent on the study (appropriate 86%, sometimes too much time 14%). Recruitment and retention rates were used to inform the proposed power calculations (see c3. Power). **Findings support the feasibility of the proposed combined lifestyle intervention and study protocol in overweight/obese pregnant Hispanic women.**

Study Design and Methods

9

The Study Design and Methods section in a proposal (sometimes called the Approach section) immediately follows the Background and Significance section. A well-written Background and Significance section will implicitly justify the study design and methods. Whether you are writing a dissertation proposal or a grant proposal, I find the following **outline** to be useful for this section of the proposal.

Study Design and Methods: Outline

   a. Study Design
   b. Study Population
      i. Setting
      ii. Subject ascertainment
      iii. Eligibility criteria/Exclusion criteria
   c. Exposure Assessment
      i. How exposure data will be collected
      ii. Exposure parameterization
      iii. Validity of exposure assessment
   d. Outcome Assessment
      i. How outcome data will be collected
      ii. Outcome parameterization
      iii. Validity of outcome assessment
   e. Covariate Assessment
      i. How covariate data will be collected
      ii. Covariate parameterization
      iii. Validity of covariate assessment
   f. Variable Categorization Table

Below, I provide strategic tips for each of the above subsections from A to F.

9.1 GOALS OF THE STUDY DESIGN AND METHODS SECTION

The Study Design and Methods section should describe the (1) overall strategy, (2) methodology, and (3) statistical analyses to accomplish the specific aims of the project. This chapter will address the first two of these three components, overall strategy and methodology, while Chapter 10, *Data Analysis Plan*, will describe strategies for writing the Data Analysis section.

9.2 OVERALL STRATEGY

In Chapter 1, *Ten Top Tips for Successful Proposal Writing*, I emphasized the importance of being *kind* to your proposal reviewer. One way of being kind is to insert a brief summary paragraph at the very beginning of the "Study Design and Methods" section that encapsulates all the key features of the study design. This paragraph would state the sample size, study population, study design (e.g., prospective cohort case–control study, cross-sectional study), assessment tools (e.g., self-reported questionnaire, plasma samples, medical record data), and any other key features. This paragraph will remind the reviewer of your overall methodology. In addition, having such a synopsis will help the reviewer to concisely present your study to the review panel. You may have already written such a brief synopsis for your abstract and/or specific aims page. If space permits, it is useful to repeat it here.

The following example overall strategy corresponds to a proposal to evaluate the association between physical activity, psychosocial stress, and risk of gestational diabetes.

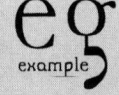

> **e.g.** *example*
> **Overall Strategy**
>
> Using a prospective cohort design, 2300 Latina (predominantly Puerto Rican) prenatal care patients will be recruited from Valley Medical Center at their first prenatal care visit. At this time, bilingual interviewers will obtain detailed information on physical activity patterns (household/childcare, occupational, and sports/exercise) as well as psychosocial stress (life events, perceived stress, anxiety, depression, and self-esteem). Information on pregravid BMI, diet, cigarette smoking, substance abuse, medical and obstetric history, acculturation,

and sociodemographic factors will also be queried. A biomarker for stress, salivary cortisol, will be collected, and weight and waist circumference will be measured. Two subsequent interviews, conducted in the second and third trimesters of pregnancy, will update information on these variables and repeat the cortisol collection. Laboratory reports and medical records will be abstracted for gestational diabetes. Logistic regression will be used to assess the relationship between physical activity, psychosocial stress, and gestational diabetes risk. Salivary cortisol will be analyzed in a nested case–control fashion on GDM cases and a matched 4:1 sample of controls (Figure 4).

9.3 IDENTIFY BENCHMARKS FOR SUCCESS

The Study Design and Methods section should identify benchmarks for success anticipated to achieve the aims. This text can be accompanied by a figure (see Figure 9.1).

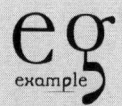

Overall Intervention Goal

Figure 9.1 shows the mean observed MET-hours/week of recreational physical activity in the study population in the first and second trimester.[108] Based upon prior literature[23,24] and our preliminary studies,[2,108] women participating in 10 MET-hours/week of recreational activity experience a clinically significant 30% reduction in risk of gestational diabetes. This proposal will test an intervention designed to increase MET-hours/week among eligible pregnant women. To achieve our goal of 10 MET-hours/week by the end of the second trimester (24–28 weeks) would require that the intervention lead to an increase in 3.8 MET-hours/week of recreational activity, which represents 0.19 of a standard deviation or a "small effect" according to Cohen's effect size.[124] In practical terms, this translates to an additional hour per week or 10 min per day of brisk walking. The following sections of the proposal demonstrate that the exercise intervention will be well capable of achieving this increase.

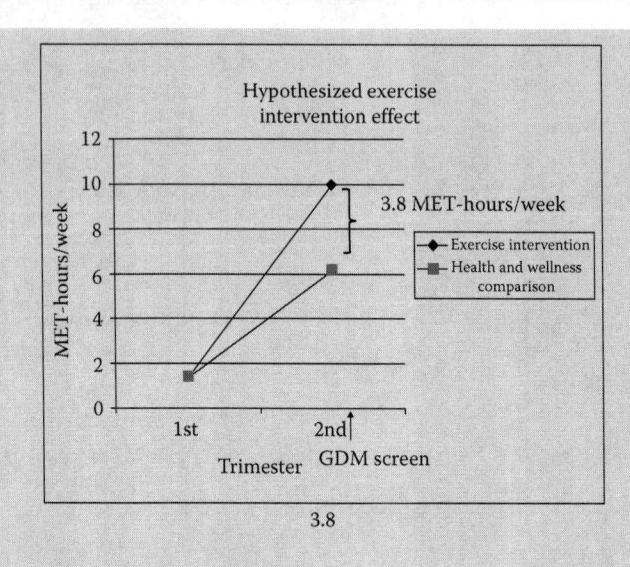

FIGURE 9.1 Benchmarks for success.

9.4 SECTION a: WHAT IS YOUR STUDY DESIGN?

After a brief synopsis of your overall strategy and benchmarks for success, the Study Design and Methods section should clarify your study design. Before writing this section of the proposal, it is critical to consider what study design you are planning to utilize. This often seems like an easy question, but there are opportunities for confusion.

For example, let's say that you are proposing to use data from an existing study. While this existing study (also known as the *parent study*) may have one study design, this does not necessarily mean that your project shares the same design. For example, the parent study may be a prospective cohort study, but you may be proposing to conduct a nested case–control study, case–cohort, or cross-sectional design within that cohort.

Other typical areas of confusion include, but are not limited to, distinguishing between case–control studies vs. retrospective cohort studies and distinguishing between cross-sectional studies vs. case–control studies. Consulting an introductory epidemiology textbook is recommended if there is any confusion with your study design.

TABLE 9.1 Typical epidemiologic and preventive medicine study designs

- Cohort study
  - Prospective
  - Retrospective
- Case–control study
- Cross-sectional study
- Ecologic or correlational study
- Other types
  - Case–cohort
  - Case–crossover

Table 9.1 is a listing of typical study designs.

In the examples below, one sentence is efficiently used to convey the study design, the association of interest, and the dates of the study:

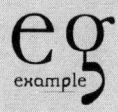

eg example
- Using a retrospective cohort design, we propose to assess the association between provider type and occurrence of episiotomy from July 1, 2013 to December 31, 2016.
- The proposed cross-sectional study will evaluate the association between breast cancer survivors' perceived recurrence risk and health behavior change using data from the Breast Cancer Survivorship Study from 2005 to 2010.

9.4.1 Consider a Study Design Figure

As noted in Chapter 1, *Ten Top Tips for Successful Proposal Writing*, I have never met a proposal with too many tables and figures. In the Study Design section, in particular, I would strongly suggest including a study design figure to complement the text.

The following Specific Aims and Figures 9.2 through 9.4 correspond to the proposal to evaluate the association between physical activity, psychosocial stress, and risk of GDM presented in Section 9.2.

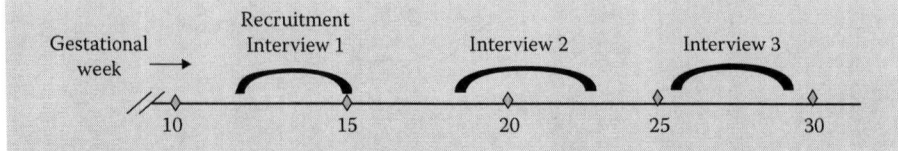

FIGURE 9.2 Timing of assessments.

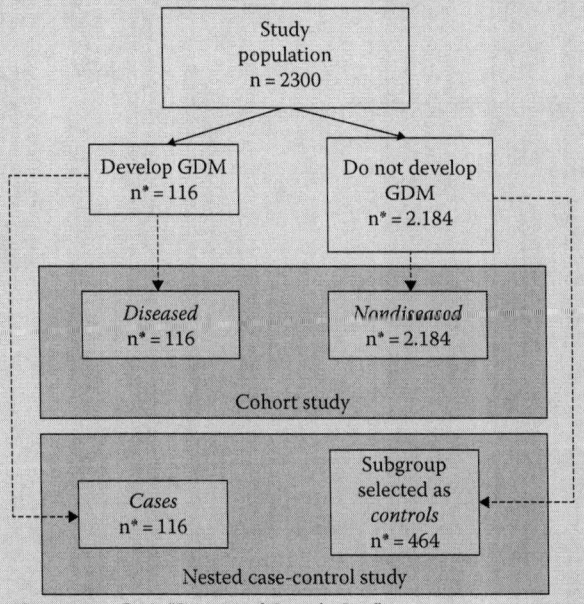

FIGURE 9.3 Study design for Aims #1 and #2.

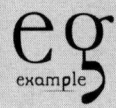

*See section D12. "Power and Sample Size"

Specific Aims

Specific Aim 1. To determine whether physical activity is prospectively associated with risk of GDM using a prospective cohort study design

Specific Aim 2. To determine whether psychosocial stress measured via cortisol is prospectively associated with risk of GDM using a nested case–control study design

Secondary Aims

Specific Aim 3. To determine whether physical activity and psychosocial stress are prospectively associated with risk of adverse birth outcomes among women with elevated screening glucose

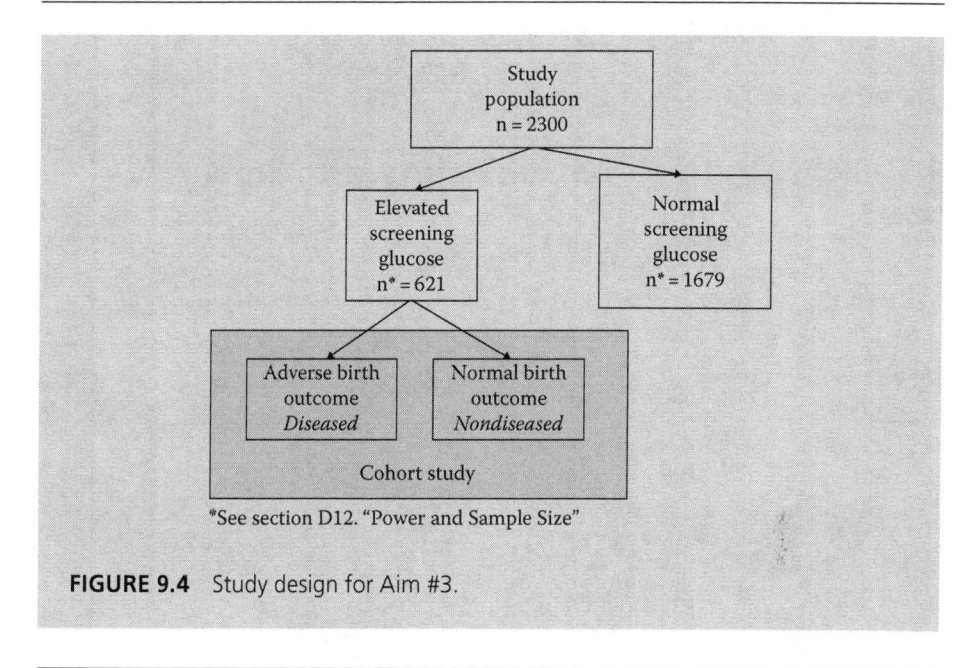

```
                    Study
                  population
                   n = 2300
                  /         \
        Elevated              Normal
        screening             screening
        glucose               glucose
        n* = 621              n* = 1679
        /      \
Adverse birth   Normal birth
  outcome        outcome
  Diseased       Nondiseased
        Cohort study
```
*See section D12. "Power and Sample Size"

FIGURE 9.4 Study design for Aim #3.

9.5 SECTION b: STUDY POPULATION (SETTING, SUBJECT ASCERTAINMENT, AND ELIGIBILITY)

After describing the study design, the proposal should next concisely describe (1) the setting for the proposed study, (2) subject ascertainment techniques, and (3) the eligibility criteria/exclusion criteria.

In describing the **study setting**, your goal is to provide the reviewers with adequate information such that they can picture your *study base*. A study base, also called a **reference population**, is a defined population whose experience during some period of time is the source of the study data. This population gives rise to study outcomes. Typically, the study base is defined by a geographical area or some other identifiable entity like a health delivery system or a cohort study.

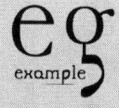

eg example
The study will be based at Jones Medical Center, a large, tertiary care teaching hospital in New York State, with 4500–5000 births annually. Jones Medical Center serves an ethnically and socioeconomically diverse population and is the perinatal transfer center for the region. Among the pregnant population, 22% are Hispanic (predominantly Puerto Rican), 11% are African American, 65% are non-Hispanic white, and 2% are other ethnicity. A third of the patients who deliver at Jones Medical Center are Medicaid insured.

The above example provides the name of the recruitment site, its geographic location, a sense of the size, and key sociodemographic factors about the study base. The reviewer can now *envision* the study base.

9.5.1 How to Describe Subject Ascertainment

In describing **subject ascertainment**, your goal is to describe how you will locate and enroll the participants in your study. For example, will you post fliers or advertise in some other manner? Will you enroll patients in a hospital? Will you be using participants from an existing database? Below are several examples:

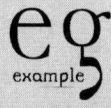

> *example*
> - From the population of all seniors enrolled in high schools in the Los Angeles Unified School District, we will select 250 at random.
> - The Labor and Delivery Log will be used to identify all patients with vaginal deliveries.
> - The proposed study will use data from the 2007 National Survey of Children's Health (NSCII).

If you are conducting a **case–control** study, it will be important to describe how you will ascertain cases as well as controls. If you are conducting a **matched** case–control study, this section should also specify your matching factors. Matching is a design technique typically used in case–control studies whereby cases are matched to controls on several key confounding factors (e.g., age, gender, study site). In this way, the cases and controls will not differ on these factors, and in turn these factors cannot be responsible for the observed association between exposure and disease (see Chapter 10, *Data Analysis Plan*, for more details on the use of matching).

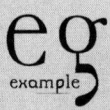

> *example*
> The cancer registry will be used to identify all bladder cancer cases from 2000 to 2010. Control group participants will be identified from lists of licensed drivers in the state during the same time period and matched to cases on age, race, and family history of breast cancer.

9.5.2 How to Describe Eligibility Criteria

In describing **eligibility criteria**, your goal is to describe who will be eligible to participate in your study. This involves describing both inclusion and exclusion criteria. Typically, inclusion criteria are listed first.

Examples of inclusion criteria include specifying

- Age range
- Gender

- Race/ethnicity
- Geographic area
- Dates

Examples of exclusion criteria include specifying

- Prevalent disease (for a prospective cohort study)
- Comorbidities

The example below is excerpted from a proposal designed to evaluate the association between provider type (i.e., certified nurse midwife vs. obstetrician) and episiotomy use.

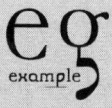

> **eg** *example* The study population will consist of all women having spontaneous vaginal delivery of a living, singleton, vertex-presenting fetus of 35 weeks gestation at the Valley Hospital from July 2013 to December 2016. We will exclude forceps and vacuum extraction deliveries, vaginal breech and multiple gestation deliveries, and preterm fetuses <35 weeks gestation as certified nurse midwives rarely are involved in delivery decisions in these cases, and these delivery situations have historically involved an increased indication for episiotomy.

A strength of the above example is that the writer provided a brief justification for the exclusion criteria of <35 weeks gestation. This can be helpful for the reviewer, particularly when the reason for the exclusion criteria is not self-evident.

Also note that, in most proposals, you will not yet know the number of participants who will be eligible or whom will fit each exclusion criteria. However, for the purposes of ensuring feasibility, it will be critical to estimate these numbers in the section on power and sample size (see Chapter 11, *Power and Sample Size*).

9.6 SECTION c: EXPOSURE ASSESSMENT

This section focuses on your **exposure of interest**.

c. Exposure Assessment
 i. How exposure data will be collected
 ii. Exposure parameterization
 iii. Validity of exposure assessment

9.6.1 How Your Exposure Data Will Be Collected

The first step is to describe how you plan to collect your exposure data. This section should briefly describe the tools you will use to assess your exposure of interest.

Examples of such tools could include questionnaires, medical records, biomarkers, or other methods. If you will be using a preexisting dataset, describe how the exposure data were originally collected regardless of the fact that you will not be collecting it yourself.

If your exposure is assessed via questionnaire, describe the following:

- Name of the questionnaire
- Number of questions
- Scale used

In describing the exposure assessment tool, provide some details about the instrument. In other words, if a questionnaire is to be used, it is not sufficient to simply state the name of the questionnaire without giving a sense of the number of questions and the scale used. On the other hand, it is too detailed to restate every single question on the questionnaire. Stating a question verbatim is only warranted if your exposure was assessed via one or two specific questions and these were so complex that it would help the reviewers to see them, in their entirety, in the proposal. According to the most recent NIH guidelines, data collection instruments such as surveys and questionnaires may be included in the Appendix of the proposal, so that reviewers can access these if necessary.

> **eg** *example*
>
> Attitude toward school was measured with the Jones Attitude Survey (Appendix A). The survey contains nine questions. The first three questions measure attitudes toward academic subjects; the next three questions measure attitudes toward teachers, counselors, and administrators; the last three questions measure attitudes toward the social environment in the school. Participants will be asked to rate each statement on a five-point scale from one (strongly disagree) to five (strongly agree).

The example above follows the guidelines by providing not only the name of the questionnaire but also a sense of the types of questions and the numerical range of responses.

If your exposure is assessed via biomarker, describe the following:

- Collection methods (e.g., phlebotomist)
- Processing methods
- Assay used
- Laboratory name

If blood and/or tissue samples will be taken, you will want to provide the name of the assay used to assess your biomarker of interest, as well as the name and location of the laboratory where the assays will be conducted. According to the most recent NIH guidelines, clinical protocols may be included in the Appendix of the proposal, so that reviewers can access these if necessary.

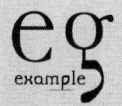

> **eg** *example*
>
> **Biomarker Assessment:** Fasting samples will be collected at home visits by study assessors at 6 months and 1 year. Assessors will collect whole blood and centrifuge the samples either immediately (to obtain plasma) or after allowing the blood to clot (to obtain serum). Samples will then be placed on dry ice and brought daily to the Franklin Laboratory and immediately stored at −80°C in a dedicated freezer with a temperature monitor, alarm, and backup power system. Samples will be assayed by Dr. Smith (Department of Laboratory Medicine, Johnson University, Boston, MA) (letter of collaboration attached). **Fasting glucose** (FG) will be measured enzymatically on the Roche P Modular system using Jones Diagnostics reagents (Boston, MA).[1] Glucose at the concentrations of 90 and 312 mg/dL are determined in Dr. Smith's laboratory with a day-to-day variability of 1.7% and 1.6%, respectively.

9.6.2 Exposure Parameterization

The second step in describing exposure assessment is providing information on how your exposure will be parameterized for analysis. That is, whether you will be using a **categorical** (i.e., two or more categories) or **continuous** scale for your exposure variable. It is also possible to propose that you will use several exposure scales (e.g., both categorical and continuous). However, it is important to note that the latter approach will have implications for your Data Analysis section in terms of the number and type of analyses that you will have to conduct/present (as described in Chapter 10, *Data Analysis Plan*).

9.6.3 How to Parameterize Your Variable

One important factor in deciding how to parameterize your exposure variable is the state of science in the field. For many variables, cut points are already established. For example, the accepted World Health Organization (WHO) cut point for obesity is a BMI ≥30 kg/m². Look over the prior literature in your proposed area to see how prior studies have parameterized your exposure variable. The advantage of following suit with these prior studies is that by using the same scale, you will be able to compare your findings to those of these prior studies.

If you are proposing to use an existing dataset, you will likely have little choice in how to parameterize your exposure variable and will be limited to the derived variables within the dataset. Or, you may be proposing to use an existing questionnaire that only asks respondents to check off categorical responses instead of asking them to write in actual numerical values.

However, in most cases, you will have some flexibility. For example, it may be possible to categorize continuous exposure variables **as well as** evaluate them continuously. For example, you could categorize BMI (e.g., underweight, normal weight, overweight, obese) **and** also evaluate BMI continuously (kg/m^2). The categorical variable has the advantage of generating findings that are translatable into public health messages (e.g., the impact of being obese on your outcome). The continuous variable, in contrast, allows you to assess if a one unit increase in BMI has an influence on your outcome in a dose–response manner. However, note that assumptions of linearity should be assessed first (e.g., utilizing a continuous variable assumes a linear dose–response relationship between your exposure and outcome, such that each unit change in exposure is associated with the same increment of increased risk). This should be discussed with your statistician.

Other possibilities, in the absence of established published cut points, are to divide your exposure variable into quartiles, quintiles, or tertiles. Ideally, this division should be based upon the exposure distribution among the nondiseased. In other words, exclude cases of your outcome when deriving cut points. This approach has the disadvantage of being data dependent, in that the cut points will be dependent on the distribution of the data in your study population. On the other hand, if you are conducting your study in a new study population, it may actually be preferable to have the cut points be study specific.

Ultimately, the decision for how to parameterize your exposure of interest will depend upon your sample size and corresponding power to detect an effect. Power will be influenced by the type of parameterization you choose and this is discussed in Chapter 11, *Power and Sample Size*.

9.6.4 Validity of Exposure Assessment

In this section, your goal is to establish the validity of the technique that you will be using to assess your exposure. This is important whether you are using subjective measures (e.g., questionnaire-based) or using objective measures (e.g., blood samples, medical records).

In the case of **subjective measures**, this section should cite prior validation studies of the assessment tool. Ideally, you will want to cite those validation studies conducted in a study population as similar as possible to your own. For example, let's say you are proposing to evaluate diet in Asian youth. Ideally, you would want to cite studies showing that the questionnaire was not only valid among children but also among Asian children.

When validation studies are available, provide the reviewer with the specific **magnitude** of findings for validity and reliability as opposed to simply their statistical significance.

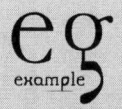

> **eg** *example* — Overall psychological distress as well as three subdimensions of psychological distress were measured by a 30-item version of the Strauss Symptom Checklist.[5] Jones et al. reported internal consistency reliability coefficients ranging from 0.84 to 0.87 for each of the three subtests and test–retest reliability estimates ranging from 0.75 to 0.82 over a 1-week interval.[6]

In the case of **objective measures** such as biomarker assessment, provide the laboratory coefficient of variation as in the example below. You may additionally specify how you will assess lab performance, such as by including blinded quality control samples and by indicating that the laboratory will be blinded to case and control status (in the context of a case–control study).

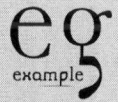

> **eg** *example* — CRP will be measured using a high-sensitivity assay with latex-enhanced nephelometry on a nephelometer at the University of Washington Medical Center, Seattle, Washington. Day-to-day coefficients of variation range from 4.93 to 7.84. Quality control for specimen handling will be performed monthly by the head lab technician.

Biomarkers may also have other limitations. For example, they may not reflect the etiologically relevant time period for the impact of your exposure on your outcome of interest. Degradation over time in frozen samples could reduce their validity. In addition, the biomarker may not be truly reflective of your exposure of interest—or may be influenced by other factors. For example, blood levels of vitamin D are not only influenced by diet but also by sunlight exposure. Therefore, the validity section should provide evidence reducing these concerns when relevant, as in the example below.

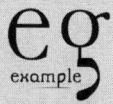

> **eg** *example* — Plasma vitamin D levels will be determined by laboratory assay of the participants' stored plasma samples for levels of 25-(OH)D_3. We chose to analyze 25-(OH)D_3 rather than its metabolite, 1,25-dihydroxyvitamin D_3 for several reasons. First 25-(OH)D_3 better reflects combined exposure from sunlight and dietary intake and is more easily influenced by behavioral interventions than its metabolite.[1] Second 25-(OH)D_3 is less closely regulated by other hormones and exists at substantially higher concentrations in the blood than its metabolite.[2] Finally, the 25-(OH)D_3 assay requires less plasma than does the assay for its metabolite.[3]

This section on validity is relevant even if your exposure assessment is based on a *gold standard*. For example, obtaining exposure information via medical record abstraction is often considered a gold standard. However, medical records may be completed by a variety of personnel including residents, attending physicians, and nurse midwives. Any of these personnel can make an error in recording key information in the medical record or selecting the appropriate code. There may also be error associated with the technique used to abstract data from the medical record.

In summary, it is critical to provide as much information to support the validity of your measures as possible. Later, in Chapter 13, *How to Present Limitations and Alternatives*, I provide tips on how to strategically describe the limitations of these measures. In this way, you will indicate to the reviewers that you have carefully weighed both the strengths and limitations of your selected exposure assessment technique.

9.6.5 What to Do If There Are No Prior Validation Studies

There are several strategies for addressing the absence of prior validation studies:

- Conduct your own validation study.
- Search for prior validation studies in similar study populations.
- Search for prior validation studies in any study population.
- Cite prior studies showing significant associations **between** your exposure measured via your proposed assessment tool and your outcome of interest.

If you find that there are no prior validation studies on your measures of interest, you may want to consider conducting such a validation study yourself. Indeed, a seed grant or foundation grant to support such validation work is often a key first step toward applying for a larger grant designed to use the questionnaire to evaluate associations with an outcome of interest.

If time constraints or other limitations prevent you from conducting your own validation study, search the literature for prior published validation studies in a study population as similar as possible to your own. In the absence of such work, the last item on the list above provides a *last-ditch* way to reassure the reviewers of the validity of your exposure assessment tool. In brief, try to find prior studies that found significant associations between your exposure, as measured via your proposed tool, and your outcome of interest. Such studies can help to reassure reviewers that your tool has sufficient precision to predict disease; but it is still not a substitute for the presence of an actual validation study.

The example below is from a proposal examining the association between food insecurity and risk of diabetes. The proposal writer found no validation studies of the food security survey to be used. However, prior studies measuring food insecurity via the same survey found significant associations with diabetes.

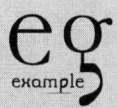

> **e.g.** *example* — While there are no published data on the validity of the 6-item Smith Food Security Survey, food insecurity measured by this survey was predictive of incident diabetes in previous studies.[3,10]

9.7 SECTION d: OUTCOME ASSESSMENT

This section focuses on your **outcome of interest**. The structure and content of the Outcome Assessment section mirrors that of the Exposure Assessment section but instead focuses on your outcome of interest.

    d. Outcome Assessment
        i. How outcome data will be collected
        ii. Outcome parameterization
        iii. Validity of outcome assessment

First, describe how your outcome data will be collected. Specifically, in this section, describe the tools by which you are assessing your outcome variables and provide relevant citations. Such tools could include all of those possible tools listed in the Exposure Assessment section (e.g., medical record abstraction, questionnaires).

If you are conducting a **case–control** study, delineate clear diagnostic criteria that you will use to identify disease outcomes (e.g., based on published consensus guidelines). Stating that diagnoses will be confirmed by an MD or medical review panel through the review of medical record and/or pathology reports will strengthen this section. Clarify how the controls will be defined as well.

The decision for how to parameterize your outcome variable will affect your choice of regression model (see Chapter 10, *Data Analysis Plan*). For a case–control study, your outcome variable will be dichotomous (case vs. control), while for other study designs, there may be several options for how to parameterize your outcome variable (e.g., continuous). Regardless, the outcome parameterization should be specified in this section of the proposal.

Finally, the **validity** of the Outcome Assessment section, as with the validity of the Exposure Assessment section, will cite relevant studies and their findings as to the validity of the tool used to assess your proposed outcome. The same cautions with both subjective and objective measures apply.

> **e.g.** *example* — Breast cancer cases will be confirmed through medical record review by a study physician; invasive vs. *in situ* and hormone receptor status will be abstracted from the medical record. Controls will be those with no personal history of breast cancer.

9.8 SECTION e: COVARIATE ASSESSMENT

The Covariate Assessment section mirrors the section on exposure and outcome assessment but is typically briefer. In the covariate section, state which variables you will consider as possible confounders of your exposure–outcome relationship. Remember that to qualify as a confounder, the variable must be independently associated with both the exposure and disease and not be on the causal pathway between exposure and disease. See Figure 9.5.

In general, you will always want to consider prior established risk factors for your outcome of interest as potential confounding factors (see Chapter 10, *Data Analysis Plan*, for more details on addressing confounding). Provide a citation supporting that these variables are indeed established risk factors for your outcome—a review article can be a useful reference. Ideas for other potential confounders to consider can be gleaned from your **summary table** of the literature created as part of Chapter 4, *Conducting the Literature Search*. Scan through this summary table and consider covariates that were included in the prior studies of your exposure–outcome relationship. In this way, you will be sure not to miss any key covariates that prior studies included, and by adjusting for them, your findings may be more comparable to those of the prior studies.

The example below is an excerpt from a proposal designed to evaluate the association between provider type (certified nurse midwife vs. obstetrician) and episiotomy use.

> *eg example*
>
> We will consider established risk factors for episiotomy in the prior literature such as parity, fetal distress, and maternal compromise.[1] These variables will be abstracted from the medical record. Prior studies have indicated that parity is the strongest predictor of episiotomy use.[10] Fetal distress and maternal compromise are considered clinical indications for shortening second stage and, hence, episiotomy use.[11]

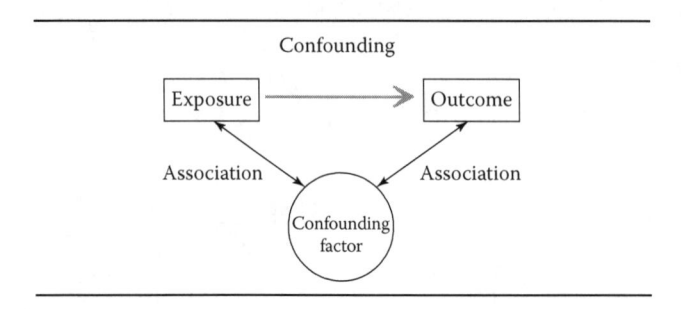

FIGURE 9.5 Confounding diagram.

A strength of the example above is that it provides a brief justification and citations for the proposed covariates.

If you plan to consider any of your covariates as possible effect modifiers of the relationship between your exposure and disease, it will be important to specify those variables in this section, as well as how they will be parameterized.

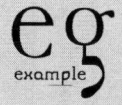

> **e.g.** *example*
> We will investigate established risk factors for type 2 diabetes as potential effect modifiers.[1] These include study site, BMI (i.e., normal weight vs. overweight/obese), and age (i.e., <40, ≥40 years of age).

9.9 SECTION f: VARIABLE CATEGORIZATION TABLE

A variable categorization table is a table that lists your key study variables (exposure, outcome, and covariates) corresponding to each specific aim. The table can also include additional details as relevant (e.g., assessment tool, timing of variable collection). Including such a table in a grant proposal is an example of being kind to your reviewer. It demonstrates to the reviewer that you have *a priori* thought through your variables of interest and have an organized plan. It removes any concerns that you will be conducting a *fishing expedition*.

Regardless whether you include such a table in your proposal, you will find that the act of creating such a table helps to ensure that you don't include extraneous variables that are not directly relevant to your analysis and, vice versa, that your proposal does not omit any variables integral to your analysis. After the proposal is approved, the variable categorization table continues to be useful by serving as a *cookbook* for your data analysis.

Table 9.2 is an example variable categorization table for a **grant proposal** designed to evaluate the association between stress and risk of hypertensive disorders of pregnancy. Note that the variable names are listed underneath the corresponding specific aims according to assessment time period. Table 9.3 is an example variable categorization table for a **doctoral proposal** designed to evaluate the association between stress and risk of hypertensive disorders of pregnancy. Note that this doctoral proposal variable categorization table is more detailed than the grant proposal example—due to the lack of space constraints. The table has three columns. **Column #1** of Table 9.3 is the name of each variable and its code name for analysis. **Column #2** of Table 9.3 provides the definition of the variable and displays each parameterization of the variable—note that there are different rows for categorical vs. continuous versions of the same variables (e.g., stress). Column #2 also shows the number that each category is

TABLE 9.2 Variable categorization table for a grant proposal to evaluate the association between stress and risk of hypertensive disorders of pregnancy

VARIABLES COLLECTED AT ASSESSMENT TIME POINTS	PREGNANCY			DELIVERY	POSTPARTUM		
	10 WEEKS	24–28 WEEKS	32–34 WEEKS		6 WEEKS	6 MONTHS	1 YEAR
Aim #1: GWG and postpartum weight loss							
GWG (kg)	x	x	x	x			
Rate of GWG	x	x	x	x			
Compliance with IOM guidelines	x	x	x	x			
Area under the GWG curve (AUC)	x	x	x	x			
Postpartum weight loss	x				x	x	x
Physical activity (actigraph, PPAQ)	x	x	x		x	x	x
Dietary intake (Hispanic FFQ)	x	x	x		x	x	x
Aim #2: Glycemia and associated biomarkers of insulin resistance							
Glucose (mg/dL)	x	x	x		x	x	x
Insulin (pmol/L)	x	x	x		x	x	x
HbA$_{1c}$	x	x	x		x	x	x
Adiponectin (μg/mL)	x	x	x		x	x	x
Leptin (ng/mL)	x	x	x		x	x	x
HOMA	x	x	x		x	x	x

Aim #3: Offspring outcomes

Birth weight-for-gestational age z-score [fetal growth]			x	x	x	x	x	x	x	x	
Ponderal index (g/cm³)				x	x	x	x	x	x		
Weight-for-length z-score (WFL-z)				x	x	x	x	x			
Weight-for-age z-score (WFA-z)				x	x	x	x	x			
Length-for-age z-score (LFA-z)				x	x	x	x	x			
Sum of skinfolds, ratio of skinfolds				x	x	x	x	x			
Waist circumference (cm)				x	x	x	x	x			
Head circumference (cm)				x	x	x	x	x			

Covariates

Clinical characteristics of current pregnancy	x	x
Medical history	x	
Sociodemographic factors	x	
Smoking (cotinine) and substance use	x	x
Depression	x	x
Sleep	x	x
Breast-feeding		

TABLE 9.3 Variable categorization table for a doctoral proposal to evaluate the association between stress and risk of hypertensive disorders of pregnancy

NAME	DESCRIPTION	TYPE
Outcome variables		
HDIS	Hypertensive disorder of pregnancy 0 = no 1 = yes	Dichotomous
PREEC	Preeclampsia 0 = no 1 = yes	Dichotomous
GHTN	Gestational hypertension 0 = no 1 = yes	Dichotomous
Exposure variables		
ESTRESS1	Early pregnancy stress 0 = low stress, at or below median l = high stress, above median	Dichotomous
ESTRESS	Early pregnancy stress 1–14	Continuous
Covariates		
AGECAT2	Age at enrollment in study 1 = 15–19 2 = 20–24 3 = 25–29 4 = 30–40	Categorical
BMI_C	Prepregnancy BMI, IOM categories 1 = BMI < 19.8 2 = BMI 19.8–26.0 3 = BMI > 26.0–29.0 4 = BMI ≥ 29.0	Categorical
EDU_GRP	Education groups 1 = less than high school 2 = high school/trade or technical school 3 = at least some college experience	Categorical
INC_GRP	Income groups 1 = ≤$15,000 2 = >$15,000–30,000 3 = >$30,000 4 = "missing" 5 = "refused/don't know"	Categorical

TABLE 9.3 (continued) Variable categorization table for a doctoral proposal to evaluate the association between stress and risk of hypertensive disorders of pregnancy

NAME	DESCRIPTION	TYPE
BRTHPLAC	Birthplace 1 = United States 2 = others	Dichotomous
LANG2	0 = English only 1 = both Spanish and English 2 = Spanish only	Categorical
PARCAT	Number of live births 1 = 0 births 2 = 1 live birth 3 = ≥2 live births	Categorical

assigned, for example, 0 = *low stress*. **Column #3** describes the parameterization of the variable:

- *Categorical* = a categorical variable with two or more categories
  - *Dichotomous* = a categorical variable with two categories (e.g., *male, female*)
- *Continuous* = a variable with values ranging from x to x

9.10 PITFALLS TO AVOID

As you can see, the high level of detail required for the Study Design and Methods section underscores the importance of being focused in your specific aims. That is, a large number of specific aims typically translate into a potentially large number of variables. Each exposure and outcome of interest needs to be justified in your Background and Significance section and carefully described in the Study Design and Methods section (e.g., assessment tool, parameterization, validation). Therefore, the decision to include multiple exposure and outcome variables should be made with caution, as their inclusion quickly whirlpools throughout the proposal resulting in multiple analyses and tables. As mentioned in Chapter 1, *Ten Top Tips for Successful Proposal Writing*, one of the classic pitfalls of doctoral students and early-career investigators is to be overly ambitious in this manner.

Another small, but important, pitfall to avoid is to ensure that your text description of your methods does not contradict the information included in your tables and figures. For example, I have seen proposals that list key variables in tables that are not mentioned in the text or, vice versa, that mention key variables in the text that cannot be found in the tables.

9.11 EXAMPLES

9.11.1 Example #1

A Proposal to Examine the Association between Psychosocial Stress and Hypertensive Disorders of Pregnancy: Study Design and Methods

Study Design and Methods

Overall Strategy

Using data from the Salud Study, we will prospectively assess the association between psychosocial stress and hypertensive disorders of pregnancy. The Salud Study is a prospective cohort of 2300 Latina prenatal care patients conducted from 2004 to 2009. Participants were recruited from Taylor Medical Center at their first prenatal care visit (8–12 weeks gestation). Taylor Medical Center has the 25th largest obstetrical service in the United States; approximately 5000 infants are delivered annually. Among the Taylor prenatal care population, approximately 45% are Latina (predominantly from Puerto Rico), 11% are African-American, 42% are non-Latina white, and 2% are of other ethnicity. At baseline, bilingual interviewers obtained detailed information on psychosocial stress (life events, perceived stress, anxiety, depression, and self-esteem). Information on pregravid BMI, diet, cigarette smoking, substance abuse, medical and obstetric history, acculturation, and sociodemographic factors were also queried. A biomarker for stress, salivary cortisol, was collected and weight and waist circumference was measured. Two subsequent interviews, conducted at 18–20 weeks of gestation and 24–28 weeks of gestation, updated information on these variables and repeat the cortisol collection (study design Figure 1). Logistic regression will be used to assess the relationship between psychosocial stress and risk of hypertensive disorders of pregnancy.

Study Population

Women who self-identify as Latina and are less than 24 weeks gestation were recruited by trained, bilingual (English/Spanish) interviewers. Study exclusions included the extremes of childbearing age (younger than 16 or older than 42), multiple gestation, chronic hypertension, preexisting diabetes, heart disease, and chronic renal disease. For the purposes of the proposed analysis, we will also exclude women with preterm birth or spontaneous abortion.

Exposure Assessment

Psychosocial stress was measured using the 14-item Perceived Stress Scale, a validated and widely used measure of perceived stress.[1] The scale includes questions such as the following: "How often have you felt you were unable to control the important things in your life?" and "How often have you felt difficulties were piling up so high that you could not overcome them?" The scale was interviewer-administered so literacy and/or language barriers were minimized. This measure will be dichotomized at the median for this analysis, as has been done by others (variable categorization Table 1).[2] Perceived stress scores will also be analyzed continuously to evaluate a dose–response effect.

Validity of Exposure Assessment
The Perceived Stress Scale has been shown to have adequate reliability (r = 0.78) and to be correlated with physical symptoms (r = 0.52–0.70) and depressive symptoms (r = 0.65–0.76).[3] Additionally, in a random sample of adults residing in the United States, there was little variance between responses when questions were analyzed by sex, race, and/or education suggesting that the test provides a meaningful measure regardless of these factors.[4] The Spanish version of the Perceived Stress Scale (10-item version of the questionnaire) validated in a Spanish population has been shown to have adequate reliability (a = 0.82, test–retest, r = 0.77, p < 0.001) and validity (r = 0.71 for distress score and r = 0.66 for anxiety score).[5]

Outcome Assessment
Hypertensive disorders of pregnancy were diagnosed using ACOG criteria.[6] Cases were identified through postdelivery review of medical records, as well as through International Classification of Disease (ICD) codes. Further, all cases identified through these mechanisms were then confirmed and classified into a subgroup (gestational hypertension or preeclampsia) by the study obstetrician.

Gestational hypertension is defined as two blood pressure measurements greater than 140/90 after 20 weeks gestation in previously normotensive women, with no lab evidence or symptoms of preeclampsia. Preeclampsia is defined as blood pressure greater than 140/90 on two occasions, with proteinuria, also after 20 weeks gestation and in women who were previously normotensive.[7] Women with gestational hypertension and preeclampsia will be analyzed together as hypertensive disorders of pregnancy, and subgroup analyses will be performed for gestational hypertension and preeclampsia independently to determine whether the effect of psychosocial stress varies among these subgroups (variable categorization Table 1).

Validity of Outcome Assessment
A trained medical record abstractor abstracted diagnosis of hypertensive disorders that were then confirmed by the study obstetrician. A reliability study of medical record abstractors at Taylor Hospital conducted in 2002 using a random sample of 100 medical records found coefficients of 0.77 across abstractors for hypertensive disorders of pregnancy.

Covariate Assessment
Data for covariates were collected via self-report as well as through postdelivery medical record abstraction (variable categorization Table 1). Specifically, education, income, smoking and drug use, and acculturation were all obtained via interview. Physical activity data were assessed via the Frances Physical Activity Survey.[8] Acculturation was measured via both language preference (English or Spanish), as well as through birthplace (United States or elsewhere). Data on physical characteristics, such as prepregnancy weight and height, and obstetric and medical history, such as parity, were abstracted from the medical record.

9.11.2 Example #2

A Proposal to Examine the Association between Coffee Consumption and Risk of Cutaneous Melanoma: Study Design and Methods

Study Design and Methods

Study Design and Population
To examine the association between coffee and tea intake and risk of cutaneous melanoma, we propose to conduct a prospective cohort study utilizing data from the Mediterranean Observational Study (MOS). MOS recruited women at five centers in the Mediterranean between 2005 and 2006 (1). Postmenopausal women aged 50–79 who had expected survival time greater than 3 years were eligible to participate in MOS.

A total of 1425 participants were enrolled in the study. Participants were screened at baseline for physical measurements (height, weight, blood pressure, heart rate, waist and hip circumferences), collection of blood specimens, and medication/supplement inventory and completed a questionnaire detailing medical history, lifestyle/behavioral factors, and quality of life. In addition, participants completed a questionnaire regarding other exposures such as residency, smoking status, early life exposures, physical activity, weight, and occupational history. FFQs were administered at baseline screening. The participants were mailed annual FFQs and questionnaires to update selected exposures and ascertain medical outcomes. Participants were followed for an average of 4 years until 2010. Women will be excluded from our study if they had history of prior cancers, including nonmelanoma skin cancer, or if they had dropped out prior to first follow-up. Follow-up time was accrued from enrollment to date of diagnosis, death, or date of last follow-up.

Exposure Assessment
Data on coffee consumption were collected at baseline and updated annually using FFQs. Participants were asked "Do you usually drink coffee each day?" Those who answered "yes" further indicated separately the number of cups of coffee per day. We will create a categorical coffee consumption variable: none, 1 cup/day, 2 cups/day, 3 cups/day, or 4+ cups/day.

Validation of Exposure Assessment
Smith et al. assessed the validity of the FFQ used to collect coffee and tea intake using four 24 h diet recalls and one 4-day food record (2). The authors compared 30 nutrients estimated from FFQ with means from 24 h recalls and the 4-day food records. The authors found that most nutrients estimated by the FFQ were within 10% of the records or recalls. The precision of FFQ used for MOS was similar to that of other FFQs (3).

No study has assessed the validity of the self-report of coffee intake in the MOS. However, a validation study by Taylor et al. found a high correlation coefficient between self-reported FFQ and two 7-day diet records for coffee in the Women's Health Study, a cohort similar in terms of dietary consumption to MOS (4). Correlation coefficients of 0.78 and 0.93 were reported for coffee and tea, respectively.

Outcome Assessment

Melanoma cases were defined as women who had an adjudicated diagnosis of melanoma (over the duration of follow-up). Potential cases were identified through self-reported annual questionnaires on various medical outcomes including melanoma. The outcome will be categorized as melanoma (yes, no).

Validity of Outcome Assessment

All diagnoses were centrally adjudicated at the Clinical Coordinating Center. Specifically, cancer epidemiologists and physicians reviewed hospital records, operative reports, history and physical examination, radiology, and oncology consultation reports. If a case was adjudicated, the physician recorded ICD codes, date of the diagnosis, and tumor behavior (invasive, *in situ*, or borderline).

Covariate Assessment

Physical measurements and medical history data on all participants were collected at baseline. Lifestyle factors were collected at baseline as well as during follow-up. Dietary data were collected by the FFQ at baseline and updated during annual follow-up. We will consider the following categorical variables as potential covariates: age (50–54, 55–59, 60–69, 70–79), alcohol intake (no/yes), smoking status (no/yes), race (white, black, Hispanic, etc.), skin reaction to sun, and past sun exposure (Table 1). Continuous variable covariates include BMI and total minutes of physical activity per week (Table 1).

Data Analysis Plan   10

The goal of this chapter is to provide you with **strategies and tips** for writing the data analysis plan of your proposal. This chapter is not meant to take the place of a statistics textbook that would provide detailed information on statistical techniques for hypothesis testing. Instead, this chapter is designed to provide you with (1) a **framework** for writing a typical data analysis plan for a dissertation or grant proposal in the field of epidemiology and preventive medicine, (2) a sense of the **scope and depth** required for the data analysis plan, and (3) *best practices* that should be addressed in a robust data analysis plan.

This chapter also includes an **example data analysis plan** for a dissertation proposal accompanied by mock tables (also known as *dummy tables*) for illustrative purposes. However, note that while recommended for a dissertation proposal, a grant proposal will rarely have space for mock tables.

Ultimately, this chapter will position you well to know the right questions to ask when meeting with your collaborating statistician, a statistical consulting center, or data analysis core.

10.1 PART I: FRAMEWORK FOR THE PROPOSED DATA ANALYSIS PLAN

10.1.1 Start the Data Analysis Plan by Repeating Your Specific Aims Verbatim

The overall goal of the data analysis plan for a proposal is to demonstrate how you plan to directly answer the questions (aka hypotheses) that you asked in your specific aims. By tightly tying the data analysis plan to the specific aims, this chapter will show you how to avoid the common pitfalls that often occur in the data analysis plan of a proposal.

Therefore, well-written data analysis plans repeat the specific aims verbatim immediately prior to describing each corresponding data analysis plan (see Table 10.1). Repeating the specific aims in the data analysis plan has several advantages. First, it makes the proposal more organized and falls under the rubric of being *kind* to your reviewers by reminding them of your specific aims. Secondly, and most importantly, it ensures that you do not accidentally omit the data analysis plan for any of your aims. Similarly, it ensures that you do not include extraneous analysis plans that do not address one of your aims.

TABLE 10.1 Template for Data Analysis section of a proposal

DATA ANALYSIS PLAN

- Specific Aim #1
  - Data analysis plan
- Specific Aim #2
  - Data analysis plan
- Specific Aim #3
  - Data analysis plan

Repeating the specific aims in the data analysis plan is not only critical for a grant proposal but also for a dissertation proposal. Remember as discussed in Chapter 2, *Starting a Dissertation Proposal*, that it is useful to view the dissertation proposal as a *contract* between you and your dissertation committee. The more your data analysis plan is tied to your specific aims, the greater protection you will have from committee members who ask you to conduct additional analyses (or ad hoc analyses) late in the stages of your dissertation.

An editorial note One important caution is to carefully check that the wording of the specific aims in the data analysis plan exactly matches the wording of the aims as originally written in the specific aims. Sometimes, in revising the proposal, you may change the wording or even the scope of your specific aims. Be sure to make those changes in the data analysis plan too! Nothing can be more disconcerting to a reviewer than seeing new aims in this plan or aims that contradict those on the Specific Aims page.

10.1.2 What if All Your Aims Require the Identical Data Analysis Plan?

Often, the data analysis plan is similar for each specific aim. Imagine a proposal evaluating the independent association between 3 exposure variables on one common outcome, for example, *to evaluate the association between age, education, and marital status on risk of knee injury*. In this situation, it may be repetitive and not an efficient use of space to repeat the same data analysis plan under each aim. Instead, in this case, it is fine to list all your aims together and then insert the relevant data analysis plan below (Table 10.2).

Or, as an alternative, the data analysis plan for Aims #2 and #3 can refer back to the plan for Aim #1 and simply state if there are any modifications or additions (Table 10.3).

TABLE 10.2 Template for Data Analysis section of a proposal with similar analyses for each Specific Aim

DATA ANALYSIS PLAN

- Specific Aim #1, #2, #3
  - Data analysis plan

TABLE 10.3 Alternative template for Data Analysis section of a proposal with similar analyses for each Specific Aim

DATA ANALYSIS PLAN

- *Specific Aim #1*
  - Data analysis plan
- *Specific Aim #2*
  - Refer to data analysis plan for Aim #1 with any modifications
- *Specific Aim #3*
  - Refer to data analysis plan for Aim #1 with any modifications

In this alternative data analysis plan, you are free to specify, when relevant, any minor differences in data analysis techniques that might be unique to each aim.

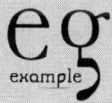

> *example*
>
> For Aim #2, we will use the same data analysis methods described for Aim #1. However, for Aim #2, we will also exclude participants with preexisting disease.

10.2 PART II: SCOPE AND DEPTH OF PROPOSED ANALYSES

10.2.1 Step #1: Are Your Specific Aims Descriptive or Analytic?

As described in Chapter 6, *Specific Aims*, the majority of dissertation and grant proposals in epidemiology and preventive medicine aim to identify an association between an exposure of interest and an outcome of interest. Therefore, addressing these aims typically requires the calculation of a measure of association. These types of specific aims are *analytic*.

> *example*
>
> Specific Aim #1: To evaluate the **association** between age and incidence of Lyme disease.

This analytic aim evaluates the association between age (an exposure) and Lyme disease incidence (an outcome).

However, some of your aims, particularly in pilot studies, will simply be *descriptive*:

- To measure the frequency of an outcome, regardless of its association with an exposure
- To measure the frequency of an exposure, independent of its association with an outcome
- To calculate recruitment and retention rates

> **e.g. example** Specific Aim #1: To estimate seasonal **trends** in the prevalence of tick-borne diseases during 2007–2011 in the northeastern United States.

In the example above, the descriptive aim simply describes the prevalence of an outcome (i.e., tick-borne diseases) regardless of its association with an exposure (e.g., age).

Your data analysis plan will differ depending on whether your aim(s) is descriptive or analytic. If you have a mixture of both types of aims, the data analysis plan should have subsections corresponding to each type of aim. Therefore, the first step is to be clear on the types of aims you are proposing.

10.2.2 Step #2: How Will You Parameterize Your Variables?

The second step in developing your data analysis plan is to consider how your variables of interest will be parameterized. You have already considered this in Chapter 9, *Study Design and Methods*, when you created your Exposure and Outcome Assessment sections and corresponding variable categorization table. In this table, you specified whether your variables will be categorical or continuous. These decisions will impact the type of statistics that you propose to calculate in your data analysis plan.

A potential pitfall to avoid The importance of referring back to your variable categorization table and corresponding Exposure and Outcome Assessment sections cannot be understated. A common pitfall is to propose to use a dichotomous exposure variable in your Exposure Assessment section but, then in your data analysis section, plan to propose to calculate means and SDs for a continuous exposure variable. It is very important that the proposal be internally consistent.

10.3 OUTLINE FOR A BASIC DATA ANALYSIS PLAN

Table 10.4 includes a simple outline for a basic data analysis plan. Typically, descriptive aims will require only univariate analyses. Analytic aims will require univariate, bivariate, **and** multivariable analyses. The data analysis plan to accomplish each of these analyses is described below.

Throughout the remainder of this chapter, we will apply this basic plan to an example proposal designed to evaluate the association between **hemorrhage size (the exposure)** and **mortality (the outcome)**. This example plan will be accompanied by mock tables for illustrative purposes. However, note that, unlike a dissertation proposal, a grant proposal will rarely have room for mock tables.

10.3.1 Univariate Analysis Plan

A univariate analysis plan is relevant for proposals with either descriptive or analytic aims.

The goal of the univariate analysis plan is to describe:

- Your response rates, retention rates, and any other relevant **feasibility** rates
- The distribution (and frequency) of any **exposure** variables of interest
- The distribution (and frequency) of any **outcome** variables of interest

The statistics you choose for the univariate plan will depend upon the parameterization of your exposure and outcome variables:

- For categorical variables
  - Number (N) and percent (%)

TABLE 10.4 Template Data Analysis Plan

DATA ANALYSIS PLAN

- *Specific Aim #1*
  - Data analysis plan
    » Univariate analysis plan
    » Bivariate analysis plan
    » Multivariable analysis plan
    » Other statistical issues as relevant
- *Specific Aim #2*
  - Same as above
- *Specific Aim #3*
  - Same as above

- For continuous variables
  - If normally distributed: mean and SD
  - If not normally distributed: median and 25th and 75th percentile interquartile range (IQR)

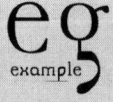

> **eg** *example*
>
> Imagine a proposal titled "Project Health" to evaluate the association between hemorrhage size and mortality. In this study, the exposure is considered both as a categorical (i.e., small vs. large hemorrhage size) and continuous variable. The outcome is a categorical variable (3-month mortality—yes or no).
>
> **Data Analysis Plan**
> *Specific Aim #1. To evaluate the association between hemorrhage size and risk of 3-month mortality*
> **Univariate Analysis**
> We will present the number and percent of subjects who refused and were excluded (Table 10.5). We will calculate the number and percent of those with large and small hemorrhage size as well as the mean and SD of hemorrhage size (Table 10.6) as well as the number and percent of patients with 3-month mortality (Table 10.7).

TABLE 10.5 Response rates; Project Health, 2010–2011

	N	%
Original study sample	N	%
Refused		
Excluded	N	%
Age <60 years	N	%
Prior hemorrhage	N	%
Nonwhite ethnicity	N	%
Lost to follow-up	N	%
Final study sample	N	%

TABLE 10.6 Distribution of hemorrhage size; Project Health, 2010–2011

HEMORRHAGE SIZE	TOTAL	
Categorical		
Small	N	%
Large	N	%
Total	N	%
Continuous	Mean	SD

TABLE 10.7 Distribution of 3-month mortality; Project Health, 2010–2011

3-MONTH MORTALITY	N	%
Yes	N	%
No	N	%
Total	N	%

10.3.2 Bivariate Analysis Plan

A bivariate analysis plan is typically only relevant for proposals with analytic aims. The goal of the bivariate analysis plan is to cross-classify two variables:

- To assess if your exposure is related to your outcome variable **prior** *to* adjusting for any confounding factors (e.g., unadjusted analysis)
- To assess if covariates are related to your exposure and outcome variables (e.g., to assess for the presence of confounding)

The statistics you choose for the bivariate plan will depend upon the parameterization of your exposure and outcome variables:

- To cross-classify categorical variables
  - Chi-square test or Fisher's exact test (if small sample size) and corresponding p-values
- To cross-classify continuous variables
  - If normally distributed: e.g., t-tests or ANOVA or Pearson correlations and corresponding p-values
  - If not normally distributed: e.g., Wilcoxon rank-sum tests or Spearman correlations and corresponding p-values

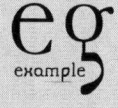

> *example*
>
> Continuing our prior example of a proposal to evaluate the association between hemorrhage size and mortality; the exposure is considered both as a categorical dichotomous variable (i.e., small vs. large hemorrhage size) and a continuous variable. The outcome is a dichotomous variable (3-month mortality—yes or no). The covariates to be considered are age and ancestry.
>
> **Data Analysis Plan**
> *Specific Aim #1. To evaluate the association between hemorrhage size and risk of 3-month mortality*
> **Bivariate Analysis**
> We will evaluate the unadjusted relationship between our exposure (hemorrhage size) and our outcome (3-month mortality) by cross-tabulating these variables (Table 10.8). We will then assess covariates as potential confounders by cross-tabulating them with both the exposure (Table 10.9) and outcome variables (Table 10.10).

TABLE 10.8 Distribution of hemorrhage size according to the 3-month mortality; Project Health, 2010–2011

	3-MONTH MORTALITY		
HEMORRHAGE SIZE	YES	NO	p-VALUE[a]
Categorical			
Small	N (%)	N (%)	
Large	N (%)	N (%)	
Total	N (%)	N (%)	
Continuous	Mean (SD)	Mean (SD)	

[a] p-values derived from chi-square tests for categorical variables and from two sample t-tests for continuous variables.

TABLE 10.9 Distribution of covariates according to hemorrhage size; Project Health, 2010–2011

	HEMORRHAGE SIZE		
CHARACTERISTICS	LARGE	SMALL	p-VALUE[a]
Age	mean (SD)	mean (SD)	
Ancestry			
S. European	N (%)	N (%)	
Scandinavian	N (%)	N (%)	
Other white	N (%)	N (%)	
Nonwhite	N (%)	N (%)	

[a] p-values derived from chi-square tests for categorical variables and from two-sample t-tests for continuous variables.

TABLE 10.10 Distribution of covariates according to 3-month mortality; Project Health, 2010–2011

	3-MONTH MORTALITY		
CHARACTERISTICS	YES	NO	p-VALUE[a]
Age	Mean (SD)	Mean (SD)	
Ancestry			
S. European	N (%)	N (%)	
Scandinavian	N (%)	N (%)	
Other white	N (%)	N (%)	
Nonwhite	N (%)	N (%)	

[a] p-values derived from chi-square tests for categorical variables and from two-sample t-tests for continuous variables.

> Chi-square tests will be used to calculate p-values for categorical variables. For tables with small cell frequencies, Fisher's exact tests will be used. For continuous variables, p-values will be derived from two sample t-tests.

10.3.3 Multivariable Analysis Plan

A multivariable analysis plan is only relevant for proposals with analytic aims and is typically the focal point of the analysis plan for such aims. The multivariable analysis plan should

- A. Select an appropriate **model**
- B. Specify how the model will adjust for **potential confounding factors** (i.e., covariates)
- C. Specify how you will evaluate **potential effect modifiers** (i.e., interaction) if *a priori* included as a specific aim

10.3.3.1 A. Select an appropriate model

The type of multivariable analysis that you will propose depends upon the parameterization of your outcome variable. In addition, each model requires a set of **assumptions** that you will want to discuss with a statistician. Below is a list of some of the most common multivariable models:

- If your outcome variable is dichotomous:
  - Multiple logistic regression and corresponding odds ratio (OR) and 95% CI
- If your outcome variable is categorical with more than two categories:
  - Multinomial logistic regression and corresponding OR and 95% CI
- If your outcome variable is continuous:
  - Multiple linear regression and corresponding beta coefficient and standard error (SE)
- If your outcome variable is time to an event:
  - Cox proportional hazards models and corresponding hazards ratio (HR) and 95% CI
- If your outcome variable is count data:
  - Poisson regression and corresponding rate ratio (RR) and 95% CI

In general, **dichotomous outcome variables** tend to be the most common in epidemiology and preventive medicine as we are often evaluating the incidence of disease diagnosis (e.g., diabetes diagnosis: yes or no), and therefore many proposals will propose to use multiple logistic regression. The multiple logistic regression model will generate an OR and corresponding 95% CI. The OR can be used as an approximation of the RR in certain contexts.

Continuous outcomes are also fairly common (e.g., weight, blood pressure, cholesterol levels) and therefore it is also common to see multiple linear regression models. Linear regression requires that the outcome variable be normally distributed or be transformed to be normally distributed. The linear regression model will generate a beta coefficient and a corresponding SE and p-value. The beta coefficient can be interpreted as the expected mean difference in the outcome variable given a unit change in your exposure variable; for example, the mean difference in blood pressure with each year increase in age.

A potential pitfall to avoid As you will note in the table above, the scale of your **outcome** variable dictates the type of regression model that you will propose use. It is common to become confused on this point and believe that the scale of the exposure variable dictates this choice. However, that is not correct. For example, a logistic regression model for a dichotomous outcome, such as diagnosis of diabetes, can include all scales of exposure and covariate variables including continuous variables (e.g., total calories) and dichotomous variables (e.g., gender: male, female).

10.3.3.2 B. Specify how the model will adjust for potential confounding factors (i.e., covariates)

There are many techniques for regression model building and your proposal should delineate a thoughtful plan for how potential confounding variables (which you listed in the Covariate Assessment section) will be considered. The goal of this analysis plan is to evaluate the independent impact of your exposure on your outcome while adjusting for **potential confounding factors** (i.e., covariates).

A statistician will be an excellent resource in this area, as will be the state of the science in your proposed topic of interest. In general, however, epidemiologists and researchers in preventive medicine tend to rely less upon *automated* forward- and backward-selection model building approaches. These techniques rely more heavily on p-values for inclusion of particular covariates in the model as opposed to an understanding of the underlying physiology. You may recall that p-values are influenced by many factors including the size of the study and the variability of your exposure of interest. Instead, epidemiologists and those in preventive medicine usually take an approach that puts a greater emphasis on biological mechanisms as well as **prior established risk factors** for their outcome of interest. Your summary table of the prior epidemiologic literature (created as part of Chapter 4, *Conducting the Literature Search*) will come in handy in identifying risk factors that prior studies included in their models.

Stratification is a technique to assess confounding. It involves comparing the measures of association in the overall sample (the crude estimate) to those same measures of association within strata of a possible confounder. If the stratified measures of association are similar to each other, but different from the overall sample, it suggests that the factor is a confounder and should be addressed using, for example, the additional techniques outlined below.

Many investigators propose to include covariates in their models that they find to be statistically significantly **associated with both their exposure and outcome** variables of interest in bivariate analysis. The data analysis plan would propose to cross-tabulate the potential confounding variables by the exposure and then by the outcome variables. Remember that to qualify as a confounder, the variable has to be independently associated with the exposure as well as the outcome and not be on the causal pathway between the exposure and outcome.

An approach commonly used in epidemiology and preventive medicine is the **change-in-estimate** method of covariate selection. In this method, a potential confounder is included in the model if it changes the coefficient, or effect estimate, of the primary exposure variable by 10%. This method has been shown to produce more reliable models than variable selection methods based on statistical significance.

Directed acyclic graphs. Directed acyclic graphs (DAGs) have recently been used in medical research. They are a set of arrows drawn along a timeline, characterizing causal and temporal relationships between variables (Figure 10.1). These diagrams are a quick, visual way to assess confounding that can aid in variable selection and can complement the above more traditional methods of evaluating confounding.

A potential pitfall to avoid One important point to keep in mind is that the ability to control for covariates will be limited in part by your proposed sample size. A multivariable regression model adjusting for many covariates may not run successfully in the scenario of a smaller sample size. Therefore, it will be important that your proposal outline a clear plan for thoughtful inclusion of covariates, recognizing this limitation. In addition, adjusting for many covariates can reduce your statistical power to detect an association even if it truly exists. Therefore, depending upon your calculated statistical power, you may consider only including those covariates that are found to be confounding variables within your dataset regardless of findings in the prior literature. Or, you could consider only including the major established risk factors for your outcome.

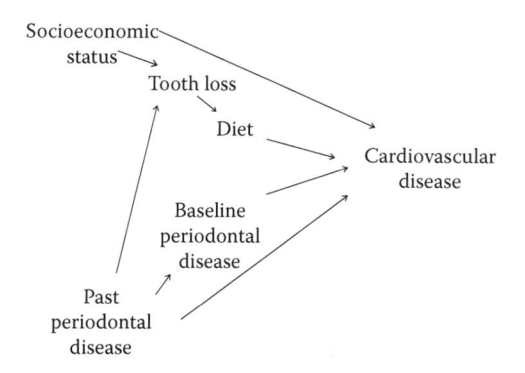

FIGURE 10.1 Example directed acyclic graph (DAG).

TABLE 10.11 Unadjusted and multivariable RR and 95% CI of 3-month mortality by hemorrhage size; Project Health, 2010–2011

	CASES		UNADJUSTED		MULTIVARIABLE[a]	
	N	%	RR	95% CI	RR	95% CI
Hemorrhage size						
Small	N	%	1.0	Referent	1.0	Referent
Large	N	%	RR	95% CI	RR	95% CI

[a] Multivariable model includes age, ancestry, and location of hemorrhage.

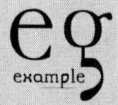

---

eg *example*

Continuing our prior example of a proposal to evaluate the association between hemorrhage size and mortality:

Data Analysis Plan
Specific Aim #1: To evaluate the association between hemorrhage size and risk of 3-month mortality
Multivariable Analysis
Multiple logistic regression will be used to model the relation between hemorrhage size and 3-month mortality (Table 10.11). Those covariates that caused a 10% change in the coefficient for hemorrhage size will be considered confounding factors and included in the model. Because prior studies have shown location of hemorrhage to be strongly associated with mortality, we will also include this variable in the model. We will calculate unadjusted and multivariable RRs and 95% CIs.

10.3.3.3 C. Specify how you will evaluate potential effect modifiers

You may be interested in determining whether the relationship between your exposure and your outcome is consistent or different across levels of **potential effect modifiers** (i.e., interaction). Often, there is confusion between confounding and effect modification. Confounding is considered a *nuisance factor* that can be reduced via study design techniques and with careful multivariable modeling. In contrast, effect modifier reflects a different physiological association between your exposure and outcome variables of interest across subgroups and should be highlighted. Therefore, the data analysis plan for each is different. The concepts of confounding are discussed in more detail in Chapter 12, *Review of Bias and Confounding*.

In the data analysis plan, one standard approach for evaluating effect modification is to propose to include multiplicative interaction terms in the multivariable models and assess their statistical significance. If the terms are statistically significant, then you would propose to repeat your multivariable analysis within strata of potential effect modifiers.

A potential pitfall to avoid   As mentioned in Chapter 6, *Specific Aims*, if you are proposing to evaluate the presence of effect modification (i.e., interaction), it is important to include this *a priori* as a study aim or hypothesis. This will help to assure your reviewers that you will not be *data dredging* for statistically significant findings if you fail to observe an overall association between your exposure and outcome of interest.

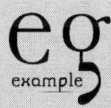

> **example** Continuing our prior example of a proposal designed to evaluate the association between hemorrhage size and mortality:
>
> **Data Analysis Plan**
> *Specific Aim #2. To assess if the association between hemorrhage size and 3-month mortality differs according to gender*
> **Multivariable Analysis—Continued**
> To assess whether gender modifies the relationship between hemorrhage size and 3-month mortality, we will include an interaction term (gender x hemorrhage size) in a multivariable logistic model. If this term is statistically significant at $p < 0.05$, we will present results (RR and 95% CIs) for men and women separately (Table 10.12).
>
> **TABLE 10.12** Multivariable RR and 95% CI of 3-month mortality by hemorrhage size according to gender; Project Health, 2010–2011
>
> | | CASES | | UNADJUSTED | | MULTIVARIABLE[a] | |
> |---|---|---|---|---|---|---|
> | GENDER | N | % | RR | 95% CI | RR | 95% CI |
> | Females (n = x) | | | | | | |
> | Small hemorrhage size | N | % | 1.0 | Referent | 1.0 | Referent |
> | Large hemorrhage size | N | % | RR | 95% CI | RR | 95% CI |
> | Males (n = x) | | | | | | |
> | Small hemorrhage size | N | % | 1.0 | Referent | 1.0 | Referent |
> | Large hemorrhage size | N | % | RR | 95% CI | RR | 95% CI |
>
> [a] Multivariable model includes age, ancestry, and location of hemorrhage.

10.3.4 Exploratory Data Analyses

The decision to include exploratory data analyses depends upon whether you have decided to include exploratory aims in your specific aims (see Chapter 6, *Specific Aims*). This is not to say that you cannot include exploratory analyses but instead that they need to be tied to exploratory aims or hypotheses.

10.3.5 Mock Tables

Mock tables are tables, such as those included in this chapter, which do not contain data but are otherwise complete with titles, row, and column headings. The process of creating such tables is useful regardless of whether you are writing a dissertation proposal or a grant proposal. However, simply due to the restrictive page requirements of grant proposals, mock tables are typically only included in the body of dissertation proposals. However, for both a dissertation and grant, you will be glad you have these tables once your proposal is approved and you have generated your data.

Mock tables provide a *home* for all the results generated by your proposed data analysis. Creating these mock tables now, at the proposal writing stage, will save you time later after your proposal has been approved and you have conducted your data analysis.

More importantly, the process of creating mock tables will crystallize your understanding of your data analysis plan—making it concrete. You will be able to visualize the statistics that your data analysis plan will generate and whether the plan is feasible. The process of creating mock tables, therefore, may lead you to revise and refine your specific aims and perhaps even your study design.

For example, if you find yourself generating multiple tables to house the data for one aim, you may decide that this aim is too broad. Broadly defined aims are one of the most common mistakes of early-career investigators. On the other hand, having little data to present in a table might indicate that your aims are too narrow or that your data collection plan is inadequate.

Creating mock tables also helps to firm up the dissertation proposal as a *contract* between you and your dissertation committee. By having the committee *sign off* on these tables, you help to reduce the risk of requests for additional ad hoc analyses.

A pitfall to avoid If you are including mock tables in the data analysis plan, you should refer to these by table number within the data analysis text (see the examples throughout this chapter). Do not fall into the trap of only including mock tables without a corresponding narrative in your data analysis plan. Without such a narrative, the reader will not know how your analysis plan corresponds to the mock tables.

10.4 PART III: BEST PRACTICES

In addition to your proposed plan to address your specific aims, reviewers will be looking for evidence of *best practices* in your data analysis plan. Most typically, these include plans to address

1. Model assumptions
2. Model diagnostics
3. Missing data
4. Multiple comparisons
5. Sensitivity analyses to address potential biases

Model Assumptions
All regression models have underlying assumptions and the proposal should note how you will ensure that these assumptions are met. For example, there are four principal assumptions that justify the use of linear regression models for purposes of prediction. These include linearity of the relationship between dependent and independent variables along with such issues as independence of the errors, constant variance of the errors, and normality of the error distribution. If any of these assumptions are violated, then the findings generated by the model may be biased or misleading. A statistician can assist you in describing how model assumptions will be addressed.

Model Diagnostics
Once a regression model has been constructed, the proposal should briefly describe techniques to determine how well the model fits the data. The techniques vary according to the type of regression model that you propose to utilize (e.g., linear, logistic) and include such techniques as Hosmer–Lemeshow goodness-of-fit tests, R-squared (R^2) statistics, likelihood ratio test statistics, and ROC curves.

Missing Data
Missing data are issues faced by nearly all studies in epidemiology and preventive medicine. It is important that your proposal address, even briefly, how you plan to address missing data. There are a variety of approaches available, and a statistician can assist you in selecting which approach best fits your proposed dataset.

Simply excluding those with missing data may raise reviewer concerns about biased estimates or reduced power to detect your association of interest. Other approaches fill in or *impute* missing values. A variety of imputation approaches are available and range from extremely simple to rather complex depending upon the reasons for the missing data and whether you anticipate that it will be missing at random. Imputation methods retain your full sample size, which can be advantageous in terms of reducing potential for bias and increasing precision; however, they can yield different kinds of bias themselves.

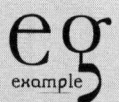

> **eg** *example*
>
> Imagine a proposal to conduct a cohort study:
>
> Accounting for Missing Data: Although every effort will be made to avoid missing data, participants with missing data will be compared to participants with complete data to describe potential bias due to differential loss of data. We will also explore methods for imputing missing data, using propensity score multiple imputation techniques, and apply these in the presence of incomplete and missing data.

Multiple Comparisons
Multiple comparisons arise when a statistical analysis encompasses a number of formal comparisons, with the presumption that attention will focus on only the strongest differences among all comparisons that are made. For example, the practice of considering a large number of variables, without thought, as potential exposures,

confounders, or effect modifiers may raise reviewer concern that some variables will appear to be statistically significant based on chance alone. This limitation is termed *multiple comparisons*. Techniques have been developed to control the false-positive error rate associated with performing multiple statistical tests and should be addressed in a proposal if multiple comparisons are proposed. Alternatively, careful consideration of the biologic plausibility of observed findings can also be proposed.

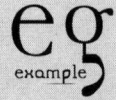

> **eg** *example*
> Multiple Comparisons: It is also important to note that we cannot rule out chance as explanation for the observed positive findings given the multiple comparisons performed. We will address this issue by carefully considering the biologic rationale of any observed associations.

Sensitivity Analyses to Address Potential Biases
Sensitivity analyses can be included in a data analysis plan to address potential biases. See Chapter 12, *Review of Bias and Confounding*, for a listing of sources of potential bias.

Outlining such sensitivity analyses, along with their rationale, in the data analysis plan will help assure the reviewers that you have a plan to address potential biases in your proposal. For a graduate student, carefully spelling out these sensitivity analyses shows your committee the full breadth of work that you will be conducting and again helps to avoid *ad hoc* analyses that might be suggested later.

Examples of sensitivity analyses to address potential bias:

- Comparing characteristics of participants to nonparticipants
- Comparing characteristics of participants lost to follow-up vs. not lost to follow-up
- Comparing baseline characteristics of each arm in a randomized trial
- Comparing characteristics of cases vs. controls

Comparing characteristics of **participants vs. nonparticipants** can help to detect the presence and potential magnitude of selection bias. The data analysis plan would simply propose to cross-classify participants vs. nonparticipants according to covariates (i.e., using the statistical techniques described above in *bivariate analysis*). However, it is important to note that with HIPAA protections regarding Protective Health Information (PHI), such detailed data on nonparticipants may not be available to you.

> **eg** *example*
> We will present the characteristics of participants as compared to nonparticipants (Table 10.13).

TABLE 10.13 Characteristics of respondents vs. nonrespondents; Project Health, 2010–2011

CHARACTERISTICS	PARTICIPANTS	NONPARTICIPANTS	p-VALUE[a]
Sample size	N (%)	N (%)	
Age	Mean (SD)	Mean (SD)	
Ancestry			
S. European	N (%)	N (%)	
Scandinavian	N (%)	N (%)	
Other white	N (%)	N (%)	
Nonwhite	N (%)	N (%)	

[a] p-values derived from chi-square tests for categorical variables and from two-sample t-tests for continuous variables.

Comparing the baseline characteristics of those **lost to follow-up vs. those not lost to follow-up**, in the context of a cohort study, would help to address the presence and potential magnitude of selection bias (also termed differential loss to follow-up and described in detail in Chapter 12, *Review of Bias and Confounding*).

Comparing the baseline characteristics of each study arm in a randomized trial will help to assess whether the randomization was successful.

Comparing the characteristic of **cases vs. controls**, in the context of a case–control study, can help to assess whether the control population adequately represents the source population that led to the cases. Remember not to include your exposure of interest in this table, as you would not want or expect it to be similar between the two groups. Instead, evaluating whether the exposure odds differ between the cases and controls addresses the primary aim of a case–control study.

10.5 EXAMPLE DATA ANALYSIS PLAN FOR A DISSERTATION PROPOSAL

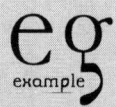

> **e.g. example**
>
> **A Proposal to Examine the Association between Psychosocial Stress and Hypertensive Disorders of Pregnancy: Data Analysis Plan**
>
> [The variable categorization table for this proposal (Table 10.14) also appears in Chapter 9, *Study Design and Methods*]
>
> *Data Analysis Plan*
> *Specific Aim #1: We propose to evaluate the association between early pregnancy stress levels and risk of hypertensive disorders of pregnancy in a population of Latina women.*

Univariate Analysis
The number and percent of subjects included in the study population prior to exclusions will be presented (Table 10.15), as well as the distribution of early pregnancy stress (Table 10.16) and the distribution of hypertensive disorders of pregnancy (Table 10.17).

Bivariate Analysis
Covariates will be cross-tabulated with outcome (Table 10.18) and exposure variables (Table 10.19) to evaluate potential confounders. Cross-tabulations will be evaluated through the chi-square test to determine whether the observed distribution fits the expected distribution when the cell size is sufficient. When the cell size is not sufficient, Fisher's exact test will be used to evaluate whether the observed distribution fits the expected distribution. p-values reflecting the differences in distributions will be presented for all of the covariates. We will use a DAG to examine the relationships between the covariates and the exposure and outcome.

Multivariable Analysis
We will model the relationship between early pregnancy stress and hypertensive disorders of pregnancy (Table 10.20) using multivariable logistic regression. ORs and 95% CI will compare participants with high levels of stress to those with low levels of stress. Additionally, we will run the model with stress scores entered continuously to evaluate a dose-response relationship.

Confounders will be evaluated by running all models with and without the suspected confounder. Any covariate that changes the estimate for early pregnancy stress by 10% or greater will be retained in the model as a confounder.

Sensitivity Analysis to Address Potential Bias
We will compare characteristics of women missing delivery information to those with complete delivery information to determine whether there are any significant differences between these groups (Table 10.21).

TABLE 10.14 Variable categorization table; Salud Study (n = 2300), 2004–2009

NAME	DESCRIPTION	TYPE
Outcome variables		
HDIS	Hypertensive disorder of pregnancy 0 = no 1 = yes	Dichotomous
PREEC	Preeclampsia 0 = no 1 = yes	Dichotomous
GHTN	Gestational hypertension 0 = no 1 = yes	Dichotomous
Exposure variables		
ESTRESS1	Early pregnancy stress 0 = low stress, at or below median I = high stress, above median	Dichotomous
ESTRESS	Early pregnancy stress 1–14	Continuous
Covariates		
AGECAT2	Age at enrollment in study 1 = 15–19 2 = 20–24 3 = 25–29 4 = 30–40	Categorical
BMIC	Prepregnancy BMI, IOM categories 1 = BMI < 19.8 2 = BMI 19.8–26.0 3 = BMI > 26.0–29.0 4 = BMI ≥ 29.0	Categorical
EDUGRP	Education groups 1 = less than high school 2 = high school/trade or technical school 3 = at least some college experience	Categorical
INCGRP	Income groups 1 = ≤$15,000 2 = >$15,000–30,000 3 = > $30,000 4 = "missing" 5 = "refused/don't know"	Categorical

(continued)

TABLE 10.14 (continued) Variable categorization table; Salud Study (n = 2300), 2004–2009

NAME	DESCRIPTION	TYPE
BRTHPLAC	Birthplace 1 = United States 2 = others	Dichotomous
LANG2	0 = English only 1 = both Spanish and English 2 = Spanish only	Categorical
PARCAT	Number of live births 1 = 0 births 2 = 1 live birth 3 = ≥ 2 live births	Categorical

TABLE 10.15 Response Rates; Salud Study (n = 2300), 2004–2009

	N	%
Original Study Sample		
Refused		
Excluded		
<16 years or > #42 years		
Multiple gestation		
Preexisting disease		
Preterm birth		
Spontaneous abortion		
Final study sample		

TABLE 10.16 Distribution of early pregnancy perceived stress among study participants; Salud Study (n = 2300), 2004–2009

	N	%
Perceived stress		
Low		
High		
	Mean	SD
Perceived stress (continuous score)		

TABLE 10.17 Distribution of hypertensive disorders of pregnancy among study participants; Salud Study (n = 2300), 2004–2009

	N	%
Hypertensive disorder		
Yes		
No		
Total		

TABLE 10.18 Distribution of covariates according to hypertensive disorders of pregnancy; Salud Study (n = 2300), 2004–2009

	\multicolumn{4}{c}{HYPERTENSIVE DISORDER OF PREGNANCY}	
	YES N	YES %	NO N	NO %	p-VALUE
Age					
15–19					
20–24					
25–29					
30–40					
Prepregnancy BMI					
<19.8					
19.8–26.0					
>26.0–29.0					
≥29.0					
Education					
Less than H.S.					
H.S./trade/tech. school					
Some college					
Income					
≤$15,000					
$15–29,999					
≥$30,000					
Birthplace					
United States					
Other					
Language preference					
English only					
Both Spanish and English					
Spanish only					
Parity					
0 live births					
1 live birth					
≥2 live births					

TABLE 10.19 Distribution of covariates according to early pregnancy stress; Salud Study (n = 2300), 2004–2009

| | PERCEIVED STRESS |||| |
| | HIGH || LOW || |
	N	%	N	%	p-VALUE
Age					
15–19					
20–24					
25–29					
30–40					
Prepregnancy BMI					
<19.8					
19.8–26.0					
>26.0–29.0					
≥29.0					
Education					
Less than H.S.					
H.S./trade/tech. school					
Some college					
Income					
≤$15,000					
$15–29,999					
≥$30,000					
Birthplace					
United States					
Others					
Language preference					
English only					
Both Spanish and English					
Spanish only					
Parity					
0 live births					
1 live birth					
≥2 live births					

TABLE 10.20 ORs of hypertensive disorders of pregnancy by early pregnancy perceived stress; Salud Study (n = 2300), 2004–2009

	CASES		UNADJUSTED		MULTIVARIABLE	
	No	%	OR	95% CI	OR	95% CI
Hypertensive disorders						
Low perceived stress			1.0	Referent	1.0	Referent
High perceived stress						
			$p_{trend} =$		$p_{trend} =$	
Continuous perceived stress						

TABLE 10.21 Characteristics of participants according to presence of delivery information; Salud Study (n = 2300), 2004–2009

	\multicolumn{4}{c}{DELIVERY INFORMATION}	
	\multicolumn{2}{c}{NOT MISSING}	\multicolumn{2}{c}{MISSING}	
	N	%	N	%	p-VALUE
Age					
15–19					
20–24					
25–29					
30–40					
Prepregnancy BMI					
<19.8					
19.8–26.0					
>26.0–29.0					
≥29.0					
Education					
Less than H.S.					
H.S./trade/tech. school					
Some college					
Income					
≤$15,000					
$15–29,999					
≥$30,000					
Birthplace					
United States					
Others					
Language preference					
English only					
Both Spanish and English					
Spanish only					
Parity					
0 live births					
1 live birth					
≥2 live births					

Power and Sample Size 11

Power is a critical component of any proposal. In my role as a member of an NIH review panel, I was surprised to see how many proposals, including those submitted by senior investigators, failed to include a Power and Sample Size section. Alternatively, some proposals included power for some, but not all, of their specific aims. Failing to include power calculations is often considered a **fatal flaw** by a grant review panel and is one of the most common reasons for reviewers to streamline (e.g., triage) a proposal (see Chapter 19, *Review Process*).

This chapter is designed to give you an applied view of power for the most common study designs in epidemiology and preventive medicine: cohort studies, cross-sectional studies, and unmatched case–control studies. The chapter discusses the factors that influence power, the study design strategies that you can use to maximize your power, user-friendly approaches to calculating power, and how to best display your power calculations in a proposal. Throughout the chapter, I include annotated examples with strategies and tips.

Finally, it is important to note that this chapter is not designed to take the place of a power and sample size chapter in a statistics textbook. In writing a proposal in epidemiology and preventive medicine, it is always best to consult with a statistician, statistical consulting center, or data analysis core for the sections on power and sample size. This chapter will make you an informed participant in that conversation.

11.1 TIMELINE

As noted in Chapter 1, *Ten Top Tips for Successful Proposal Writing*, after drafting your aims, the next step in the proposal writing process is to calculate your statistical power to achieve these aims. This will help you to answer the question, "Will your sample size provide you with sufficient power to detect a difference between groups, if there is truly a difference?"

FIGURE 11.1 Possible study outcomes.

Investigator's decision	Reality: Groups are not different	Reality: Groups are different
Conclude that groups are not different	Correct decision	Type II error probability = beta
Conclude that groups are different	Type I error probability = alpha	Correct decision probability = 1− beta (power)

11.2 WHAT IS POWER?

Power is the probability of statistically detecting a difference between groups when a difference indeed exists. For the purposes of proposals in epidemiology and preventive medicine, power is most often the likelihood of observing a statistically significant difference in an **outcome** between an **exposed** and **unexposed** group, when there is indeed a difference. So, even the most beautifully designed proposal will be irrelevant if it can't detect what it is designed to detect.

In Figure 11.1, *reality* reflects what truly exists while *investigator's decision* reflects the decision that you as an investigator will make based on your observed findings.

Focusing on the last column of Figure 11.1, you will see that there are two possibilities when the groups are, in reality, truly different. We might conclude, in error, that the groups do not differ (*type II error*). Or we might conclude, correctly, that the groups differ (*power*). This probability, 1− beta, is the power of our study. In epidemiology and preventive medicine, power of 80% is generally considered acceptable. In other words, your proposal should have **at least 80% power** to detect a difference between exposed and unexposed groups if it indeed exists.

11.3 KEY CHARACTERISTICS OF POWER

There are several key principles to be cognizant of when calculating power.

- Key characteristic #1: The larger the sample size, the larger the power.
  In other words, simply due to the fact that you have more people in your study, and therefore greater precision to estimate an effect, you will be more likely to detect a difference between groups given that there truly is a difference. This does not mean, however, that the effect that you detect will be

clinically significant but simply that you will be able to detect even small differences between exposure groups.
- Key characteristic #2: The larger the true difference between groups, the easier it will be to have power to detect it.

It is always easier to detect large differences between groups than small differences. Therefore, power increases as the expected true differences between groups get larger. Vice versa, power decreases as the differences between groups get smaller. In other words, it is always harder to find a needle in a haystack than an elephant in the room.

11.4 WHEN IS IT OK NOT TO INCLUDE A POWER OR SAMPLE SIZE CALCULATION?

The typical purpose of a feasibility study, or pilot study, is to generate rates upon which you will base subsequent power calculations for the purposes of a larger proposal. For example, feasibility studies are critical in generating anticipated recruitment rates, eligibility rates, and retention rates—all necessary for subsequent power calculations. Therefore, including a statement in your proposal reminding the reviewers that you have not included power calculations because this is a pilot/feasibility study is usually sufficient.

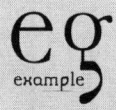

> **eg** *example*
>
> **A Feasibility Study for a Behavioral Intervention**
>
> Specific Aim #1: Assess process measures related to the administration of the intervention. These include the rates of recruitment and rates of follow-up.
>
> **Corresponding section on power:** Findings from this pilot study will serve as the basis for power calculations to support a larger prospective cohort study designed to investigate the effects of iron levels on diabetes risk in older Asians.

A potential pitfall to avoid
As a graduate student or an early-career investigator, you will often find yourself proposing to conduct a secondary data analysis of an **existing dataset**. Some investigators may inadvertently believe that because their sample already exists, and their sample size is *fixed*, they do not have to include a section on Power and Sample Size. However, even if you are using an existing dataset (e.g., NHANES, NHIS, or BRFSS), it is still critical to include a Power and Sample Size section. This section will tell the reviewers, for the purposes of your analysis, how many participants will have complete data on your key variables of interest and whether you will be making additional exclusions to the dataset. If you are proposing to

use data from an **ongoing** study, and are relying upon future participant recruitment, it will be even more important to include a section on sample size as your power to make meaningful inferences will depend upon the success of those future projected recruitment and retention rates.

11.5 STEP #1: ESTIMATE YOUR SAMPLE SIZE

Your proposed sample size will be one of the primary factors influencing the costs of conducting your study as it is associated with so many aspects of study operations (e.g., number of participant incentives, number of assays to be run). Also, ask yourself whether it is feasible to actually recruit this number of participants. For example, if you are proposing to conduct a hospital-based study, find out if the hospital actually sees that number of patients per day/week/year? Are that many patients likely to be eligible *and* agree to participate? Such questions of feasibility can be answered by your own preliminary work, that of your coinvestigators, or that by other investigators at your proposed study site.

Therefore, the Sample Size section of the proposal should include your projected eligibility, recruitment, and retention rates as well as your final expected sample size for analysis. A corresponding Table 11.1 can be included as well.

11.5.1 Basis for Sample Size Estimation

In proposals to conduct a new study and recruit new participants, you will likely not yet know all these figures in Table 11.1. However, for the purposes of ensuring feasibility, it will be critical to estimate these numbers in the section on Sample Size.

Such estimation can be based on

- Your own pilot study or one conducted by your research team
- Prior studies published in the literature

TABLE 11.1 To estimate your sample size, you will need to project the number of:

- Eligible participants
- Those who will agree to participate
- Participants who will remain at the end of follow-up (if a prospective study)
- Participants who will have complete data for analysis

The ideal option is listed first. A **pilot study**, at the same study site as your proposal, will be the best way to assure the reviewers that you have a well-grounded basis for your expected recruitment and retention rates and therefore the corresponding sample size. This highlights the need, as discussed in Chapter 1, *Ten Top Tips for Successful Proposal Writing*, to conduct a pilot or feasibility study prior to proposing a larger grant.

However, if such pilot data are not available, there are still reasonable alternatives. Prior studies conducted by your research team including your coinvestigators and/or mentor can also provide evidence to support your proposed rates. Ideally, these prior studies were conducted at your study site, but if not, then clarify in the proposal how you expect the rates might change in your own setting.

Finally, if prior studies by your research team are not available, then look to the prior literature. Base your recruitment and retention rates upon a published study at a site as similar as possible to your own in terms of sociodemographic status and other key variables.

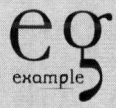

> **eg** *example*
>
> **Imagine a proposal to assemble a prospective cohort of older Asian patients:**
>
> Proposed Sample Size: Taylor Health Clinic sees approximately 4040 patients per year, of which approximately 37% are older Asians (>50 years of age). We expect 1495 (85.7%) of older Asians to agree to participate, 1181 (79% of those who agree) to be eligible, 1075 (91% of eligible participants) to be followed through the end of the study, and valid questionnaires to be completed by 1000 (93% of the final sample). The above rates are based on (1) recruitment figures observed in prior studies conducted among the older Asian population at Taylor Hospital and (2) the rates reported by a prior study conducted in a similar setting.[1]

11.6 STEP #2: CHOOSE USER-FRIENDLY SOFTWARE TO CALCULATE POWER

There are several software packages commonly used by investigators in epidemiology and preventive medicine to calculate power, some of which are free and publically available.

Examples of free software packages include the following:

- EpiInfo—available for download on the CDC website (www.cdc.gov/epiinfo/). The software has a *statcalc* function that includes power calculations for typical study designs in epidemiology and preventive medicine.
- G*Power (www.psycho.uni-duesseldorf.de/aap/projects/gpower).

Examples of software *not* currently free of charge include the following:

- PASS software (http://www.ncss.com/) from NCSS statistical software
- nQuery Advisor software (http://www.statistical-solutions-software.com/nquery-advisor-nterim/)
- Statistical analysis software such as SAS (www.SAS.com) to calculate power

These software packages take the intimidation factor out of power calculations. With this software in hand, you will be empowered to *play* with your power calculations. The programs let you experiment with different *inputs* (e.g., projected sample size and anticipated outcome rates). By experimenting with these *inputs*, you will observe the impact on your subsequent power and sample size needs. In this way, such software not only facilitates the calculation of your power but can provide vital information on the robustness of your intended inferences.

11.7 STEP #3: REMIND YOURSELF OF YOUR MEASURE OF ASSOCIATION

The type of test that you will use to calculate power will depend upon the measure of association that you proposed to calculate in your Data Analysis section.

Below are two common measures of association in epidemiology and preventive medicine. Look back at your Data Analysis section and remind yourself of the measure you selected to calculate:

A. **Ratio measures of association:** Measures of association in which relative differences between groups are being compared
   i.e., If your outcome is dichotomous and you proposed to calculate odds ratios (ORs) (e.g., via logistic regression)
B. **Difference measures of association:** Measures of association in which absolute differences between groups are being compared
   i.e., If your outcome of interest is continuous and you proposed to calculate mean absolute differences between exposed and unexposed groups (e.g., via linear regression)

In general, **dichotomous outcomes** tend to be the most common in epidemiology and preventive medicine as we are often comparing the incidence of disease diagnosis (e.g., diabetes diagnosis: yes or no) between exposed and unexposed groups. For these proposals, your measure of association will typically be a ratio such as a relative risk (RR) (i.e., an OR, rate ratio, or risk ratio).

Continuous outcomes are also fairly common. For these proposals, your measure of association will typically be mean differences in an outcome variable (e.g., fasting glucose levels, blood pressure, cholesterol levels) between exposed and unexposed groups.

11.8 STEP #4: CALCULATE AND PRESENT YOUR POWER FOR RATIO MEASURES OF ASSOCIATION (i.e., RELATIVE RISKS)

The following sections will focus on the data that you will need to gather to use the typical power software packages for RRs (e.g., risk ratios, rate ratios, ORs).

An RR is a comparison of proportions between groups. To detect this difference in proportions between an exposed and unexposed group, power is typically based on a **chi-square test**.

The *inputs* that you will need to enter into the software package will vary according to your proposed study design. The sections below are divided into **cohort study and cross-sectional study and unmatched case–control study**.

11.8.1 A. For Cohort and Cross-Sectional Studies

For all study designs, the generally accepted confidence level is 95% (Table 11.2). If you are using an existing dataset, you can calculate the *ratio of unexposed to exposed* directly from the dataset. If not, the best approach is to use data from a pilot study or find prior literature that evaluated your exposure of interest. Note that relevant studies only need to have evaluated your exposure of interest—regardless of whether they evaluated your outcome of interest. In searching the prior literature, prioritize studies with a study population and setting most similar to your own.

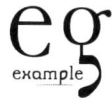

eg example Imagine a proposal to conduct a study of iron levels measured via serum ferritin (i.e., your exposure of interest) and risk of type 2 diabetes (i.e., your outcome of interest) in older Asians in Washington State. You plan to categorize participants as having high or low ferritin levels according to a national standard. To determine your anticipated ratio of exposed to unexposed, you would search the prior literature for studies of the distribution of serum ferritin among older Asian adults in Washington State. If you cannot find these specific studies, you can broaden your search step by step—only going as broad as you have to: ferritin levels in Asian adults of similar socioeconomic status in other geographic regions, ferritin levels in younger Asian adults, or ferritin levels in older adults of any race.

TABLE 11.2 Data needed for power calculations for cohort and cross-sectional studies with RRs as the measure of association

- Confidence level (95%)
- Sample size
- Ratio of unexposed to exposed
- Frequency of disease in the unexposed
- Risk ratio

The closer you can get to your proposed study population, the more relevant your ultimate power calculations will be. In addition, it will be key to **cite the sources** upon which you are basing your exposure distribution. These citations will demonstrate your thoughtful, quantitative, literature-based approach to calculating power.

The next piece of information asked for by statistical software packages is the **frequency of disease in the unexposed**. This is the disease rate in those without the exposure of interest. Using our example above, this would be the percent of older Asian adults with type 2 diabetes who had low ferritin levels. However, such information will be very difficult to find as diabetes rates may not be published among such specific subgroups, particularly if you are looking at a novel exposure. Instead, it is considered acceptable to use the overall frequency of disease (diabetes) in a study population as close to the characteristics of your sample as possible. Again, you will want to **cite the source** of your disease frequency rates.

If you cannot find disease frequency rates in a study population similar to your own, you may need to calculate a **weighted estimate of disease frequency**. Disease frequency will vary according to sociodemographic characteristics such as gender and age. Therefore, the calculation of a weighted disease frequency simply involves multiplying the percent of your study population with that characteristic by the disease frequency among people with that characteristic.

Weighted disease incidence rate (IR) = (% sample with characteristic #1 * IR among those with characteristic #1) + (% sample with characteristic #2 * IR among those with characteristic #2) + etc.

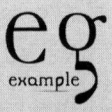

---

eg example

Continuing our proposal to study the association between ferritin levels and type 2 diabetes:

We expect our study population to have the following gender distribution: 39% male and 61% female. We have calculated the expected diabetes rates using a weighted average of this gender distribution multiplied by the best available data on diabetes rates in Asian older adults. These are 15% for men[11] and 10% for women.[12] This weighted disease incidence rate is therefore 12%.

- Weighted diabetes rate = men [0.39 * 15%][11] + women [0.61 * 10%][12] = 0.12

Next, the software will ask you for the **risk ratio** that you would like to detect. If you have not conducted a pilot study, search for prior literature that has evaluated the relationship between your exposure and outcome of interest and enter their observed risk ratios.

Again, you will want to **cite the source** of these risk ratios. Your goal is to demonstrate that you will have adequate power (>80%) to detect risk ratios that have been observed by the prior literature. If no prior studies have been published on your exposure–outcome relationship, it is also sufficient to choose a range of clinically meaningful risk ratios.

11.8.2 B. For *Unmatched* Case–Control Studies

Because case–control studies are designed to compare exposure odds in the cases to exposure odds in the controls, a different formula is used for power calculations and there are some key differences in the data that you will need to gather and *input* (Table 11.3).

Instead of entering the ratio of exposed to unexposed as you would for a prospective cohort study or a cross-sectional study, you will enter the **ratio of controls to cases**.

Next, instead of inputting the disease prevalence in the unexposed, you will enter the **percent of controls who are exposed**. However, it is often quite unusual to find exposure rates published specifically in the subgroup among those without your disease—particularly if you are looking at a novel association. Luckily, because most diseases are fairly rare, it is generally considered acceptable to present exposure rates among a population that is as similar to your own as possible (and not be concerned about whether or not they had your disease of interest).

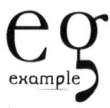

e.g. example Imagine a proposal to conduct a case–control study of ferritin levels (exposure) and type 2 diabetes (outcome) in older Asian adults in Washington State. Your cases have diabetes and your controls do not. You would need to enter the percent of those without type 2 diabetes (your controls) who have high levels of ferritin (your exposure). As you can imagine, it is unlikely that ferritin levels will be published only among adults without diabetes. Instead, it would be acceptable to display the percent of people with high ferritin levels in a population that is as similar to your own as possible (and not be concerned about whether or not they had diabetes). **Cite the source** of these percentages.

Lastly, similar to prospective cohort studies and cross-sectional studies, you will need to enter the measure of association (i.e., the OR) that you wish to detect. Again, if you have not conducted a pilot study, search for prior literature that has evaluated the relationship between your exposure and outcome of interest and enter their observed ORs, citing the source. If no prior studies have been published on your exposure–outcome relationship, it is also sufficient to choose a range of clinically meaningful ORs.

TABLE 11.3 Data needed for power calculations for case–control studies with ORs as the measure of association

- Confidence level (95%)
- Sample size
- Ratio of controls to cases
- Percent of controls exposed
- Odds ratio

11.8.3 C. How to Display Your Power in the Proposal

The choice of table to display your power depends on whether your sample size is fixed (e.g., you are proposing to use an existing dataset) or flexible (e.g., you are proposing to recruit a new sample).

When you have a **fixed sample size**, your proposal should include a table that displays the calculated power for a range of RRs given your sample size (Table 11.4).

How to choose which range of RRs to display in a power table:

- The **range of RRs or ORs** that prior studies of your exposure–disease relationship have observed
- The **smallest RR or OR** that your study has the power to detect

If your study has the power to detect RRs comparable to those observed by other studies, this will be considered a study strength. If, on the other hand, you don't have power to detect comparable RRs to prior studies, it will not be fruitful to try to hide this fact. Instead, reviewers will be looking for an explanation for why your study will still be worth conducting.

Therefore, the text accompanying the table describes the implications of the table to the reviewer.

Items to mention in the text accompanying the power table:

- The name of the **statistical test** used to calculate the displayed power and its corresponding citation
- The **smallest RR** that you will have the power to detect
- A comment upon the **degree of observed power** (e.g., adequate, insufficient, excellent) given your sample size
- A comment on the **clinical significance** of these power calculation findings

It is true that the reviewer may be able to deduce this information from the table, but you want to be kind to the reviewer and do this work for them. Remember that the smaller the RR that you can detect, the better.

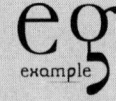

> **eg** *example*
>
> **For a Prospective Cohort Study:**
>
> Based on our pilot study,[1] we anticipate that 50% of our study population will have high ferritin levels and 50% will have low ferritin levels for a 1:1 ratio of the exposed to the unexposed groups. Based on state surveillance data, we chose 12% as the diabetes incidence rate among the unexposed.[2] Given our sample size of 1000 participants, a two-group chi-squared test with a 0.05 two-sided significance level will be able to detect an RR of at least 1.5 with 80% power and 95% confidence (Table 11.4). This RR is clinically significant[3] and is comparable to prior studies of ferritin levels and diabetes risk in which RRs ranging from 1.3 to 1.8 have been observed.[4–6]

TABLE 11.4 Power and RR for total study, N = 1000 (exposed = 500, unexposed = 500) assuming 12% disease frequency in unexposed

RR[a]	POWER (%)
1.6	88
1.5	80
1.4	58
1.3	38

[a] Rounded to one decimal place.

Note in the table above that larger power is needed to detect smaller RRs.

An alternative presentation Depending upon the dataset you will be using, you may be unsure of the ratio the unexposed to exposed or the frequency of disease. In this situation, including a table that displays power for a **range of exposure distributions and outcome frequencies** may be preferable, as in the following example.

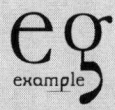

eg example Table 11.5 shows the power to detect an RR of 1.5 given a range of exposure distributions and disease frequencies based on a two-group chi-squared test[2] with a 0.05 two-sided significance level and a fixed sample size of 1000. For example, given a diabetes prevalence of 15%, we will have 80% or greater power to detect an RR of 1.5 if the prevalence of high ferritin levels is 40% or above. Given a higher diabetes prevalence (20% or greater), we will have >80% power to detect an RR of 1.5 if the prevalence of high ferritin is 30% or greater.

TABLE 11.5 Power to detect an RR of 1.5 for diabetes with 95% confidence based on a sample size of n = 1000

OUTCOME PREVALENCE (e.g., DIABETES) AMONG THE UNEXPOSED	EXPOSURE PREVALENCE (e.g., HIGH FERRITIN)		
	30%	40%	50%
10%	56%	63%	67%
12%	66%	73%	76%
15%	77%	83%	86%
20%	91%	94%	95%

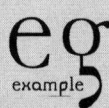

> **A Prospective Cohort Study:**
>
> Based on an expected incidence rate of diabetes of 12% and a 1:1 ratio of exposed to unexposed, a two-group chi-squared test[2] with a 0.05 two-sided significance level will have 80% power to detect the RRs displayed in Table 11.6 given the following sample sizes. For example, with a sample size of n = 1000, we will have 80% power to detect an RR as small as 1.5 (Table 11.6).
>
> **TABLE 11.6** RRs detected at 80% power given a range of sample sizes
>
> | RR | SAMPLE SIZE[a] |
> |---|---|
> | 2.0 | 300 |
> | 1.7 | 600 |
> | 1.5 | 1000 |
> | 1.3 | 3000 |
>
> [a] Rounded to the closest hundred.

If you are proposing to conduct a **new study**, your sample size may still be flexible. In this situation, your proposal could have a table that displays the smallest RRs that you would be able to detect at 80% power given a range of sample sizes (Table 11.6).

11.9 STEP #5: CALCULATE AND PRESENT YOUR POWER FOR DIFFERENCE MEASURES OF ASSOCIATION (i.e., CONTINUOUS OUTCOME VARIABLES)

Many proposals in epidemiology and preventive medicine will have continuous outcome variables (e.g., blood pressure, cholesterol levels, weight). If your proposal involves a **continuous outcome variable**, your measure of association will be mean differences in this outcome between exposed and unexposed groups. To detect mean differences between exposed and unexposed groups, power is typically based on a **two sample t-test**.

Proposals to detect differences in mean values of an outcome of interest between exposed and unexposed groups typically require smaller sample sizes to achieve adequate power. Indeed, given the budgetary constraints for pilot/feasibility studies and early-career awards, selecting a continuous outcome can be a very **strategic study design decision**. Note that, by definition, continuous outcomes cannot be utilized if you are proposing to conduct a case–control study.

TABLE 11.7 Data needed for power calculations for a cohort or cross-sectional study to detect differences in means

- Confidence level (95%)
- Standard deviation of the outcome variable
- Mean difference in the outcome variable that you wish to detect
- Number exposed
- Number unexposed

11.9.1 A. For Cohort and Cross-Sectional Studies

For all study designs, the generally accepted confidence level is 95% and the generally acceptable power is 80% (Table 11.7).

The best approach to finding the **standard deviation of your outcome variable** is to locate prior papers that evaluated your outcome in a study population as similar as possible to your own, regardless of whether they were interested in your exposure variable. Be sure to cite these sources.

The **mean difference in outcome** you wish to detect should be based upon clinical significance. Clinical significance can be determined by consulting with your physician collaborators on the project or published papers in the field. The bottom line is to consider what magnitude of difference in your outcome variable will have an important impact on public health.

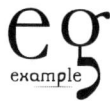

example Let's say you were interested in evaluating the association between ferritin levels (the exposure) and fasting glucose levels (a marker of insulin resistance) in older Asian adults in Washington State. You need to find data on the standard deviation of fasting glucose levels (your continuous outcome variable). If you have not conducted a pilot study, the best source is prior papers that evaluated the distribution of fasting glucose levels in older Asian adults in Washington State. If this is not available, then glucose data among older Asians in the United States could serve as a proxy. Then, you need to determine a clinically meaningful difference in fasting glucose by consulting with a physician. Or, you can search for publications that evaluated the impact of differences in fasting glucose levels on risk of subsequent diabetes. Differences in glucose levels that led to increased risk of disease would be clinically meaningful. Be sure to cite these sources.

11.9.2 B. How to Display Your Power in the Proposal

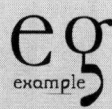

example Using a two-group t-test[1] with a 0.05 two-sided significance level and assuming a 7 mg/dL standard deviation in fasting glucose,[2] a sample size of 1000 has >99% power to detect a 9 mg/dL clinically meaningful mean difference[3] in fasting glucose (Table 11.8).

TABLE 11.8 Inputs to detect a clinically significant mean difference in fasting glucose based on a cohort of n = 1000

	FASTING GLUCOSE
Confidence level	95%
Standard deviation of fasting glucose	7 mg/dL[2]
Clinically meaningful mean difference in fasting glucose	9 mg/dL[3]
Number with high ferritin (exposed)	500
Number with low ferritin (unexposed)	500

11.10 WHAT IF YOUR POWER IS NOT ADEQUATE?

Now that you have calculated your expected power, it's time consider whether your power is sufficient to achieve your specific aims. If not, before discarding your aims, consider the factors that influence power (i.e., sample size, disease frequency, exposure prevalence) and consider whether you can make any adjustments to these factors to increase your power.

The following are examples:

- Consider selecting a population that has a higher disease incidence—for example, a group at higher risk of disease. This can be done by selecting a new study site or by changing your inclusion criteria to limit participants to those at high risk of your disease.
- Consider selecting a population with a higher prevalence of exposure. This can be done by over-enrolling exposed participants and/or selecting a study site with a higher prevalence of exposure.
- Consider extending the recruitment time as a way to increase your sample size.
- Consider adding study sites (e.g., conducting a multisite study) in conjunction with other collaborators as a way to increase your sample size.

You can then adjust your sample size upwards to allow for any of these study design changes.

The following formula is useful to calculate the number of participants that you would need to recruit to compensate for anticipated refusals to participate, exclusions, and loss to follow-up:

Sample Size * (100% ÷ [100% − Total rate of missing usable response]) *eg example* Imagine that you conduct your power calculations and determine that you require a sample size of 200 participants to have adequate power to observe an effect. However, you estimate that 8% of subjects will refuse to participate, 5% will be excluded, 4% will be lost to follow-up, and 3% will have missing data on your exposure variable of interest.

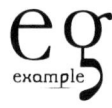

Total rate of missing usable response: 8% + 5% + 4% + 3% = 20%

- 200 * (100% ÷ [100% − 20%])
- = 200 * (100% ÷ 80%)
- = 200 * 1.25
- = 250

Therefore, you need to recruit 250 participants to have a final usable sample size of 200.

11.11 OTHER FACTORS THAT INFLUENCE POWER

This chapter has covered the main factors that influence power for traditional study designs in epidemiology and preventive medicine. However, note that there are a variety of other study design and analysis issues that may also have an influence—these will be useful to discuss with a statistician:

- Adjusting for multiple covariates
- Clustering
- Less traditional study designs: for example, complex sampling designs that use sample weights to produce nationally representative data

11.12 FINAL PEP TALK

Overall, it's important to remember that power calculations are more of an art than a science. The estimates that go into the power and sample size calculations are at best well-considered estimates of what you expect will occur in your study. Life is unpredictable, and your recruitment and retention rates, as well as disease incidence and exposure prevalence rates, may all be different than what you expect.

Review of Bias and Confounding

12

When writing a grant proposal, it is critical to try to identify as many of your study limitations as possible—before your reviewer does. Reviewers are selected because they are among the top experts in their fields (usually!). Therefore, it is not wise to try to *hide* potential limitations in a proposal. In fact, if a reviewer discovers a limitation that you have not discussed, they might believe that you are not aware of the limitation and attribute this to a lack of expertise on your part. A similar approach should be taken with a dissertation proposal with the idea that your committee members are playing the role of reviewers. This makes the dissertation proposal process an excellent opportunity to practice writing grant proposals—the ultimate focus of your career.

Remember that there is no perfect study. In addition, there exist true controversies in the field regarding the ideal study methods and designs. Therefore, this chapter provides a brief **review** of the **most common** sources of bias and confounding in epidemiology and preventive medicine studies. At the end of this chapter, you will find a section titled **Issues for Critical Reading**—this can assist you in identifying potential limitations for your selected study design.

Please note that this chapter is not meant to be a substitute for an introductory epidemiology textbook—to which you can turn for a more comprehensive review of each of these topics.

Chapter 13, *How to Present Limitations and Alternatives*, follows up where this chapter leaves off, describing strategies for presenting study limitations with a focus on techniques to minimize their impact.

12.1 FIRST: A PEP TALK

I always advise my graduate students that they will be fortunate if their master's or doctoral dissertation is fraught with limitations. In this way, they have the *opportunity* to face these limitations in the context of a supportive environment of dissertation committee members and senior advisors. What better place to practice these skills than surrounded by the mentors that accompany a graduate school experience? Once students graduate, and have embarked on their own career, they may never again have this level of support.

Imagine a student who had a simple dissertation with few, if any, study limitations. Let's say they had access to a large prospective dataset with thousands of participants and comprehensive objective data on their exposures and outcomes of interest. Once this student graduates, and finds themselves in the field creating their own line of research, they will be facing the challenging issues of bias and confounding—perhaps for the first time!

12.2 STUDY LIMITATIONS: CHANCE, BIAS, AND CONFOUNDING

The classic limitations faced by studies in epidemiology and preventive medicine are summarized in Table 12.1. These limitations can be divided into threats to **internal validity** and threats to **external validity**. In terms of the former, chance, bias, and confounding can all be considered as *alternate explanations* for a true relationship between your exposure and disease of interest. Following the proposal outline presented in Chapter 2 (Table 2.2):

TABLE 12.1 Threats to validity

a. Threats to internal validity
    i. Chance
    ii. Bias
        1. Nondifferential
            a. Nondifferential misclassification of exposure
            b. Nondifferential misclassification of outcome
        2. Differential misclassification
            a. Selection bias
            b. Information bias
    iii. Confounding
b. Threats to external validity
    i. Generalizability

12.3 CHANCE

Studies in epidemiology and preventive medicine involve samples of the population about which we wish to make inferences. Therefore, chance may affect study results simply because of **random variability** from sample to sample.

At this point, it will be helpful to revisit Figure 11.1 presented in Chapter 11, *Power and Sample Size*, and repeated here. See Figure 12.1.

In the above figure, the subheading "Reality" reflects what truly exists while *Investigator's Decision* reflects the decision that you as an investigator will make.

Focusing on the first column of this table, you will see that there are two possibilities when the groups are in reality **not different**. We might conclude, correctly, that the groups are not different (*correct decision*). Or we might conclude, in error, that the groups are different (*type I error or alpha*). Our goal is to keep this alpha value low and, by convention, it is typically set to 5% (e.g., we will only make this error less than one out of 20 times):

$p < .05$ = statistically significant
$p \geq .05$ = **not** statistically significant

Why? Because we want a small probability of observing a difference due to chance if there is in reality no difference.

Therefore, a p-value can be defined as follows:
Given that there is no difference, the probability of observing a difference or one more extreme, by chance alone.

- Interpretation of a p-value of 0.05 in words:
There is a 5% probability that the observed results are due to chance.

Potential pitfalls to avoid It is important to note that p-values that are not statistically significant (such as p = 0.20 or *a 20% probability that the observed results are due to chance*) do not mean that your findings may not be true. It just means that chance cannot be excluded as an explanation for the observed findings. On the flip side, a statistically significant p-value (of 0.001 *a one in a thousand probability that the observed results are due to chance*) does not mean that the finding is definitely not due to chance; it simply means that chance is unlikely. Therefore, statistical significance can never tell us definitively about the truth—just the likelihood.

Investigator's decision	Reality Groups are not different	Groups are different
Conclude that groups are not different	Correct decision	Type II error probability = beta
Conclude that groups are different	Type I error probability = alpha	Correct decision probability = 1− beta (power)

FIGURE 12.1 Possible study outcomes.

Even if a p-value is statistically significant (p < .05)

- Your results could still be due to bias or confounding
- Your results could lack biological importance or plausibility
- p-values give no indication of the direction or magnitude of the effect
- p-values give no information about the power of the study to detect a difference

So, even if your observed p-value is statistically significant, your proposal still needs to address the threats of bias and confounding.

12.4 BIAS

Bias is an integral aspect of study design and execution. Bias cannot generally be corrected by analytic methods and therefore it must be prevented by careful study design and execution. Bias encompasses both **nondifferential** as well as **differential** misclassification. As you will see from the descriptions below, in general, nondifferential misclassification is viewed as the lesser of these two potential threats.

12.5 NONDIFFERENTIAL MISCLASSIFICATION

Nondifferential misclassification addresses the question of whether your exposure or outcome is accurately measured. In any study, inaccuracies in the collection of data are inevitable. Nondifferential misclassification minimizes the differences between the two groups being compared, making them seem more similar than they actually are. Therefore, nondifferential misclassification typically results in an underestimate of any true association.

One should consider nondifferential misclassification both in light of the exposure of interest as well as the outcome of interest.

12.5.1 Nondifferential Misclassification of Exposure

Almost all forms of exposure assessment are subject to some degree of misclassification. Potential misclassification (error) includes inaccuracies in exposure measurement. These include reliance on proxy respondents, self-report, or recall. Even biomarkers can be subject to error. For example, samples of stored urine and blood can degrade over time. In addition, a biomarker may not be truly reflective of your exposure of interest—or may be influenced by other factors. For example, blood levels of vitamin D are not only influenced by diet (which may be your exposure of interest) but also by sunlight exposure. As you can see from Figure 12.2, nondifferential misclassification of

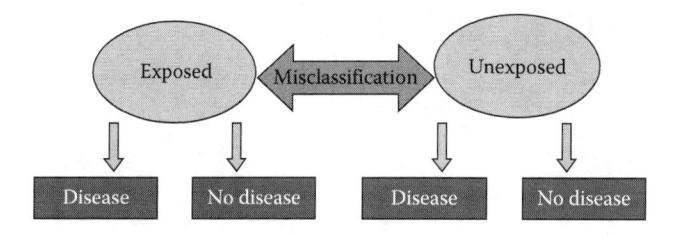

FIGURE 12.2 Nondifferential misclassification of exposure.

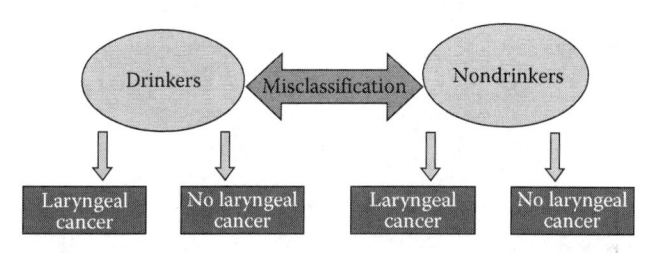

FIGURE 12.3 Nondifferential misclassification of exposure in a cohort study of alcohol consumption and laryngeal cancer.

exposure minimizes the differences between the exposed and unexposed groups, making them seem more similar in regard to their disease experience than they actually are. Therefore, nondifferential misclassification typically results in an underestimate of any true association between exposure and disease.

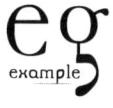

eg example Imagine a proposal to conduct a cohort study to assess the impact of alcohol consumption on laryngeal cancer (Figure 12.3). Alcohol consumption will be measured via an FFQ. An FFQ may be subject to error simply due to the difficulty faced by all participants in accurately remembering and reporting their alcohol consumption. There may also be differences in reporting of alcohol consumption between drinkers and nondrinkers (e.g., drinkers may be more likely to underestimate their alcohol consumption). All these types of error would be termed nondifferential misclassification. It mixes up the exposed (drinkers) and unexposed (nondrinkers) leading to more similar incidence rates of laryngeal cancer in drinkers and nondrinkers. This then leads to a weaker association between alcohol and laryngeal cancer than is true or a *bias toward the null*. In other words, our study might conclude that alcohol does not have an adverse impact on laryngeal cancer when indeed it does.

12.5.2 Nondifferential Misclassification of Outcome

Almost all forms of outcome assessment are subject to some degree of misclassification. Potential misclassification (error) includes inaccuracies in outcome measurement. These include reliance on proxy respondents, self-report, or recall. Even medical records or

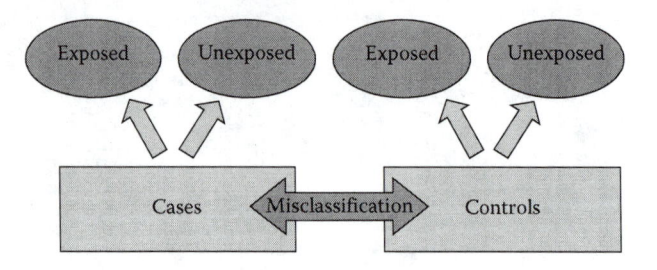

FIGURE 12.4 Nondifferential misclassification of outcome.

ICD codes, often considered a *gold standard*, are subject to error. For example, medical records may be completed by a variety of personnel including residents, attending physicians, and nurse midwives. In addition, *coders* assign ICD codes based on notes recorded in the medical record. Any of these personnel can make an error in recording key information in the medical record or in selecting the appropriate diagnostic code. There may also be error associated with the technique used to abstract data from the medical record. As you can see from Figure 12.4, nondifferential misclassification of outcome minimizes the differences between the diseased and nondiseased groups, making them seem more similar in regard to their exposure history than they actually are. Therefore, nondifferential misclassification typically results in an underestimate of any true association between exposure and disease.

example

Imagine a proposal to conduct a case–control study of strenuous exercise and risk of miscarriage (Figure 12.5). Information on miscarriage will be self-reported by women. However, miscarriages that happen very early in pregnancy may be undetected (i.e., if a woman miscarries before she recognizes that she was pregnant). Therefore, some of the controls (women reporting no miscarriages) may have been unaware that they miscarried and therefore actually may be cases (women with miscarriages). Or, some of the controls may have terminated their pregnancies and did not want to report this. Such error would be termed nondifferential misclassification of outcome. It mixes up the cases and controls leading to more similar odds of exposure (exercise) between the two groups. This then leads to a weaker association between exercise and miscarriage than is true.

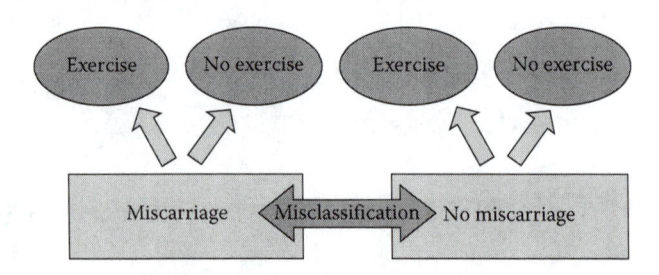

FIGURE 12.5 Nondifferential misclassification of outcome in a case–control study of exercise and miscarriage.

12.6 SELECTION BIAS

Selection bias is bias in the **selection** of your study population. It can be viewed as a biased way in which participants come into your study. Selection bias is a differential bias and, unlike nondifferential misclassification, can lead to either an **overestimate** or an **underestimate** of the true association between your exposure and outcome of interest. Therefore, it is typically considered a more serious study limitation by reviewers. Once a study is faced with selection bias, no analysis can alleviate it.

This type of bias is generally more of a concern for a case–control study or a cross-sectional study than for a prospective cohort study. Why? Because in a case–control and cross-sectional study, both the outcome and exposure have already occurred at the time the investigator initiates the study. Because of this timing, it is possible that having the exposure and the disease can influence a person's decision to participate in the study. This becomes dangerous when the presence of exposure differentially influences the selection of diseased and nondiseased people into the study.

12.6.1 Selection Bias in a Case–Control Study

As you can see in Figure 12.6, in a case–control study, selection bias occurs when **selection** of cases and controls is influenced by their exposure status.

e.g. example: Imagine a proposal to conduct a case–control study of the association between multiple sexual partners and risk of human papillomavirus (HPV) (Figure 12.7). People who have HPV (cases) **and** who have had multiple sexual partners (exposed) may be more motivated to participate because they are concerned that their HPV infection was caused by their having had multiple sexual partners. In other words, the cases' knowledge of their exposure influences their decision to participate in the study. This results in an overestimate of the number of cases with multiple partners, and therefore a stronger association between having multiple sexual partners and HPV than is true.

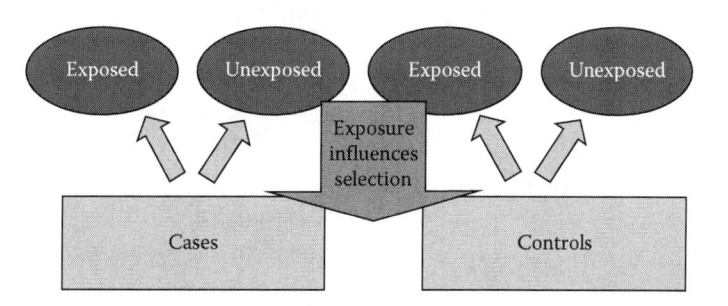

FIGURE 12.6 Selection bias in a case–control study.

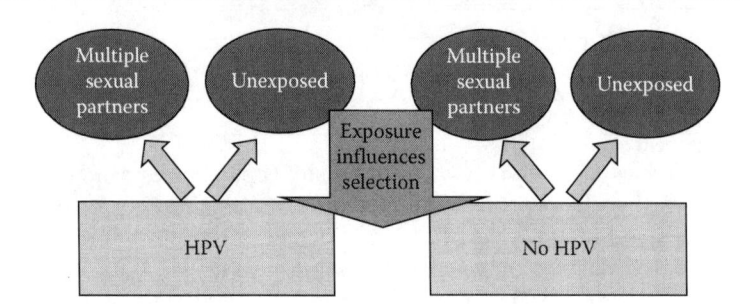

FIGURE 12.7 Selection bias in a case–control study of multiple sexual partners and HPV.

12.6.2 Selection Bias in a Cohort Study

Recall that a cohort study enrolls participants who do not have your disease of interest and follows them for disease incidence. Therefore, the disease (outcome) of interest is unknown at the beginning of the study (baseline) and should not influence selection of participants into exposed and unexposed groups.

However, instead, selection bias is possible in a prospective study through **differential loss to follow-up**. Just as participants who do not agree to participate will not be in your final dataset, participants who are lost to follow-up will also not be present in your final dataset. That is why loss to follow-up in a prospective cohort study can also be viewed as a type of **potential** selection bias. I use the term *potential* because not all loss to follow-up is differential and therefore not all loss to follow-up meets the criteria for selection bias.

For example, if women lost to follow-up were more likely to develop our disease of interest **and** be in our exposed group, this would constitute selection bias and bias our results toward the null. One way to assess this possibility is to compare characteristics of those lost to follow-up vs. those not lost to follow-up.

12.7 INFORMATION BIAS

Information bias is bias in the collection of **information**. There are several subtypes of information bias (e.g., recall bias, interviewer bias, and surveillance bias). As noted in the Table 12.2, depending upon your proposed study design, your proposal may be particularly susceptible to certain subtypes of information bias.

TABLE 12.2 Types of information bias

STUDY DESIGN	TYPE OF INFORMATION BIAS
Case–control or cross-sectional	
	Recall bias
	Interviewer (observer) bias
Cohort	
	Surveillance (detection) bias

12.7.1 Information Bias in a Case–Control or Cross-Sectional Study

Case–control and cross-sectional studies are particularly susceptible to recall bias and interviewer bias. Why? Because in these study designs, the outcome of interest has already occurred at the time that exposure information is collected. So, it is more likely that a participant's disease status will influence the collection of information on their exposure.

In a case–control study, information bias occurs when *collection of information* on exposure is performed differently among cases than controls, as shown in Figure 12.8.

Recall bias occurs when having the disease influences the way that information is *recalled*. Most typically, cases tend to remember or report exposures differently than controls. For example, if I've been diagnosed with a disease, I may overreport my history of a particular exposure because I suspect that it may have caused my disease. Recall bias is even more likely when the hypothesis of a potential association between exposure and disease is well known.

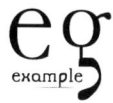

example Imagine a proposal to conduct a case–control study of the association between infant conjunctivitis and risk of infant mortality (Figure 12.9). Mothers of cases (infants who died) may be more likely to recall information on conjunctivitis than mothers of healthy children (controls). That is, due to the infant's death, case mothers are likely to think back more carefully on every single exposure that occurred and therefore are more likely to recall and report conjunctivitis than mothers of healthy children. This results in an overestimate of the frequency of conjunctivitis among the cases and therefore a stronger association between having conjunctivitis and infant mortality than is true.

Interviewer (observer) bias occurs when interviewers ascertain exposure information differently among the cases as compared to the controls. For example, if interviewers are aware of the study hypothesis, they may probe and prompt cases more for information on exposures than they do for controls.

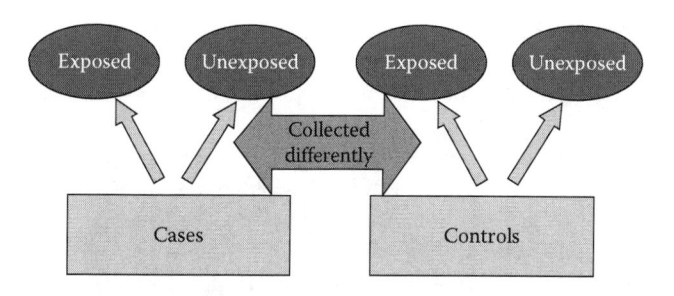

FIGURE 12.8 Information bias in a case–control study.

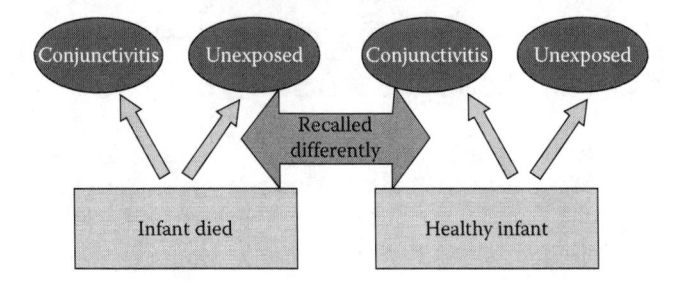

FIGURE 12.9 Recall bias in a case–control study of conjunctivitis and infant mortality.

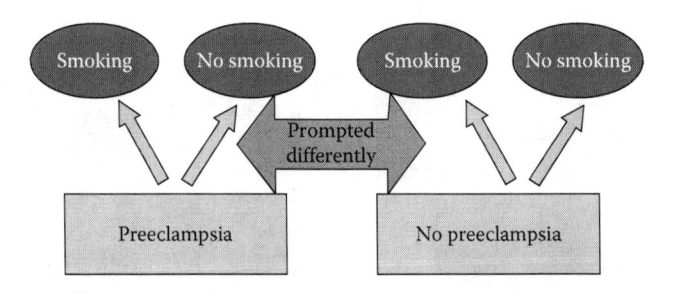

FIGURE 12.10 Interviewer bias in a case–control study of smoking and preeclampsia.

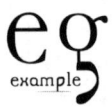

e.g. example Imagine a proposal to conduct a case–control study of smoking during pregnancy on risk of preeclampsia (Figure 12.10). The interviewers are aware of this study hypothesis and may prompt women with preeclampsia (cases) more for smoking information than they do for controls. This would lead to an overestimate of the smoking rate among cases and the findings of a stronger effect of smoking on preeclampsia than is actually true.

12.7.2 Information Bias in a Cohort Study

Recall bias and interviewer bias are less of a concern for prospective cohort studies. Why? Because in a prospective cohort study, the collection of information on exposure happens **before** the outcome (disease) has occurred. So, the disease, by definition, cannot influence collection of information on the exposure.

However, over the course of follow-up, exposed groups may be monitored more closely for disease than unexposed groups—this is called surveillance bias and is a particular concern for cohort studies.

Surveillance bias (detection bias) is a form of information bias typically faced by cohort studies. Most commonly, it occurs when information on the disease (outcome) of interest is collected differently among exposed participants than among unexposed participants. That is, if the person collecting information on the outcome is aware of the participant's exposure status and of the study hypothesis, they may be more motivated to search for incident disease. For example, a medical record

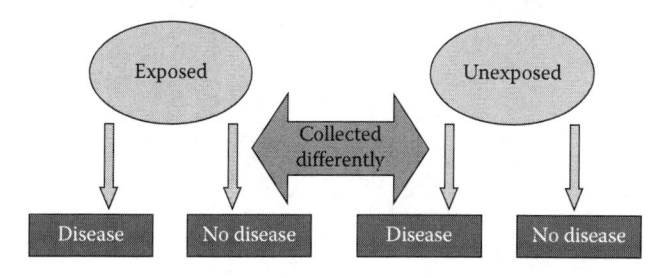

FIGURE 12.11 Surveillance bias (detection bias) in a cohort study.

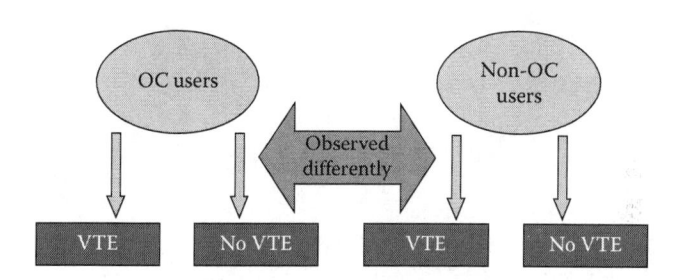

FIGURE 12.12 Surveillance bias (detection bias) in a cohort study of OCs and risk of VTE.

abstractor may search the medical records of exposed participants more thoroughly for signs of the disease (outcome) than they do for unexposed participants (Figure 12.11).

e.g. example Imagine a proposal to conduct a cohort study of oral contraceptives (OCs) and risk of venous thromboembolism (VTE) (Figure 12.12). OC users must attend regular medical appointments in order to have their prescriptions continued. In contrast, women not on OCs would likely not be attending doctors' visits in such a regular fashion. Therefore, VTEs are more likely to be detected among OC users because they are monitored more closely than nonusers of OCs who may have the same symptoms. This leads to a stronger association between OCs and VTE than is actually true.

12.8 CONFOUNDING

Confounding distorts the true relationship between exposure and disease. Confounding can be considered a *confusion of effects* between the exposure under study and another variable (the confounder).

Confounding is an important concern for most study designs, with the exception of randomized trials (as discussed later in this chapter). To qualify as a confounding factor, the

```
        Exposure  ━━━━▶  Disease
              ↖        ↗
               Confounder
```

FIGURE 12.13 Diagram of confounding.

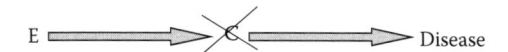

```
      E ━━━▶ ╳ ━━━▶ Disease
```

FIGURE 12.14 A confounder must not be in the causal pathway between the exposure and disease; E = exposure, C = confounder.

potential confounder must be independently associated with both the exposure and outcome (Figure 12.13):

- A confounder must be a risk factor for the disease of interest.
- A confounder must be associated with the exposure of interest.
- A confounder must *not* be in the causal pathway between the exposure and disease.

In other words, the confounder cannot be on the physiologic pathway for how the exposure potentially causes the disease (Figure 12.14).

eg example Imagine a proposal to study the impact of a high-fat diet (exposure) on risk of myocardial infarction (MI). High cholesterol would not qualify as a potential confounder even though it is associated with both high-fat diets and MI. In other words, cholesterol is likely on the physiologic pathway (mechanism) by which high-fat diet causes an MI (Figure 12.15).

A pitfall to avoid A common mistake is to forget that both the left and right sides of the above triangle in Figure 12.13 are necessary to qualify as a potential confounder. Imagine a study of coffee (exposure) and risk of bladder cancer (disease). If coffee drinkers differ from noncoffee drinkers in terms of their height, but we know that height is not associated with bladder cancer, then height cannot be a potential confounder of the association between coffee and bladder cancer! In this example, the right side of the triangle is missing.

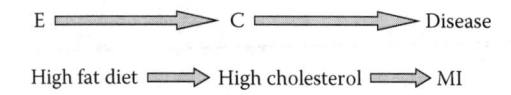

```
        E ━━━▶ C ━━━▶ Disease
  High fat diet ━━▶ High cholesterol ━━▶ MI
```

FIGURE 12.15 Example causal pathway between high-fat diet and MI; E = exposure, C = confounder.

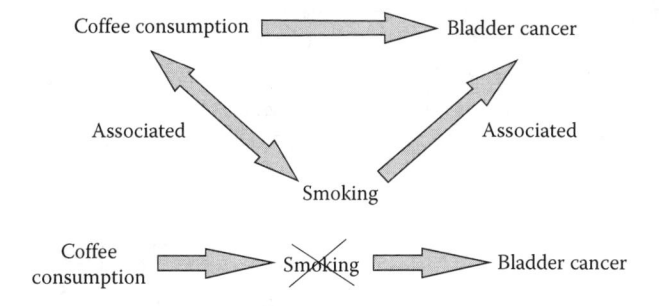

FIGURE 12.16 Smoking as a confounder of the relationship between coffee consumption and bladder cancer.

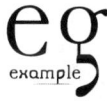

e.g. example Imagine again a proposal to conduct a study of coffee drinking and risk of bladder cancer (Figure 12.16). You are concerned that cigarette smoking might be a confounding factor. Smoking is associated with both your exposure (coffee drinking) and with your disease (bladder cancer). In addition, smoking is not on the causal pathway between coffee drinking and bladder cancer. That is, coffee drinking doesn't *cause* smoking. Therefore, smoking does indeed qualify as a potential confounding factor for this study.

12.8.1 Confounding in Randomized Trials

Typically, confounding is not a concern in a randomized trial. Due to the randomization, not only is the exposure randomized between study arms, but both **known** and **unknown confounding factors** are also randomized. The one caveat to this rule is the setting of a small trial. Depending upon the sample size, randomization may not always successfully work. Therefore, it is always wise to propose to check that baseline characteristics (potential confounding factors) are similar between the study arms after you have conducted the randomization.

12.8.2 Difference between Confounding and Effect Modification

Unlike confounding, which is a nuisance effect that distorts the true relationship between an exposure and disease, effect modification is a characteristic of nature. Most simply, effect modification is a true physiological difference in the relationship between your exposure and outcome of interest among different subgroups (e.g., age groups, gender groups).

While confounding can be controlled through careful study design and analysis, you do not want to control effect modification. Instead, you want to display the effect of your exposure on your outcome **within that particular subgroup**.

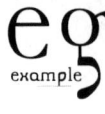

eg *example* Imagine our prior example of coffee drinking and risk of bladder cancer. You believe that age might be a potential effect modifier. That is, the physiological effect of coffee on bladder cancer may differ between young and older people. In this situation, you would want to present the association between coffee drinking and bladder cancer separately among young people and among older people.

12.8.3 Will You Be Missing Information on Any Potential Confounding Factors?

In writing a proposal, it is important to consider if there are any potential confounders that you will be unable to address. This is a critical exercise, again with the idea of preempting potential concerns from reviewers or from dissertation committee members at a dissertation defense. Identify these potential uncontrolled confounders and then clarify how lack of control for these factors may influence your study findings.

Figures 12.17 and Tables 12.3 and 12.4 describe the potential impact of uncontrolled confounding on your exposure–outcome relationship (Figure 12.17).

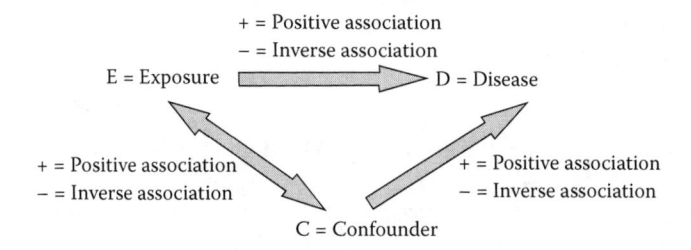

```
                + = Positive association
                − = Inverse association
    E = Exposure ══════════════▶ D = Disease
         ╲                              ╱
    + = Positive association    + = Positive association
    − = Inverse association     − = Inverse association
                 C = Confounder
```

FIGURE 12.17 Schematic of potential confounding.

TABLE 12.3 Impact of uncontrolled confounding on the relative risk given a hypothesized *positive* association between exposure and disease (RR > 1)

E-C (+)	C-D (+)	Unadjusted RR is incorrectly overestimated. For example, unadjusted RR = 1.5; true RR = 1.2.
E-C (−)	C-D (−)	Unadjusted RR is incorrectly overestimated. For example, unadjusted RR = 1.5; true RR = 1.2.
E-C (+)	C-D (−)	Unadjusted RR is incorrectly underestimated. For example, unadjusted RR = 1.2; true RR = 1.5.
E-C (−)	C-D (+)	Unadjusted RR is incorrectly under estimated. For example, unadjusted RR = 1.2; true RR = 1.5.

E, exposure; C, confounder; D, disease; RR, relative risk.

12 • Review of Bias and Confounding   233

TABLE 12.4 Impact of uncontrolled confounding on the relative risk given a hypothesized *inverse* association between exposure and disease (RR < 1)

E-C (+)	C-D (+)	Unadjusted RR is incorrectly underestimated (closer to the null value of 1.0). For example, unadjusted RR = 0.8; true RR = 0.5.
E-C (−)	C-D (−)	Unadjusted RR is incorrectly underestimated (closer to the null value of 1.0). For example, unadjusted RR = 0.8; true RR = 0.5.
E-C (+)	C-D (−)	Unadjusted RR is incorrectly overestimated (further away from the null value of 1.0). For example, unadjusted RR = 0.5; true RR = 0.8.
E-C (−)	C-D (+)	Unadjusted RR is incorrectly over estimated (further away from the null value of 1.0). For example, unadjusted RR = 0.5; true RR = 0.8.

Referring back to the above example, let's say you are hypothesizing a positive association between coffee and bladder cancer (i.e., that coffee consumption increases risk of bladder cancer). Prior studies have found that coffee drinkers are more likely to smoke (E-C [+]) and that smoking increases risk of bladder cancer (C-D [+]). Therefore, failure to control for smoking would lead to an unadjusted RR that is incorrectly overestimated (Table 12.3, row 1).

The impact of confounding is always a bit more challenging to envision if you are hypothesizing an inverse or protective association between your exposure and disease.

eg example

Imagine that you are proposing to conduct a cohort study of fruit and vegetable intake and risk of lung cancer. Prior cross-sectional studies have found that individuals who eat five or more servings of fruits and vegetables have a 50% lower risk of developing lung cancer than those who eat fewer servings of fruits and vegetables. In addition, you know from the previous literature that individuals who consume five or more servings of fruits and vegetables are less likely to smoke than those who consume less of these foods (E-C [−]). Cigarette smoking is a known risk factor for lung cancer (C-D [+]). In this situation, you are hypothesizing that the unadjusted exposure–outcome (fruit/vegetable–lung cancer) relationship is inverse. If you fail to adjust for smoking, (Table 12.4, last row) the inverse association will be artificially low (further away from the null value of 1.0). That is, some of the health benefit that you will be attributing to a healthy diet will actually be due to the fact that these people are less likely to smoke.

12.9 OTHER LIMITATIONS SPECIFIC TO CROSS-SECTIONAL AND CASE–CONTROL STUDIES

Survivor bias: Survivor bias is typically only a concern in cross-sectional and case–control studies. It can occur when high levels of your exposure lead to death from your outcome of interest or, in a less severe example, when high levels of your exposure lead to inability to participate (e.g., due to illness from your outcome). Therefore, these people cannot be recruited into your study. Survivor bias results in an underestimate of the impact of your exposure upon your outcome.

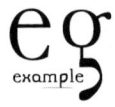

e.g. example Imagine a proposal to conduct a cross-sectional study of weight and risk of MI. Those who were of the heaviest weights (e.g., obese) may be more likely to die from an MI and therefore would not be available to participate in your study at the time of enrollment. This would result in an underestimate of the true association between weight and MI.

Temporal bias: Temporal bias is another typical concern faced by cross-sectional and case–control studies. Because both the exposure and outcome of interest have already occurred at the time the investigator launches the study, we cannot ensure that the exposure indeed led to the disease. Instead, the disease may have led to the exposure. Thus, temporal bias is often referred to as *reverse causality*.

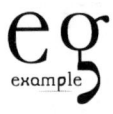

e.g. example Imagine a proposal to conduct a case–control study of vitamin D deficiency and risk of cancer. You enroll cases of cancer, and controls who are cancer-free, and take blood samples to measure plasma vitamin D. Temporal bias is a concern because the cancer itself may have led to the vitamin D deficiency, as opposed to the vitamin D deficiency leading to the cancer. In other words, the disease has led to the exposure, instead of vice versa.

12.10 GENERALIZABILITY

In my experience, students and early-career faculty are often too conservative in generalizing their study findings. In contrast, the more that you can generalize your study findings to other populations, the greater **potential public health impact** and **potential for funding** your proposal will have.

The main question to answer in determining generalizability is the following:

- **"Assuming causality**, to what larger population may the results of this study be generalized?"

What do I mean by *assuming causality*? Generalizability is an issue of external validity. It should only be considered after thoroughly considering all the threats to internal validity discussed above (bias, confounding, misclassification). At this point, you want to suspend disbelief and assume that your study is internally valid.

In generalizing, we are assuming that our exposure causes our outcome.

- *The decision to generalize should be based primarily upon physiology.* "Assuming that there is a true independent association between your exposure and outcome, will the **physiological relationship** between exposure and outcome differ among groups not represented in the study?"

If you do not generalize to certain groups, the burden is on you to justify why—based on a physiologic rationale. If you don't expect the physiologic impact of the exposure on the risk disease to be any different in these groups, then you should definitely generalize.

Try this in a stepwise fashion:

- Can you generalize to those of a different race/ethnicity than your study sample?
- Can you generalize to those of different ages than your study sample?
- Can you generalize to those of different gender than your study sample?
- Can you generalize to those of different geographical locations than your study sample?

To answer each of these above questions, ask yourself if the physiologic association between your exposure and disease would differ in those groups.

e.g. example: Imagine a proposal to conduct a case–control study of cigarette smoking and lung cancer among white males in a developed country. Based on the postulated physiologic mechanism between smoking and lung cancer, you must judge whether the findings can be generalized to

- Nonwhite males
- Females
- Individuals in developing countries

I would propose that you can indeed generalize to these groups because *being male and white and from the United States is irrelevant to the carcinogenic action that smoking has on lung tissue.*

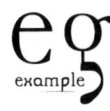

> **example:** Imagine a proposal to conduct a study of hair dye and risk of breast cancer among a large cohort of female nurses in 25 states in the United States. Based on the postulated physiologic mechanism between hair dye and breast cancer, you must judge whether the findings can be generalized to

- Nurses in the other 25 states
- Women in the United States who are not nurses
- Women in other countries

If you presume that *being a nurse and being from the United States is irrelevant to the carcinogenic action that hair dye has on the breast*, then yes, you can generalize your findings to each of these three groups.

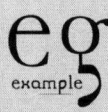

> **example:** Imagine a proposal to conduct a study of eating disorders and weight loss:
>
> Women who volunteer to participate may not be representative of women who live in other parts of the country. Perhaps those women who agree to participate in the study will be less likely to use hair dye than those who decline to participate. However, there is little basis for believing that the biological relation between hair dye and breast cancer observed in this study population of nurses would be substantially different from that in most American women.

A pitfall to avoid: **Do not** base the generalizability of study findings upon the **representativeness** of your study sample. Study populations should be selected to maximize internal validity, and not to maximize representativeness. The issue of representativeness does not impact the generalizability of study findings. Instead, the generalizability of findings is based on the question of whether the physiologic mechanism between your exposure and outcome would be the same in other groups.

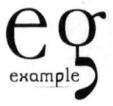

> **example:** Imagine a proposal to conduct a study of eating disorders on risk of dental disease. You will recruit a convenience sample of volunteers. Women who volunteer to participate may not be representative of women who live in other parts of the country—they may have fewer eating disorders, be older, or be of different race/ethnic groups. However, because there is little basis for believing that the physiological relation between eating disorders and dental disease would be different in women of different sociodemographic groups, you can still generalize to all US women.

12.10.1 Reasons to Limit Generalizability

While the overall theme is to encourage generalizing, there are three situations in which you should limit generalizability.

Reason #1 (discussed above): Difference in expected physiologic association between your exposure and outcome in a different population.

Reason #2: Differences in the content of the exposure between your study population and the population to which you hope to generalize.

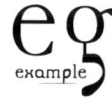

eg example Imagine a proposal to conduct a study of OCs and risk of breast cancer among women in the United States. One potential reason for not generalizing to European populations would be the difference in European formulations of OCs as compared to OCs used in the United States. In other words, because the OCs (the exposure) are not chemically the same, European OCs may have a different physiologic impact on the breast.

Reason #3: Nonoverlapping range of exposure between your study population and the population to which you hope to generalize.

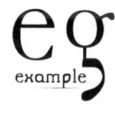

eg example Imagine a proposal to conduct a study of exercise on risk of preterm birth in Hispanic pregnant women. National figures show that Hispanic women are less active, in general, than non-Hispanic white women. The range of exercise participation in your Hispanic sample may not overlap with the range of exercise in a more active non-Hispanic sample. That is, your most active Hispanic women may be even less active than the most sedentary women in an active non-Hispanic white population. Therefore, you would not generalize your findings to an active non-Hispanic white population.

12.11 EXERCISES

1. In a case–control study of condom use and risk of human papillomavirus (HPV), you suspect that the cases were more likely to remember that they had used a spermicide-coated condom than were the control women. This is:
   a. Nondifferential misclassification of exposure
   b. Nondifferential misclassification of disease
   c. Information bias
   d. Selection bias
   e. Confounding

2. A study of alcohol intake and heart disease was performed among 80,000 male health professionals. The authors classified the men as regular drinkers (≥5 drinks/week) or nondrinkers (<5 drinks/week). Men were followed 4 years for development of heart disease.
   The investigators suspect that men may not tell the truth about their alcohol consumption. Some may say they do not drink when they actually do.

Others may misunderstand the question and say that they are regular drinkers when they are not. This is:
a. Nondifferential misclassification of exposure
b. Nondifferential misclassification of disease
c. Information bias
d. Selection bias
e. Confounding

3. A case–control study of exercise (regular vs. irregular) during pregnancy and preeclampsia reports a relative risk of 1.5. The investigators suspect that smoking is a confounder. In their sample, smoking is inversely associated with preeclampsia but not associated with exercise. Is smoking a confounder of the relationship between exercise and preeclampsia?
a. Yes
b. No

4. A prospective study of risky sexual behavior and risk of human immunodeficiency virus (HIV) was performed among young men who were inducted into military service in northern Thailand. The authors classified the men as having visited a commercial sex worker (CSW) or not having visited a CSW. Men were followed for 2 years for development of HIV infection.
The investigators suspect that military men may not tell the truth about their HIV status. This is:
a. Nondifferential misclassification of exposure
b. Nondifferential misclassification of disease
c. Information bias
d. Selection bias
e. Confounding

5. In a case–control study of condom use and risk of urinary tract infection (UTI) in young women, the investigators reported a relative risk of 2.4 for the association between use of a spermicide-coated condom in the previous month and UTI.
You suspect that the case women were more likely to agree to participate in the study if they knew that they used spermicide-coated condoms. This is:
a. Nondifferential misclassification of exposure
b. Nondifferential misclassification of disease
c. Information bias
d. Selection bias
e. Confounding

Answers: 1c, 2a, 3b, 4b, 5d

12.12 ISSUES FOR CRITICAL READING

12.12.1 Cohort Studies

POTENTIAL PROBLEM	IMPLICATION	SOURCE OF PROBLEM	EXAMPLE
Nondifferential misclassification of exposure	Results underestimated	Poor indicator/ inaccurate	Will you use an inaccurate way to measure exposure, for example, proxy respondents, self-report, unstable urine levels, and recall?
Nondifferential misclassification of outcome	Results underestimated	Poor indicator/ inaccurate	Will you use an inaccurate way to define the outcome? For example, will there be clear diagnostic criteria for the disease such as ICD codes? Will self-report be used instead?
Selection bias	Results biased	Noncomparable selection	None if prospective cohort.
		Loss to follow-up	Will diseased people be lost to follow-up? If so, will they be more likely to be exposed?
Information bias	Results biased	Recall bias	None if prospective cohort.
		Surveillance bias	Will the disease be measured more carefully in the exposed group? For example, will the exposed group be screened for disease more often than the unexposed group? Or, will the exposed be more likely to visit the doctor?
Confounding	Results biased	Confounding	Will you adjust for confounders? For example, other characteristics of the exposed people that may lead to their developing the disease.

(continued)

(continued)

POTENTIAL PROBLEM	IMPLICATION	SOURCE OF PROBLEM	EXAMPLE
Generalizability	Limited application	Restricted selection/ selective attrition	Who will the study be limited to? Who can you generalize to? For example, you can generalize to people in whom we could expect the same physiologic relationship between exposure and disease.

12.12.2 Randomized Trials

POTENTIAL PROBLEM	IMPLICATION	SOURCE OF PROBLEM	EXAMPLE
Nondifferential misclassification of exposure	Results underestimated	Poor indicator/ inaccurate	Will you use an inaccurate way to measure who takes the drug? For example, will you rely on self-report or will you test blood levels?
Nondifferential misclassification of outcome	Results underestimated	Poor indicator/ inaccurate	Will you use an inaccurate way to define the outcome? For example, will there be clear diagnostic criteria for the disease such as ICD codes? Will self-report be used instead?
Selection bias	Results biased	Noncomparable selection	None.
		Loss to follow-up	Will diseased people be lost to follow-up?
Information bias	Results biased	Recall bias	None.
		Surveillance bias	Will the disease be measured more carefully in those that receive the drug? For example, will the drug group be screened for disease more often than the control group? Will the drug group be more likely to visit the doctor?

(continued)

POTENTIAL PROBLEM	IMPLICATION	SOURCE OF PROBLEM	EXAMPLE
Confounding	Results biased	Confounding	None, but propose to demonstrate in a table that all relevant variables will be randomized (equally distributed between the drug and the placebo group).
Generalizability	Limited application	Restricted selection/ selective attrition	Who will the study be limited to? Who can you generalize to? For example, you can generalize to people in whom we could expect the same physiologic relationship between exposure and disease.

12.12.3 Case–Control and Cross-Sectional Studies

POTENTIAL PROBLEM	IMPLICATION	SOURCE OF PROBLEM	EXAMPLE
Nondifferential misclassification of exposure	Results underestimated	Poor indicator/ inaccurate	Will you use an inaccurate way to measure exposure, for example, proxy respondents, self-report, unstable urine levels, and recall?
Nondifferential misclassification of outcome	Results underestimated	Poor indicator/ inaccurate	Will you use an inaccurate way to define cases? For example, will there be clear diagnostic criteria for the cases such as ICD codes? Will self-report be used instead?
Selection bias	Results biased	Noncomparable selection	Will cases who have been exposed be more likely to be motivated to participate?
		Loss to follow-up	None.
Information bias	Results biased	Recall bias	Will cases be more motivated to remember exposure than controls? Will the interviewers probe the cases more for exposure than the controls?
		Surveillance bias	None.

(continued)

(continued)

POTENTIAL PROBLEM	IMPLICATION	SOURCE OF PROBLEM	EXAMPLE
Confounding	Results biased	Confounding	Will you adjust for confounders? For example, will the cases and controls differ in other characteristics that may lead to their developing the disease?
Generalizability	Limited application	Restricted selection/ selective attrition	Who will the study be limited to? Who can you generalize to? For example, we can generalize to people in whom we could expect the same physiologic relationship between exposure and disease.

12.13 EXAMPLES

Note that each of these examples will be repeated in Chapter 13, *How to Present Limitations and Alternatives*, with the addition of techniques to minimize these threats to validity.

12.13.1 Example #1

A Proposal to Conduct a Case–Control Study of Maternal Heat Exposure and Congenital Heart Defects

Study Limitations

Nondifferential Misclassification of Exposure
Mothers of cases and controls will be asked to recall the period of early pregnancy 3–8 years after delivery has occurred. While women's memory of their pregnancy might be better than for other life periods, inaccuracy is likely to result from the extended time lapse and difficulty in estimating average hours per week of heat exposure, over a several-month time period, in the past.

Another possible source of nondifferential misclassification is in the definition of heat exposures, which requires some judgment by participants. No objective heat exposure measures will be available in this study. However, misclassification resulting from poor participant recall or inaccurate exposure measurement is likely to be nondifferential (i.e., misclassification will not significantly differ between cases and controls), biasing results toward the null value.

Nondifferential Misclassification of Outcome
Congenital cardiovascular malformations will be abstracted from the New York birth defects registry. Inaccuracies in classifying birth defects as congenital cardiovascular malformations are possible, and such misclassification would bias our findings toward the null.

Selection Bias
In our pilot study, the response rate was 55.4% due to the difficulty in locating study subjects. Respondents were significantly different from nonrespondents with regard to age, race, ethnicity, and geographic location of residence within New York State. This raises the concern of selection bias, leading to an under or overestimate of our findings.

Information Bias: Recall Bias
In searching for possible causes for their children's heart defects, mothers of cases may more carefully report exposures as compared to mothers of controls. This recall bias would result in an overestimation of the association between heat exposure during pregnancy and congenital cardiovascular malformations.

Information Bias: Interviewer Bias
Because exposure information will be collected by an interviewer, it is possible that an interviewer will prompt case mothers differently from control mothers, resulting in an overestimate of the association between physical exposures and congenital cardiovascular malformations.

Confounding
The questionnaire will include information on all known risk factors for congenital cardiovascular malformations, including maternal chronic diabetes, binge drinking during pregnancy, fever during pregnancy, sex of the infant, and family history of congenital cardiovascular malformations. As with the main study exposures, information on these variables will be obtained through self-report. For information that was difficult to recall or associated with social stigma, such as drinking alcohol during pregnancy, some women's answers may be inaccurate. Failure to adequately control these variables may lead to over- or underestimates of the association between physical exposures and congenital cardiovascular malformations. For example, prior studies have found that heat exposure during pregnancy (e.g., sauna use) is positively associated with binge drinking during pregnancy. In turn, binge drinking during pregnancy is positively associated with congenital cardiovascular malformations. Therefore, any inaccuracies in our measure of binge drinking may lead to an overestimate of the association between heat exposures and congenital cardiovascular malformations.

Generalizability
We do not expect the physiological association between pregnancy heat exposure and congenital cardiovascular malformations to differ according to race, ethnicity, or age. Therefore, inspite of the fact that study participants were African American and Hispanic youth, we will still be able to generalize our findings to pregnant women in the United States.

12.13.2 Example #2

A Proposal to Conduct a Prospective Cohort Study of Stress and Risk of Preeclampsia

Study Limitations

Nondifferential Misclassification of Exposure
Trained, bilingual interviewers will administer the Perceived Stress Scale during a structured interview in early pregnancy (mean = 15 weeks gestational age). It is possible that women will over- or underreport their perceived stress. This may occur to the extent that perceived stress may be a sensitive issue for a select group of women. This type of misclassification would bias our results toward the null, thereby reducing our effect estimate for the relationship between perceived stress and hypertensive disorders of pregnancy. We expect this misclassification to be minor.

Nondifferential Misclassification of Outcome
Cases of hypertensive disorders of pregnancy will be ascertained through medical record abstraction, as well as through a review of ICD codes for hypertension in pregnancy. Nondifferential misclassification could occur if diagnoses are missed by physicians or via the data collection methods employed. This would result in a bias of our results to the null, but we expect the effect to be minimal.

Selection Bias: Differential Loss to Follow-Up
Due to the prospective nature of this study, selection bias is unlikely to occur as exposure status (stress) will be collected before the disease (hypertension in pregnancy) occurs. However, selection bias is possible in a prospective study through differential loss to follow-up. For example, if women lost to follow-up were more likely to be in the high-stress group and also more likely to be hypertensive in pregnancy, selection bias could occur and bias our results toward the null.

Information Bias: Surveillance (Detection) Bias
Surveillance bias will be unlikely in this study because women are not monitored differently for hypertension in pregnancy according to their stress levels.

Confounding
We are not aware of any key confounders that are not available through our dataset. It is possible, however, that we measured one or more of these confounders inadequately. This residual confounding could result in a change in our effect estimate in either direction depending on the direction of the measurement error.

Generalizability
The results of this study may be generalized to pregnant women as the biological mechanisms through which stress may impact hypertension in pregnancy should not vary by race or ethnic origin.

13
How to Present Limitations and Alternatives

Now that you have identified the potential sources of bias and confounding in your proposal with the help of Chapter 12, *A Review of Bias and Confounding*, it is time to decide how to best present these limitations to your reviewers.

The Approach section of a proposal should discuss potential study limitations and alternative strategies. Therefore, this chapter describes strategies for presenting study limitations with a focus on techniques to minimize their impact. Part I of the chapter starts with a fourfold approach to strategically presenting limitations. Part II of the chapter applies this approach to the typical study limitations that you are likely to face. Part II goes on to additionally review design and analytic techniques for minimizing these threats to validity along with accompanying examples.

13.1 WHICH LIMITATIONS TO HIGHLIGHT?

One of the goals of writing a dissertation proposal is to demonstrate that you have mastery of the concepts of bias and confounding. Therefore, it is typically expected that a dissertation proposal will cover each potential study limitation listed in the "Issues for Critical Reading" tables in Chapter 12. The proposal will state why it does, or does not, face each limitation. This process demonstrates to the dissertation committee that the student has an understanding of each type of study limitation regardless of whether or not it is a serious threat to their approach.

In contrast, in the context of a grant proposal, there is no room for this type of exercise given space limitations. Instead, you are expected to comment only on the most important/major limitations of your proposal. This gives you the opportunity to address what you anticipate will be the most important threats to validity and to discuss the methods that you will use to minimize these concerns. Finally, as I will demonstrate below, you will also discuss why you dismissed alternative approaches.

13.2 PART I: HOW TO STRATEGICALLY PRESENT LIMITATIONS—A FOURFOLD APPROACH

The key principle in presenting limitations is **transparency**. As mentioned in Chapter 12, instead of trying to hide limitations, you want to identify and present them. You want to be open about your thought process and describe the pros and cons of your study design decisions. Remember that there is no perfect study. All studies face limitations, and being humble and knowledgeable about these limitations will be more impressive to reviewers than ignoring them.

A fourfold approach can be used when presenting limitations as outlined in the Figure 13.1: (1) describe the potential limitation, (2) describe the potential impact of the limitation on your study findings, (3) discuss alternatives and why they were not selected, and (4) describe the methods that you propose to minimize the impact of this limitation.

13.2.1 Step #1: Describe the Potential Limitation

For each important limitation that you identify, specify the type. For example, is it nondifferential misclassification of exposure or outcome (e.g., error), or is it a more dangerous limitation—that is, a differential bias such as selection bias, information bias, or confounding? Or, perhaps the limitation is not related to internal validity, but is instead a matter of external validity such as limited generalizability of study findings.

As a starting point, consider limitations mentioned by the prior literature on your exposure and outcome of interest. Even if you do not face the same limitations, you will want to be sure to highlight this fact as a study strength.

The most important key to success in writing a limitations section is to avoid the use of professional jargon without an accompanying explanation. *Professional jargon* refers to the use of such terms as *selection bias, information bias, nondifferential misclassification,* and *confounding*. Additionally describing your study limitations in a direct manner using simple terms will show the reviewers that you have a clear grasp

---
Step 1: Identify the limitation
Step 2: Describe the impact on your findings
Step 3: Discuss alternatives
Step 4: Describe methods to minimize

FIGURE 13.1 A fourfold approach for presenting study limitations in a proposal.

of these limitations—this may be somewhat counterintuitive but it is true. For NIH grant proposals, this is even more important, as not all of your reviewers will have training in epidemiology and preventive medicine; some will have expertise in other pertinent fields.

> **e.g. example** Imagine a proposal to conduct a prospective study of postmenopausal hormones (hormone replacement therapy [HRT]) on risk of breast cancer.
>
> **Original Version**
> This proposal may face detection bias.
> **Improved Version**
> One potential source of bias in our study is detection bias. In other words, those who are taking HRT are more likely to have mammograms and thus more likely to be diagnosed with breast cancer than those women not taking HRT. This would lead to an overestimate of the association between HRT and breast cancer.

Note that the improved example still includes professional jargon (i.e., *detection bias*) but then goes on to define it. To further save space, the term *detection bias* could be removed entirely from the improved example to avoid altogether the use of jargon.

13.2.2 Step #2: Describe the Potential Impact of the Limitation on Your Study Findings

For each limitation, it is important to try to project the:

- Likelihood
- Magnitude
- Direction of the limitation on your study findings

Remember, as discussed in Chapter 12, that some limitations are more likely to bias your findings toward the null value, while others are more likely to bias your findings away from the null. Other limitations may have an unpredictable impact on your findings.

In general, limitations that lead to a bias toward the null are considered less dangerous than limitations that cause a bias away from the null. On the other hand, limitations that lead to a conclusion that your exposure impacts your outcome when it does not (i.e., a bias away from the null) are often considered more dangerous.

Such limitations will lead your reviewers to carefully scrutinize your methods, as well as the alternatives that you considered. The reviewers will assess whether you have minimized these limitations to the extent possible.

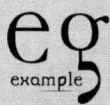

> **eg example** Imagine a proposal to conduct a cross-sectional study of acid-lowering agents (ALA) and risk of vitamin B12 deficiency. Participants in this study will be asked to self-report their ALA during a home interview.
>
> It is possible that people with vitamin B12 deficiency will be more motivated to remember ALA use than people without vitamin B12 deficiency. Such a recall bias would result in an **overestimate** of the relationship between ALA use and vitamin B12 deficiency.

Note that the example indicates the likelihood, direction, and magnitude of the study limitation—as indicated by the bold phrase.

A potential pitfall to avoid As noted earlier in this chapter, in a grant proposal, you are expected to only comment on the most important limitations of your proposal. For example, let's say that you are proposing to conduct a prospective cohort study. Given this design, it is probably not necessary to waste space by saying that this type of design reduces the risk of selection bias because participants are enrolled before the outcome occurs. However, given that your assigned reviewers may not include epidemiologists, and one of your study strengths is the prospective design, it may not hurt to point this out. On the other hand, in a doctoral proposal, you are expected to show mastery of all the potential limitations.

> **eg example** Imagine a graduate proposal that simply states the following:
>
> **Original Version**
> This study is a prospective cohort and therefore is not subject to recall bias.
>
> **Improved Version**
> This study is a prospective cohort, and as such, information on exposure is collected prior to the occurrence of the outcome. Therefore, it is unlikely that the outcome will influence the collection of information on the exposure of interest.

In this example, the first quote would not be sufficient for most dissertation committees, as it does not display that the student understands the concept of recall bias. The improved example clearly defines the concept of recall bias as it relates to the proposed study design and then dismisses it as being unlikely.

Because it is typically considered fair game to ask about any potential limitation at a dissertation defense, considering each potential limitation will provide you with a well-thought-out response for why or why not your study faces each potential limitation.

13.2.3 Step #3: Discuss Alternatives

In any proposal, there will be alternative approaches that you could have, but chose not to, propose. Discuss these alternatives—both their pros and cons—and clearly explain to the reviewer why you chose the approach that you did. In writing this section, be up to date on approaches that prior studies have used and the subsequent impact on their findings. Be sure to cite any review articles or convened panels that make particular recommendations—this can be persuasive evidence in support of the approach that you ultimately chose to take, or it can lead you to reconsider this decision. At the least, it will help you to become adept at defending your decision—both in writing and orally (e.g., most relevant for a dissertation defense).

A word of reassurance Remember that for many study design and data analysis issues, there are true controversies in the field and even established investigators may disagree on the ideal strategy to take. Therefore, be transparent about your thinking as to why you choose one type of design or analysis, in spite of its limitations, over and above other alternatives. In this manner, you will show that you have a grasp of the current state of the field and thoughtfully considered all the issues in making a final decision. While this decision may not be perfect, you are indicating to the reviewer that you are aware of the alternatives as well as the impact of your decision on the interpretation of your study findings.

13.2.4 Step #4: Describe Methods to Minimize the Limitation

In describing methods to minimize your study limitations, first consult prior studies of your exposure and outcome of interest. Did these studies use design or analysis techniques to minimize limitations that would be prudent for you to adopt as well?

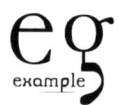

Examples of **design techniques** to minimize study limitations include:

- Choosing a prospective study design over a case–control study design—to avoid such issues as recall bias and selection bias

- Blinding interviewers in a case–control study—to avoid interviewer bias
- Incorporating repeated administrations of questionnaires over the course of follow-up—to minimize nondifferential misclassification of exposure due to changes in behaviors over time
- Use of life events calendars—to boost the accuracy of recall thereby reducing nondifferential misclassification of exposure

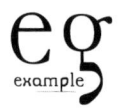

Example **analysis techniques** to minimize study limitations include:

- Comparing baseline characteristics of the experimental and standard care group in a clinical trial—to ensure that the randomization was successful
- Performing subgroup analyses among participants with and without missing data on key variables of interest—to address potential selection bias
- Conducting analyses among participants with asymptomatic disease—to address concerns regarding temporality, that is, that whether preclinical symptoms of disease may have influenced exposure

In Part II, I provide specific examples of design and analysis techniques to address each of the classic study limitations in epidemiology and preventive medicine proposals.

13.2.5 Conclusion to Fourfold Approach to Address Limitations

This fourfold approach of identifying the study limitation, describing its potential impact on study findings, discussing alternatives considered, and ending with methods to minimize limitations has a **key strategic benefit**. By ending with the steps that you are taking to minimize your limitations, you leave the reviewer with a **positive impression**. This leads us to the issue of where to place your study limitations in a grant proposal.

13.2.6 Where to Place Your Study Limitations in a Grant Proposal

In general, there are two schools of thought on where to place your study limitations in a dissertation or grant proposal. The first is to place your limitations section near or at the end of the Approach section. The second school of thought is to intermingle your limitations within each relevant subsection of the Approach. Below, I discuss the advantages and disadvantages of each technique. Regardless of which technique you choose, the Study Limitations section can be titled, *Limitations and Alternatives*. This is a key catch phrase that reviewers will search for—and will criticize proposals for failure to include.

13.2.6.1 Limitations section at the end of the approach section

This technique involves writing **one section** with a subheading titled, *Limitations and Alternatives* in which you discuss **all** the potential limitations of your proposal. For each limitation, you use the above fourfold approach—discussing the source of the limitation, the potential impact on the findings, the alternatives considered, and the methods that you will use to minimize this problem.

The advantage of this technique is that in one centralized section, you can carefully and thoroughly evaluate and discuss each potential limitation.

The first disadvantage of this technique is that, as the reviewer reads your proposal, they will be thinking of limitations in real time. However, the reviewer will be forced to wait until the end of the Approach section to see if you have addressed their concerns. A careful reviewer will be forced to keep a list of concerns as they arise in your application and will then have to cross-check this list with your limitations summary at the end. Therefore, this approach is less *kind* to reviewers.

The second disadvantage of this approach is that you are essentially ending the grant on a fairly negative note. Accumulating all study limitations in one section at the end of the Approach can inadvertently lead to a diminished enthusiasm for the proposal on the part of the reviewer. This can be particularly risky as this section comes at the end of the reviewer's reading of the application—immediately before they need to assign their score.

One way to modestly diminish this concern is to add a final section to the Approach, immediately after this *Limitations* section, titled *Summary of Significance*, where you have a few lines rehighlighting the importance of the application. However, with strict page limitations on grant proposals, it is often difficult to have space for this final upbeat note. In addition, reviewers may find it repetitive of your initial *Significance* section that already appeared earlier in the proposal.

13.2.6.2 Intermingled limitations sections

In contrast, the technique I prefer is to intersperse limitations—as they arise—throughout the Approach section. In this manner, you can address in real time concerns that arise for the reviewer and don't leave them waiting and concerned until the end of the application. This approach is kinder to the reviewer—just as they are about to put pen to paper to note a concern, you immediately address it.

For example, when you are describing the study design, you intersperse a few lines discussing limitations of your study design and your rationale for choosing it. Further on, when you discuss exposure assessment, you insert another small limitation section discussing limitations to your exposure assessment and your rationale for choosing it. In other words, each of these limitations sections is a microversion of the fourfold approach presented above—dismissing each limitation individually, as it occurs. Each of these subsections can be titled *Limitations and Alternatives*.

13.3 PART II: METHODS TO MINIMIZE CLASSIC LIMITATIONS—DESIGN AND ANALYSIS TECHNIQUES

13.3.1 How to Present Nondifferential Misclassification

There are a number of different techniques that can be used to minimize nondifferential misclassification—both via study design and via data analysis.

13.3.1.1 Design techniques to minimize nondifferential misclassification

Design techniques to minimize nondifferential misclassification of exposure can include shorter recall periods, use of validated questionnaires, interviewer administration of questionnaires, use of calendars to assist participant recall, and many other techniques. Design techniques to minimize nondifferential misclassification of outcome include the use of clear diagnostic criteria to identify disease outcomes (e.g., based on published consensus guidelines).

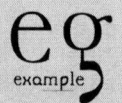

> **eg** *example*
>
> Imagine a proposal to conduct a prospective study to assess the impact of coffee on bladder cancer. In this study, coffee consumption was measured via an FFQ.
>
> - *Identify the limitation*: Women may generally underreport their coffee consumption.
> - *Describe the impact on your findings*: The effect of such misclassification, however, will be to underestimate any true association between coffee consumption and the outcome.
> - *Discuss alternatives*: We selected an FFQ, as opposed to 24 h dietary recalls, as FFQs are less prone to error due to the day-to-day variability in diet and have demonstrated relationships between dietary patterns and cancer incidence.[1]
> - *Methods to minimize*: Because we collected dietary information every year, nondifferential misclassification will likely be modest. Also, validation studies have indicated that self-reported coffee intake correlates well with true intake.[2]

Of course, in your proposal, you would write this up as one complete paragraph: Women may generally underreport their coffee intake. The effect of such misclassification, however, will be to underestimate any true association between coffee intake and the outcome. We selected an FFQ, as opposed to 24 h dietary recalls, as FFQs are less prone to error due to the day-to-day variability in diet and have demonstrated relationships between dietary patterns and cancer incidence.[1] Because we collected dietary information every year, nondifferential misclassification will likely be modest. Also, validation studies have indicated that self-reported coffee intake correlates well with true intake.[2]

13.3.1.2 Analysis techniques to minimize nondifferential misclassification

One example of an analysis technique to minimize nondifferential misclassification would be to propose to use findings from a validation study to correct for measurement error. Such a validation study may be available from your preliminary studies or from the prior published literature. Measurement error techniques are discussed in detail in several excellent textbooks on the topic, and you could consult a statistician for assistance in this regard.

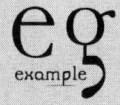

eg example
Imagine a proposal to evaluate physical activity and risk of breast cancer.

Physical activity will be based upon self-report and therefore is subject to misclassification. Due to the prospective nature of the study, this misclassification should not be differential according to breast cancer diagnosis. To the extent that nondifferential misclassification occurs, our observed odds ratios will be biased toward the null. As prior studies have observed strong relationships between self-reported physical activity and diseases such as cancer and cardiovascular disease, this threat should not be substantial. In addition, we will use data from our physical activity questionnaire validation study to evaluate the extent of measurement error (see "Data Analysis" section).

13.3.2 How to Present Selection Bias

Unlike nondifferential misclassification, selection bias cannot be removed in data analysis after it has occurred. Instead, it must be prevented in the design of the study. On the other hand, data analysis techniques such as sensitivity analyses can be used to evaluate the extent of selection bias.

13.3.2.1 Study design techniques to minimize selection bias

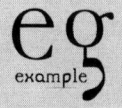

> **e.g. example** Recall the proposal to conduct a case–control study of the association between multiple sexual partners and HPV presented in Chapter 12. People who have HPV (cases) **and** who have had multiple sexual partners (exposed) may be more motivated to participate because they are concerned that their HPV infection was caused by having multiple sexual partners. The following design techniques could reduce this concern:
>
> > Participants will be identified via random sampling of medical records. In addition, we will ensure that participants are blinded to the proposed hypothesis. Finally, questions regarding sexual partners will be embedded in a long questionnaire that includes reproductive history as well as other medical and psychosocial factors.

13.3.2.2 Analysis techniques to minimize selection bias

The following sensitivity analysis could also be proposed to address the extent of selection bias:

> In addition, we will compare characteristics of cases and controls to see if they differ on sociodemographic and other medical history variables.

13.3.3 How to Present Information Bias

Just as with selection bias, information bias can only be prevented through study design approaches. Analysis techniques can, however, be used to address the extent of information bias—but cannot remove information bias once it has already occurred.

13.3.3.1 Study design techniques to minimize information bias

The best way to reduce the threat of detection or surveillance bias is to blind the assessor to the participants' exposure (in a cohort study) or to the participants' case/control status in a case–control study. For example, in a prospective cohort study, if medical record abstractors are blinded to exposure status, information on exposure cannot influence the collection of information on the outcome. Similarly, in a case–control study, if interviewers are blinded to case/control status, then information on outcome cannot influence the collection of information on the exposure of interest. In addition, bias is also reduced when the hypothesized association between the exposure and the outcome is not known to the assessor.

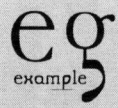

> **e.g.** *example*
>
> Imagine again our proposal to conduct a cross-sectional study of ALA and risk of vitamin B12 deficiency. Participants in this study will be asked to self-report their ALA during a home interview.
>
> It is possible that people with vitamin B12 deficiency will be more motivated to remember ALA use than people without vitamin B12 deficiency. Such a recall bias would result in an overestimate of the relationship between ALA use and vitamin B12 deficiency. **However, the home interviews were conducted by trained interviewers and participants were blinded to the study hypothesis. Additionally, vitamin B12 deficiency was ascertained by serum concentration and results were not shared with participants until after exposure quantification; thus, they were unaware of their disease status at the time of the interview.** Thus, it is unlikely that information bias occurred in this study, and if it occurred, we would expect its effect to be minor.

Note that the *bold phrases* indicate the design techniques used to minimize information bias.

13.3.3.2 Analysis techniques to minimize information bias

Sensitivity analyses can be used to examine the extent of information bias. For example, if there are concerns about detection bias or surveillance bias in a cohort study, one approach would be to compare the amount of surveillance applied to the exposed vs. unexposed groups—by comparing such factors as number of medical visits, recency of medical visits, and number of screenings. Another sensitivity analysis to address surveillance bias would be to repeat the analysis after excluding nonsymptomatic cases (i.e., *in situ* cases) as these cases would only tend to be detected during regular medical surveillance. In the examples below, the techniques to minimize information bias are *bold*.

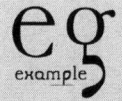

> **e.g.** *example*
>
> Imagine a proposal to conduct a prospective study of postmenopausal hormone use and risk of breast cancer.
>
> One potential source of bias in our study is the difference in the rates of mammographic screening between hormone users and nonusers. Those who are taking postmenopausal hormones are more likely to have a mammogram and thus more likely to be diagnosed with breast cancer than those women not taking postmenopausal hormones. This would lead to an overestimate of the association between postmenopausal hormones and

> breast cancer. **We will address this problem in several ways. We will compare rates of mammography screening among postmenopausal hormone users as compared to nonusers. We will also exclude in situ breast cancers because they are more likely to be diagnosed through mammography.**

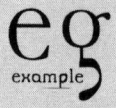

example: Imagine a proposal to conduct a prospective study of dietary factors and their impact on incident diabetes.

> Bias could arise if those with early signs of diabetes, but not a formal diabetes diagnosis, started to change their diet in response to these early indicators. This bias would cause an overestimate of the association between diet and diabetes. **To minimize this potential bias, we will perform a subanalysis only among participants without reported symptoms of diabetes.** If we observe a comparable association between diet and diabetes in this subgroup as in the overall sample, this would reduce concerns about the impact of information bias.

13.3.4 How to Present Confounding

13.3.4.1 Study design techniques to minimize confounding

There are a number of study design techniques to minimize the threat of confounding—as summarized in Table 13.1.

1. *Subject restrictions*: Design approaches to address confounding include restricting subjects to particular characteristics. Specifically, you could propose to restrict subjects to particular strata of a confounding factor such that your exposed and unexposed groups will have this factor in common. Because most study designs already limit inclusion criteria, by definition, most proposals are already taking a first step in limiting confounding!

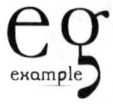

   example: Imagine that you are proposing to conduct a study of depression and risk of preterm birth. You are concerned about parity as a potential confounding factor. Therefore, you propose to restrict the study sample to nulliparous women (women who have not had prior children). In this way, parity cannot act as a potential confounder of the observed association between depression and preterm birth because all the women will have the same level of that potential confounding factor (i.e., no children). That is, having had children cannot be responsible in any part for the observed association between depression and preterm birth.

TABLE 13.1 Study design techniques to minimize confounding

- Subject restrictions
- Collect information on confounders
- Matched design
- Randomization

Even if you cannot fully restrict inclusion criteria to rule out all confounders, you can try to limit the range of a potential confounder. For example, if you were concerned about confounding by age, you could exclude extreme ages (e.g., children or the elderly). This will not remove the need to address potential confounding by age in your analysis, but will limit the potential extent of confounding.

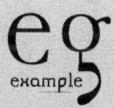

> *example*
>
> Imagine a proposal to evaluate vitamin D intake and cataract incidence. You will be using an existing dataset of dental hygienists.
>
> Although we controlled for many cataract risk factors in the analysis, we did not have information on exposure to sunlight. Because sunlight is positively associated with vitamin D, and positively associated with cataract incidence, the lack of control for sunlight may lead to an overestimate of the association between vitamin D and cataract incidence. However, because the cohort is not occupationally exposed, variation in sunlight is not likely to be as large as in a general population sample.

Note that the example ends by minimizing the threat of confounding. The last sentence points out that the study population does not vary significantly according to the level of sunlight. Remember, as described above, that if all participants do not differ according to the confounding factor (e.g., all one gender, or all one age, or in this case, all one level of sunlight exposure), then there cannot be confounding by this factor. That is, differences between participants in levels of this confounding factor will not be responsible for the observed association between vitamin D and cataract incidence. However, some residual confounding is likely to remain.

2. *Collect information on confounders*: The second approach involves designing your study to collect information on potential confounders. By having this data in hand, you will be able to adjust for these potential confounders once you get to the data analysis phase. This approach requires careful consideration of all the potential confounding factors when writing the proposal. Reviewing the prior literature will help to identify potential confounders. The construction of DAGs (see Chapter 10, *Data Analysis Plan*) is also a common approach.

The flip side of this approach is the potential for heavy participant burden. That is, collecting information on each potential confounder (e.g., either through questionnaires or biomarkers) may take up an inordinate amount of participant time or require a high amount of biomarker assessment (e.g., multiple blood draws, biopsies).

It is also important to note that this approach does not remove the potential threat of **residual confounding**, but does minimize this concern. For example, if you are concerned that sleep is a potential confounder of the relationship between depression and preterm birth, you may choose to administer a sleep questionnaire to collect information on sleep. However, if this questionnaire has some error associated with it (e.g., reliance on self-report), adjusting for sleep in your analysis will only address a portion of the confounding by sleep and some residual confounding will remain.

3. *Matching*: The third design approach to address confounding is matching participants on potential confounders. Matching is a design technique typically used in case–control studies whereby cases are matched to controls on several key confounding factors (e.g., age, gender, study site). In this way, the cases and controls will not differ on these factors, and in turn, these factors cannot be responsible for the observed association between exposure and disease. However, it is typically not feasible to match on a multitude of factors because logistical concerns come into play. For example, it may become difficult to find a control that matches your case according to a long list of matching criteria.

4. *Randomization*: The fourth design approach involves conducting a randomized trial. Randomized trials include clinical trials in which medical treatments are randomized. Randomized trials can also include behavioral interventions in which, for example, educational programs may be randomized. As long as the investigator is assigning the exposure in a random fashion, the study design qualifies as a randomized trial. Randomized trials are considered the gold standard design because the use of randomization results is not only random distribution of known confounders, but just as importantly, the randomization of unknown confounders as well.

13.3.4.2 Analysis techniques to minimize confounding

There are a variety of analysis approaches to minimize confounding and the most common are listed in Table 13.2. For a more detailed discussion of these techniques, see Chapter 10, *Data Analysis Plan*.

- *Stratification*: Stratification involves analyzing the association between your exposure and outcome separately within individual strata of your confounding variables. In other words, if you are concerned about confounding by

TABLE 13.2 Analysis techniques to minimize confounding

- Stratification
- Matched analysis
- Multivariable regression

gender, you could conduct the analysis only among your female participants and then again among your male participants. Statistical techniques are available to derive a summary measure of association that pools the measure of association across each stratum (e.g., Mantel Haenszel summary odds ratios).

- *Matched analysis*: If you choose to use matching in the design of your study, then your analysis plan has to follow suit. Typically, for a matched case–control study, conditional logistic regression is used. However, there are other approaches to handling a matched study design that can be discussed with your statistician.

- *Multivariable regression*: Lastly, the most common approach to address potential confounding in the data analysis portion of your proposal is to propose to conduct multivariable analyses. Such analyses typically involve the construction of multivariable regression models that include your confounding factors. Chapter 10, *Data Analysis Plan*, discusses techniques for incorporating confounding factors in multivariable models. Even if you have conducted a randomized trial, it will be important to assess whether the random assignment actually worked. If there are any observed differences in covariate status between the treatment groups at baseline, you could consider whether to adjust for these in multivariable analyses. The smaller your study, the more likely that these baseline characteristics will differ in spite of the random assignment of treatment arm.

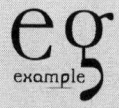

> **eg** *example*
>
> Imagine a proposal to evaluate physical activity and risk of gestational diabetes.
>
> Women who are more active during or prior to pregnancy could be healthier in some overall way that decreases their risk of gestational diabetes. We will have information on a variety of confounding factors that reflect overall health and will include them in multivariable models. In addition, the study population has excluded women with more severe diseases such as existing diabetes, hypertension or heart disease, and chronic renal disease. In addition, while healthier women may be more likely to engage in sports and exercise, they may have little choice whether to undertake occupational or household activity. Our analyses will include an assessment of the independent contribution of occupational activity and household activity, as well as sports and exercise on gestational diabetes risk.

13.3.4.3 Techniques to minimize lack of data on a confounder

There are several ways that you can address anticipated lack of data on a potential confounding variable in your proposal.

First, you can propose to adjust for a **proxy variable** in place of the confounder of interest. In our cataract example above, you could propose to adjust for geographic region (e.g., northern vs. southern latitude) as a proxy for adjusting for sunlight exposure, your confounder of interest. Or, if you are missing information on income level, you could consider adjusting for highest level of education as a proxy. While a proxy will not be a perfect substitution, it will help to reduce confounding.

A second way to propose to address lack of data on a potential confounder is to propose that you will perform a **sensitivity analysis**. For example, let's say you are conducting a study of exercise during pregnancy and risk of preterm birth but are missing information on history of preterm birth—an important confounder. In this situation, you could propose to repeat the analysis among women with no prior pregnancies (nulliparous women) who therefore have never had the opportunity for a preterm birth. By comparing these findings to those among your entire sample of nulliparous and parous women, you can assess the extent of possible confounding by history of preterm birth.

13.3.5 How to Present Survivor Bias

As described in Chapter 12, survivor bias is a concern typically faced by cross-sectional and case–control studies. It can occur when those with high levels of your exposure may have died from your outcome or are no longer available to participate in your study. This concern can be addressed by comparing survival rates among those with high vs. low levels of your exposure.

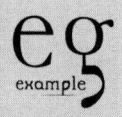

> *example*
>
> Imagine again a proposal to evaluate ALA and risk of vitamin B12 deficiency. You propose a cross-sectional design in which you will recruit participants from an outpatient clinic. Given this design, participants involved in the study will have all, by definition, survived their vitamin B12 deficiency.
>
> If those with high levels of ALA use are more likely to die of vitamin B12 deficiency, they would not be available to be included in our study. This would constitute survival bias and findings would be biased toward null. However, this is not likely to be an important concern as the consequences of vitamin B12 deficiency are not usually life threatening. Therefore, we expect the possibility of survivor bias to be minor.

13.3.6 How to Present Temporal Bias

As discussed in Chapter 12, temporal bias is another typical concern faced by cross-sectional and case–control studies. Because both the exposure and outcome of interest have already occurred at the time the investigator launches the study, we cannot ensure that the exposure indeed led to the disease and not vice versa.

This concern is minimized if you are studying immutable exposures such as blood type and eye color. For these unmodifiable risk factors, we can be sure that they definitely preceded the disease.

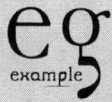

> **eg** *example*
>
> Imagine a proposal to conduct a case–control study of blood type and risk of Asperger's syndrome. You enroll cases of Asperger's syndrome and controls that do not have Asperger's and abstract medical records for their blood type.
>
> Temporal bias is not a concern because Asperger's syndrome could not have led to the blood type of the patient. Instead, we can be sure that blood type came first and diagnosis of Asperger's followed.

13.3.7 How to Present Generalizability

Generalizability was discussed in Chapter 12. Below is an approach for minimizing reviewer concerns regarding the lack of generalizability while clarifying for the reviewers the principles upon which generalizability should be based.

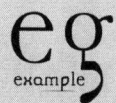

> **eg** *example*
>
> Imagine a proposal to evaluate eating disorders and risk of weight loss among Latinas. You are proposing to recruit a convenience sample of volunteers.
>
> Women who volunteer to participate may not be representative of women who live in other parts of the country. Perhaps those women who agree to participate in the study will have fewer eating disorders than those who decline to participate. However, there is little basis for believing that the biological relation between eating disorders and weight loss observed in this study will be substantially different in our population from that in most American women.
>
> Our decision to focus on one ethnicity (Latinas) is based upon both the methodologic and public health limitations of an ethnic comparison. Comparisons across ethnic groups may be limited in applicability because these groups are often profoundly different. Furthermore, ethnicity is not a modifiable risk factor. Therefore, by selecting Latinas, we will be able to examine gradient of risk within this group and findings from the study will be more closely tied to public health recommendations. Finally, Latinas are an understudied, high-risk population with little representation among the studies of weight loss.

13.4 EXAMPLES

Note that these examples extend the examples included in Chapter 12, with the addition of *techniques to minimize the limitations in bold.*

13.4.1 Example #1

Proposal to Conduct a Case–Control Study of Maternal Heat Exposure and Congenital Heart Defects

Study Limitations

Nondifferential Misclassification of Exposure
Mothers of cases and controls will be asked to recall the period of early pregnancy 3–8 years after delivery has occurred. While women's memory of their pregnancy might be better than for other life periods, inaccuracy is likely to result from the extended time lapse and difficulty in estimating average hours per week of heat exposure over a several-month time period in the past. **To minimize the possibility for such misclassification, mothers were sent individualized, multicolored calendars of their pregnancy periods, which were used as visual aids during phone interviews.**

Another possible source of nondifferential misclassification is in the definition of heat exposures, which requires some judgment by participants. No objective heat exposure measures will be available in this study. However, misclassification resulting from poor participant recall or inaccurate exposure measurement is likely to be nondifferential (i.e., misclassification will not significantly differ between cases and controls), biasing results toward the null value.

Nondifferential Misclassification of Outcome
Congenital cardiovascular malformations will be abstracted from the New York birth defects registry. Inaccuracies in classifying birth defects as congenital cardiovascular malformations are possible, and such misclassification would bias our findings toward the null. **However, a validation study conducted by the New York birth defects registry in 2010 found reasonable validity for major congenital cardiovascular malformations with Spearman correlation coefficients ranging from 0.54 to 0.76 as compared to medical record abstraction.**[1]

Selection Bias
In our pilot study, the response rate was 55.4% due to the difficulty in locating study subjects. Respondents were significantly different from nonrespondents with regard to age, race, ethnicity, and geographic location of residence within New York State. This raises the concern of selection bias, leading to an under or overestimate of our findings. **However, we compared response rates and demographics between cases and controls and found no statistically significant differences, making the possibility of selection bias unlikely.**

Information Bias: Recall Bias
In searching for possible causes for their children's heart defects, mothers of cases may more carefully report exposures as compared to mothers of controls. This recall bias would result in an overestimation of the association between heat exposure during pregnancy and congenital cardiovascular malformations. **However, the hypotheses tested in this study are not well known to the public, and there is no reason to believe that mothers will particularly suspect these exposures as possible causes of their children's heart defects.**

Information Bias: Interviewer Bias
Because exposure information will be collected by an interviewer, it is possible that an interviewer will prompt case mothers differently from control mothers, resulting in an overestimate of the association between physical exposures and congenital cardiovascular malformations. **However, interviewers will be blinded as to case/control status of the subject until the end of the interviews. Their blinded status, in addition to the structured nature of the telephone questionnaire, will help to reduce the likelihood of such interviewer bias. In addition, the questions pertaining to our study exposures will represent a minor part of the overall study questionnaire, and it is possible that neither interviewer nor participant will have preconceived notions of the effects hypothesized for those exposures.**

Confounding
The questionnaire will include information on all known risk factors for congenital cardiovascular malformations, including maternal chronic diabetes, binge drinking during pregnancy, fever during pregnancy, sex of the infant, and family history of congenital cardiovascular malformations. As with the main study exposures, information on these variables will be obtained through self-report. For information that was difficult to recall or associated with social stigma, such as drinking alcohol during pregnancy, some women's answers may be inaccurate. Failure to adequately control for these variables may lead to over- or underestimates of the association between physical exposures and congenital cardiovascular malformations. For example, prior studies have found that heat exposure during pregnancy (e.g., sauna use) is positively associated with binge drinking during pregnancy. In turn, binge drinking during pregnancy is positively associated with congenital cardiovascular malformations. Therefore, any inaccuracies in our measure of binge drinking may lead to an overestimate of the association between heat exposures and congenital cardiovascular malformations.
   However, other important covariates in this study will be less likely to be misclassified by participants, such as whether they had chronic diabetes or whether an immediate family member had congenital heart disease.

Generalizability
We do not expect the physiological association between pregnancy heat exposure and congenital cardiovascular malformations to differ according to race, ethnicity, or age. Therefore, in spite of the fact that study participants were African American and Hispanic youth, we will still be able to generalize our findings to pregnant women in the United States.

13.4.2 Example #2

Proposal to Conduct a Prospective Cohort Study of Stress and Risk of Preeclampsia

Study Limitations

Nondifferential Misclassification of Exposure

Trained, bilingual interviewers will administer the Perceived Stress Scale during a structured interview in early pregnancy (mean = 15 weeks gestational age). It is possible that women will over- or underreport their perceived stress. This may occur to the extent that perceived stress may be a sensitive issue for a select group of women. This type of misclassification would bias our results toward the null, thereby reducing our effect estimate for the relationship between perceived stress and hypertensive disorders of pregnancy. We expect this misclassification to be minor.

However misclassification will be minimized through the use of a stress questionnaire that has been validated among Hispanic women.[1] In addition, interviewers who are bilingual and/or native speakers of Spanish will assist women in completing the questionnaire.

Nondifferential Misclassification of Outcome

Cases of hypertensive disorders of pregnancy will be ascertained through medical record abstraction, as well as through a review of ICD codes for hypertension in pregnancy. Nondifferential misclassification could occur if diagnoses are missed by physicians or via the data collection methods employed. This would result in a bias of our results to the null, but we expect the effect to be minimal.

The threat of nondifferential misclassification is minimized because all cases will be confirmed by the study obstetrician. Therefore, it is unlikely that misclassification of the outcome will occur given the comprehensive nature in which diagnoses will be ascertained. Specifically, blood pressure measurements are obtained at every prenatal care visit as part of routine prenatal care, as well as regularly throughout labor and delivery. Therefore, it is unlikely that hypertension will be missed in any woman with complete delivery information. Additionally, women experiencing preeclampsia may have symptoms such as headache and visual disturbances, which would be recognized by the clinician as symptomatic of a hypertensive condition.

Selection Bias: Differential Loss to Follow-Up

Due to the prospective nature of this study, selection bias is unlikely to occur as exposure status (stress) will be collected before the disease (hypertension in pregnancy) occurs. However, selection bias is possible in a prospective study through differential loss to follow-up. For example, if women lost to follow-up were more likely to be in the high stress group and also more likely to be hypertensive in pregnancy, selection bias could occur and bias our results toward the null.

However, in our pilot study, women lost to follow-up were similar to those with complete delivery information, and therefore it is unlikely that selection bias will occur in this cohort.

Information Bias: Surveillance (Detection) Bias
Surveillance bias will be unlikely in this study because women are not monitored differently for hypertension in pregnancy according to their stress levels. The medical record abstractor will also be blinded to stress status.

To reduce the threat of detection bias, the medical record abstractor will also be blinded to stress status.

Confounding
We are not aware of any key confounders that are not available through our dataset. It is possible, however, that we measured one or more of these confounders inadequately. This residual confounding could result in a change in our effect estimate in either direction depending on the direction of the measurement error.

However, given that we are not missing information on any factors that are strongly associated with both stress and hypertensive disorders, we do not expect that uncontrolled confounding will affect our results in a meaningful way.

Generalizability
The results of this study may be generalized to pregnant women as the biological mechanisms through which stress may impact hypertension in pregnancy should not vary by race or ethnic origin.

Reproducibility and Validity Studies

14

Demonstrating the reproducibility and validity of your measures of exposure and outcome is one way of assuring your reviewers that a proposal based upon these measures will work. Remember that showing that you can *pull it off* is one of the *Ten Top Tips for Successful Proposal Writing*, as presented in Chapter 1.

A seed grant or foundation grant to support such validation work is often a key first step toward applying for a larger grant designed to use these measurement tools to evaluate etiologic associations between exposures and diseases. For this reason, a proposal to conduct a reproducibility and validity study is typically the first proposal written by a graduate student or early-career faculty.

Due to their fairly small size and delineated methods, reproducibility and validity studies are quite feasible for early-stage investigators. Furthermore, their critical role in the development of a larger project makes them particularly appealing for reviewers. In other words, such studies are the first step toward answering a larger etiologic question.

As discussed below, the need for reproducibility and validity studies remains even if the tools that you are proposing to use have been validated previously, but you are proposing to use them in a **new study population** or **modify** them in any way.

Therefore, this chapter will describe methods for designing and conducting reproducibility and validity studies, issues to consider in the analysis and interpretation of findings from these studies, as well as strategies for writing their corresponding limitations sections.

14.1 WHY CONDUCT A REPRODUCIBILITY OR VALIDITY STUDY?

The majority of proposals in epidemiology propose to measure the association between some type of exposure and risk of some outcome. These studies are termed *etiologic studies* and they rely upon tools to measure exposure and disease.

It is critical that these tools be *reliable and valid*. When tools have low reproducibility and validity, their use may lead to failure to observe an association when one indeed exists. At worse, their use may lead to the finding of a biased association between exposure and disease.

For these reasons, grant reviewers and committee members may consider a proposal to be fatally flawed if it does not provide evidence on the reproducibility and validity of the proposed measurement tools.

An important caveat
It is important to acknowledge here that in earlier, more economically advantaged times, it was considered acceptable for a large NIH R01 grant to include a reproducibility/validity study of its measurement tools as one of its specific aims. However, in the current economic climate, reviewers do not look favorably upon this approach. They naturally ask, "What if the study tools are found not to be valid? How would the principal investigator accomplish the subsequent aims of the project?" For example, imagine if aim 1 proposes to conduct a validation study of the questionnaire to be used in aims 2 and 3. If aim 1 fails to find that the questionnaire is valid, then how can the remainder of the project proceed?

14.2 WHAT IS REPRODUCIBILITY AND VALIDITY?

Reproducibility is defined as the ability of the measurement tool to produce the same results over repeated administrations. Reproducibility answers the question, "Does the questionnaire consistently provide the same results under the same circumstances?" Therefore, a *reproducibility study* is typically designed to compare data from repeated administrations of a measurement tool.

Reproducibility—the consistency of measurements

- On more than one administration
- To the same people
- At different times

A perfectly reproducible method will yield the same results on repeated administrations. However, in reality, a measurement method will always be subject to error.

In contrast, validity answers the question, "How well does the tool measure what it is designed to measure?" Therefore, validation studies are designed to compare data collected by some type of proxy measure (e.g., your proposed measurement tool) against a *gold standard*. In practice, *gold standards* often do not exist, and in their place, a superior, although typically imperfect, comparison method is utilized.

Validity—the degree to which the tool actually measures what it was designed to measure

14.3 RELATIONSHIP BETWEEN REPRODUCIBILITY AND VALIDITY

In the figures below, the *bull's-eye* center of the dartboard reflects the truth, that is, the true value that you are trying to measure. The dots represent the values observed by your measurement tool over repeated administrations of the tool. The degree of validity is indicated by the proximity of these dots to the bull's eye, while the degree of reproducibility is indicated by the proximity of these dots to each other.

Figures 14.1a and 14.1b both demonstrate high reproducibility because the dots are in a tight circle—showing that repeated measurements are consistent with each other over time. Figure 14.1a demonstrates high validity because the dots encircle the center of the circle (the truth), while Figure 14.1b demonstrates low validity because the circles do not encircle the truth.

The take-home message here is that *high reproducibility does not ensure high validity*.

Figures 14.2a and 14.2b both demonstrate low reproducibility because the dots are in a wide circle—showing that repeated measurements are not consistent with each other over time. However, Figure 14.2a demonstrates high validity because the dots

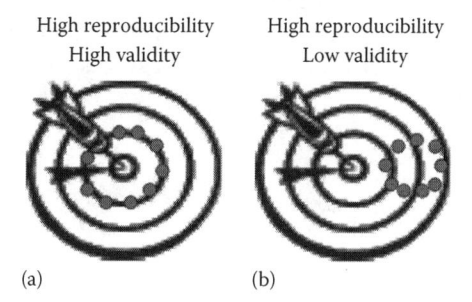

FIGURE 14.1 The relationship between reproducibility and validity: high reproducibility and high (a) and low (b) validity.

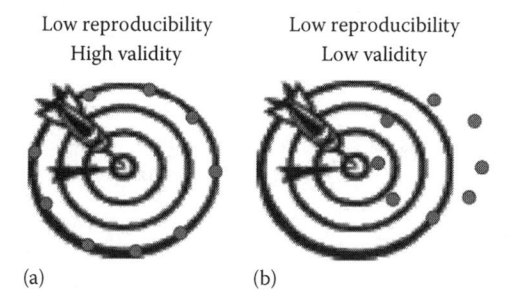

FIGURE 14.2 The relationship between reproducibility and validity: low reproducibility and high (a) and low (b) validity.

still encircle the center of the circle (the truth). Figure 14.2b demonstrates low validity because the circles do not encircle the truth.

In summary, because reproducibility studies are usually quick and inexpensive to conduct, they are an appropriate part of the measurement tool evaluation but cannot substitute for validity studies.

14.4 BOTH SUBJECTIVE AND OBJECTIVE MEASUREMENT TOOLS REQUIRE EVIDENCE OF REPRODUCIBILITY AND VALIDITY

Because there are typically no true *gold standard* measurement methods, the need for reproducibility and validity studies is critical whether you are using subjective measures (e.g., questionnaire-based) or using more *objective* measures (e.g., laboratory assays, medical records).

14.4.1 Questionnaires

Questionnaires are a common approach to measuring exposures of interest in the fields of preventive medicine and epidemiology. Indeed, questionnaires have become the primary method for measuring such behavioral and psychosocial exposures as physical activity, diet, stress, and anxiety.

Advantages of questionnaires

- Practical for large sample sizes
- Nonreactive
- Tailored to specific populations and time periods

As epidemiologic studies typically involve hundreds to thousands of subjects, questionnaires are extremely practical and cost efficient. They are easy for subjects to complete and can be self-administered or interviewer-administered, both in person or on the telephone. They can ask participants to recall past information or to report current real-time information (e.g., 24 h logs or diaries).

In addition, questionnaires are nonreactive, meaning that they tend not to interfere with the conduct of the behaviors themselves. Finally, questionnaires are malleable. They can be tailored to the characteristics of your particular study population (e.g., age, gender) or limited to a particular period of time (e.g., past week, past year, lifetime).

Disadvantages of questionnaires

- Precision

The disadvantages of questionnaires involve their precision in measuring absolute levels of the exposure of interest, due in part to their reliance upon self-report.

TABLE 14.1 When to perform reproducibility/validity studies

- For new questionnaires
- When a questionnaire is modified
- When questionnaires will be used in a different population according to:
  - Age
  - Gender
  - Culture
  - Other medical or behavioral factors

Documenting the reproducibility and validity of any new questionnaire is critical (Table 14.1). For existing questionnaires, even small changes in the design of instruments may affect their performance. Therefore, the validity and reproducibility of any modified instrument should be evaluated independently. In addition, when a questionnaire will be administered to a study population that differs from the one in which it was developed, its reproducibility and validity should again be evaluated. Questionnaires are culture-specific and their performance will differ according to the age, gender, and culture of the study population.

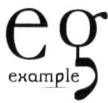

e.g. example Imagine a proposal to use a questionnaire to evaluate diet in Asian youth. Ideally, you would want to cite studies showing that the questionnaire was valid not only among children but also among Asian children. If such studies are not available, you may want to consider conducting such a validation study yourself.

14.4.2 Particular Challenge of Behavioral Questionnaires

Questionnaires have become the primary method for measuring behaviors (e.g., physical activity, diet, substance use) in epidemiologic studies. Such human behaviors are complex and difficult to measure accurately. In addition, because epidemiologic questionnaires are based upon self-reported data, documenting the reproducibility and validity of any new behavioral questionnaire is critical.

The particular challenge of behavioral questionnaires

- Behaviors have multiple components
- Reliance on self-report
- Unstructured nature of many behaviors
- Rare nature of many behaviors

Many behaviors have **multiple components** that make up the total *dose* of behavior (i.e., type, frequency, and intensity/content). Each of these individual components may vary from person to person. Furthermore, individuals rarely make clear changes in their behaviors at identifiable points in time. Instead, behavioral patterns typically evolve over periods of years.

Questionnaires designed to assess such behaviors are based upon **self-report** and therefore face the additional challenges of relying upon a participant's memory and accuracy in reporting.

Because many human behaviors are **unstructured**—they are even more difficult for subjects to report accurately. In addition, unstructured activities are less memorable than behaviors that require planning or effort.

Behaviors that are **rare** may be more or less difficult to report accurately. On the one hand, the planned nature of rare activities may make them easier to accurately report. In addition, salient events (e.g., key life events) may be more easy to recall and lead to higher estimates of validity and reproducibility as compared to routine day-to-day events. On the other hand, activities that are rarely engaged in may be more difficult to reliably recall.

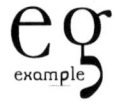

e.g. example
Physical activity is a complex behavior made up of type, frequency, duration, and intensity of activity. "Types" of physical activity can include sports/exercise, occupational activity, and household activity. Physical activity also spans different intensities including light intensity, moderate intensity, and vigorous intensity. Perceived intensity may also vary from person to person.

Studies have found that vigorous physical activity is more accurately recalled than moderate and nonvigorous activity since it may require planning or an effort that moderate activities do not require. In addition, vigorous activities like skiing or running may be reported more accurately if they are part of a participant's exercise schedule. In contrast, moderate activities such as walking and playing with children tend to be much more difficult to accurately report from memory.

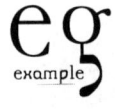

e.g. example
Dietary consumption is also a complex behavior made up of type, portion size, number of servings, and the nutrient content of the food consumed. The same food may have a different nutrient content depending upon the preparation technique and other factors. In addition, mixed foods such as casseroles and stews may contain many individual food components that are often difficult to tease apart. Unstructured behaviors such as snacking may be difficult for subjects to report accurately.

14.4.3 Objective Measures Also Require Reproducibility and Validity Studies

Objective measures are also subject to error. Examples of objective outcome measures can include biomarkers, medical records, and monitors. Each of these measures, although termed *objective*, faces potential errors as described below.

Biomarkers are measurable chemical, physical, or biological characteristics that aim to represent the severity or presence of some disease state. They are often obtained via blood or urine samples or biopsy. However, biomarkers face several limitations. First, biomarkers may not reflect the etiologically relevant time period for the impact of your exposure on your outcome of interest. For example, a cholesterol measure obtained after diagnosis of heart disease may not be representative of the cholesterol levels that preceded the heart disease. Second, degradation over time in frozen samples could reduce their validity. In addition, the biomarker may be influenced by other factors. For example, blood levels of vitamin D are not only influenced by diet but also by sunlight exposure.

Medical records or **ICD codes** are often considered a gold standard. However, medical records may be completed by a variety of personnel including residents, attending physicians, and nurses. Any of these personnel can make an error in recording key information in the medical record or in selecting the appropriate code. There may also be error on the part of the medical record abstractors in terms of their ability to abstract data.

Monitors can include physical activity monitoring systems such as actigraphs. Monitors face several sources of error. Participants may not be compliant in consistently wearing the monitors or may wear them incorrectly. Such devices can be reactive such that participants change their activity when they are wearing them. Lastly, the monitors themselves may have difficulty measuring particular types of activity. For example, waist-worn physical activity monitors have difficulty measuring upper body movements and may have to be removed during swimming.

Therefore, providing evidence for the reproducibility and validity of objective measures is just as important as doing so for subjective measures.

14.5 STUDY DESIGN OF REPRODUCIBILITY STUDIES

The goal of a reproducibility study is to assess variation in questionnaire performance from one administration to the next.

The first step in designing a reproducibility study is to consider the **time interval** between administrations of the measurement tool (Figure 14.3).

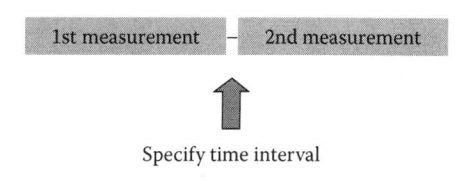

FIGURE 14.3 Reproducibility studies: consider the time interval between administrations of the measurement tool.

Both short and long time intervals have advantages and disadvantages described in more detail later in the chapter. However, briefly, these are described as follows:

Short intervals (i.e., days or weeks) between questionnaire administrations may result in participants recalling their previous responses as opposed to truly considering the questions. This will lead to artificially increased reproducibility.

Long intervals of time between questionnaire administrations (i.e., one year) may encompass true changes in behaviors and lead to reduced reproducibility.

One approach to address these problems is to administer the questionnaire over both short as well as long intervals of time to provide an estimate of both the lower as well as upper level of reproducibility.

14.6 STUDY DESIGN OF VALIDITY STUDIES

The goal of a validity study is to compare your measurement tool with a *gold standard*—a perfect measure of your variable of interest. In the absence of a true gold standard, you will want to select a superior method that has few, if any, shared sources of error with your measurement tool. Therefore, the first step in conducting a validity study is to choose your comparison measure.

All measures have error, although they differ in magnitude and type. Given that neither your measure nor the comparison measure will be perfect, the error of both should be as uncorrelated as possible to avoid falsely high estimates of validity.

14.6.1 Subjective Comparison Measures

In terms of the subjective comparison measures, a log or diaries are likely to have the least correlated errors with questionnaires. For each 15 min interval of each hour of the day, participants record either their actual behavior (e.g., diet, physical activity) or a code corresponding to the type of behavior. Unlike a self-administered questionnaire, a 24 h log or diary is filled out in real time over the course of the day (Table 14.2).

Major sources of errors associated with questionnaires are due to the restricted list of activities, memory, and misinterpretation of questions. These sources of error are not typically shared by logs or diaries that are open-ended and not reliant upon memory (i.e., activities are recorded as they occur) (Figure 14.4). Disadvantages of logs or diaries

TABLE 14.2 Examples of subjective comparison measures

- Logs or diaries
- 24-h recall
- 7-day recall
- Previous month recall
- Previous year recall

Day One			Date: / /	
Minutes → Hours ↓	1–15 min past the hour	16–30 min past the hour	31–45 min past the hour	46–59 min past the hour
12:00 PM				
1:00 PM				
2:00 PM				
3:00 PM				
4:00 PM				
5:00 PM				

FIGURE 14.4 Example excerpt from a 7-day activity diary.

involve the fact that they rely heavily on subject motivation—they are time consuming to complete. Completing them may also lead to heightened awareness that may alter normal behaviors (i.e., reactivity). Logs or diaries also share error due to self-report with questionnaires. For example, subjects are often prone to overestimate their physical activity on both questionnaires and diaries.

Table 14.2 provides examples of subjective comparison measures.

14.6.2 Objective Comparison Measures

Objective measures are often the comparison method of choice for questionnaires as they are not subject to errors associated with self-report. On the other hand, objective measures are typically more expensive to administer and can cause reactivity (i.e., changes in behavior due to the device) (Table 14.3).

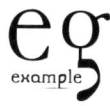

eg example Imagine that you are proposing to validate a physical activity questionnaire. Epidemiologic studies are most interested in assessing typical or long-term physical activity due to its potential association with disease. However, there are no perfect measures of typical or long-term physical activity. Examples of comparison measures for a physical activity questionnaire include both subjective measures (based on self-report) and objective measures (based on direct measurement). Subjective comparison measures can ask participants to recall past physical activity (questionnaire) or to

TABLE 14.3 Examples of objective comparison measures for physical activity

- Monitors (e.g., actigraph, heart rate monitors)
- Biomarkers
- Doubly labeled water
- Direct observation

report current physical activity (24 h logs or diaries). Objective comparison measures include markers of movement (accelerometers), physiological responses that are affected by physical activity (heart rate), direct measures of energy expenditure (doubly labeled water), and observed or videotaped activity (direct observation).

14.6.3 Number of Administrations of the Comparison Method

The next step in designing a validity study is to consider the **number of administrations** of the comparison method, which should be based upon:

- Intraindividual variation in the behavior
- The accuracy of the comparison measure
- Participant burden
- Questionnaire time frame

The greater the variation in the behavior being measured, and the lower the accuracy of the comparison measure, the more administrations you will want to consider. On the other hand, the number of administrations of the comparison method should be tempered by the burden on the participant.

eg *example* Imagine a proposal to conduct a validation study of a physical activity questionnaire whose goal is to assess usual activity over the past year. To assess reproducibility, you propose to administer the questionnaire at the beginning of the year and then repeat it at the end of the year. As a validation tool, you propose to administer four comparison measures (i.e., 7-day activity diaries) during each season throughout that year to capture day-to-day and seasonal variation in activity levels. In this way, the comparison measure covers the interval of time corresponding to the questionnaire—1 year. Each seasonal administration will include a sufficient number of days to represent average energy expenditure (i.e., 7 days) (Figure 14.5).

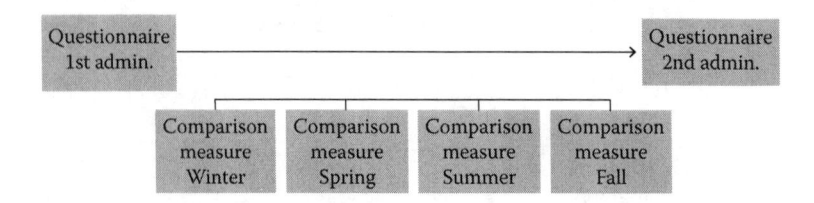

FIGURE 14.5 Study design for a reproducibility and validity study of a physical activity questionnaire.

14.7 WRITING DATA ANALYSIS SECTIONS FOR REPRODUCIBILITY/VALIDITY STUDIES

There are many statistical techniques available that can be used to assess reproducibility and validity. These include

- Kappa coefficients
- Percent agreement
- Correlation coefficients (e.g., Pearson or Spearman)
- Sensitivity
- Specificity
- Paired comparisons (e.g., paired t-test, Wilcoxon signed rank test)
- Bland–Altman plots

Ideally, these agreement statistics should be accompanied by **confidence intervals (CIs)**, which allow for the interpretation of the precision of the reported estimates.

These measures all have specific strengths and limitations and the choice of which method to use will depend upon your specific measurement tools and other characteristics of your study design and setting. Consultation with a statistician on which technique to choose is highly recommended.

For example, because kappa is prevalence dependent, it is often viewed in combination with percent agreement and sensitivity to obtain a more accurate overall interpretation of agreement. Sensitivity calculations are especially instructive when a condition is rare. In contrast, specificity may be inflated in the context of rare events as they are less likely to have false-negative findings. Correlation coefficients are largely influenced by the range of the observed values and can be high even when the measurements do not agree (e.g., when there is a systematic difference between measures).

Bland–Altman plots have been promulgated as a method that can both quantify the comparison between two measurement tools and indicate the direction of mismeasurement between the tools. Specifically, for every subject, the **difference** between the two measures (y-axis) is plotted against the **average** of the two measures (x-axis) (Figure 14.6).

> **eg** *example*
>
> Recall the previous example of a proposal to validate a physical activity questionnaire.
>
> Data analysis section: Intraclass correlation coefficients will be used to describe the reproducibility of the two questionnaires. To evaluate the questionnaire's validity, Spearman correlation coefficients will be calculated between each of the questionnaires and the comparison method (i.e., the average of the four weekly diaries). Correlations will be calculated for overall activity, as well as activity according to intensity and type.

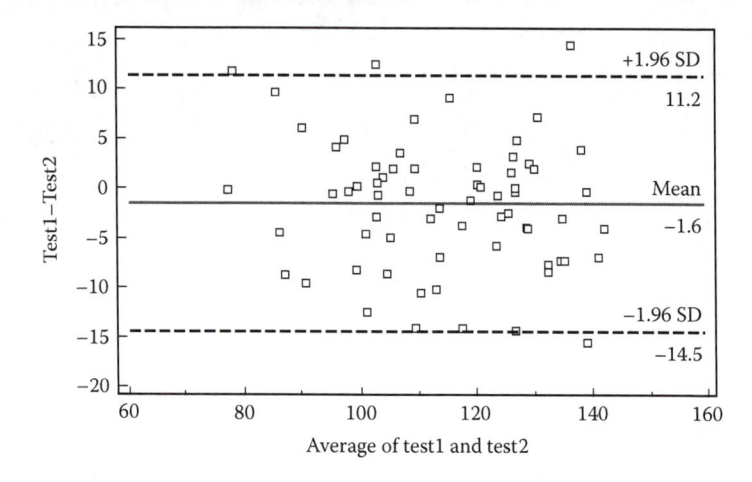

FIGURE 14.6 Bland–Altman plot.

14.8 WRITING LIMITATIONS SECTIONS FOR REPRODUCIBILITY/VALIDITY STUDIES

Limitations sections for reproducibility/validity studies differ from limitations sections for etiologic studies described in Chapter 12, *Review of Bias and Confounding*. Specifically, the limitations section for a reproducibility/validity study focuses on factors that may bias the observed measure of agreement—either between repeated administrations of your measurement tool (i.e., reproducibility) or between your measurement tool and a comparison measure (i.e., validity) (Table 14.4).

Just as described in detail in Chapter 13, *How to Present Limitations and Alternatives*, when presenting limitations in your reproducibility/validity proposal, you will want to use the same fourfold approach. Specifically, you will (1) describe the potential limitation, (2) describe the potential impact of the limitation on your study findings, (3) discuss alternatives and why they were not selected, and (4) describe the methods that you propose to minimize the impact of this limitation (Table 14.5).

TABLE 14.4 Study limitations for a reproducibility/validity study

Threats to observed reproducibility scores
- Correlated error between administrations
- True changes in behavior between administrations
- A heightened awareness of behavior after the first administration

Threats to observed validity scores
- Correlated error between the measurement tool and the comparison

Threats to generalizability

TABLE 14.5 A fourfold approach for presenting study limitations in a proposal

Step 1: Identify the limitation
Step 2: Describe the impact on your findings
Step 3: Discuss alternatives
Step 4: Describe methods to minimize

14.8.1 Threats to Observed Reproducibility Scores

There are several common threats to observed reproducibility scores as described below:

1. *Correlated error*

    Observations of high reproducibility scores for a questionnaire may be caused by consistent errors in the completion of both administrations of the measurement tool. For example, if the participants consistently **misinterpret questions** on each administration of the questionnaire, their scores would be highly (but incorrectly) correlated.

    Similarly, if the questionnaire consistently **omitted an important question**, this would also lead to incorrectly high reproducibility scores.

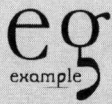

> **eg** *example*
>
> Recall our proposal above to conduct a reproducibility and validity study of a physical activity questionnaire. The questionnaire was administered at the beginning of the year. To assess reproducibility, the questionnaire was administered for a second time at the end of the year.
>
> *Identify the limitation*
> It is also possible that the 2010 questionnaire and the 2011 questionnaire would be highly correlated but not represent the actual ability of women to recall physical activity. An apparent correlation could be due to consistent errors of self-report on both questionnaires or to an error in the questionnaire itself such as omission of a common activity. It is also possible that participants may systematically exaggerate their level of physical activity.
>
> *Describe the methods to minimize the limitation*
> However, the questionnaire was developed based on a series of focus groups that used open-ended techniques to assemble a comprehensive list of activities engaged in by the study population. Therefore, we feel it is unlikely that the questionnaire will omit any important activities. In addition, the questionnaires will be interviewer-administered and interviewers will be highly trained to provide guidance on interpretation of questionnaire items and to reality-check responses with participants. Therefore, we feel that the concerns of misinterpretation and exaggeration will be minimized.

2. *True changes in behavior*

Observations of low reproducibility scores may reflect **too long a time period** between administration of the measurement tools such that there are true changes between the intervals. On the other hand, **too short a time interval** between administrations of the questionnaire may lead to respondents recalling their previous responses as opposed to truly considering the questions. This would lead to an overestimate of reproducibility between the measures.

Low reproducibility scores may also reflect *differences in the reference time period* of recall. For example, imagine a questionnaire that asks respondents to recall their behavior over the past 3 months and then is repeated 3 months later. By definition, the participants are being asked to recall behaviors over a different time period on the first administration than they are on the second administration. The participants may have truly changed their behavior over this time period and, therefore, the estimates of reproducibility will be lower due to this true variation in behavior.

This concern can be minimized in several ways:

If the measurement tool is querying **usual behavior**, this concern is reduced. For example, if the questionnaire is asking about usual dietary consumption and is repeated one week apart, then true changes in diet over that past week should not substantively influence the responses to the second administration of the questionnaire.

This is also less of a concern if the behavior tends to be **stable over time**. For example, if the respondent tends to eat the same foods from week to week, then any true changes in diet over the week are likely to be minimal.

Finally, this concern is also minimized if you will be categorizing participants in fairly **broad categories**. In this situation, for bias to occur, it would have to be substantial enough to move participants from one category of, for example, dietary consumption (e.g., the lowest quartile) to a higher category (e.g., the second or higher quartile).

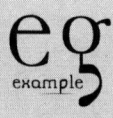

> **e.g. example**
>
> Imagine a proposal to conduct a reproducibility study of a dietary questionnaire among middle-aged men.
>
> *Identify the limitation*
>
> Random within-person error may lead to underestimates of the true reproducibility of the questionnaire.
>
> *Describe the methods to minimize the limitation*
>
> Because the questionnaire asks men to integrate diet over the course of an entire year, we expect that random within-person error will be minimal. In addition, actual dietary patterns are unlikely to change drastically for middle-aged men between questionnaire administrations. It is also unlikely that participants will have changed their dietary consumption levels so dramatically as to move from quartile 1 (lowest) to quartile 4 (highest) of total energy intake.

3. *A heightened awareness of behavior*
   Low reproducibility scores may also reflect heightened awareness of behavior due to the completion of the first administration of the questionnaire. That is, the first completion of the questionnaire may lead respondents to be more aware of their behaviors during the following time interval such that on the second administration of the questionnaire, they will report their behavior differently even if it has not changed.

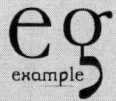

> **eg** *example*
> Imagine again a proposal to assess the reproducibility and validity of a physical activity questionnaire.
>
> *Identify the limitation*
> The experience of completing the first questionnaire may influence participants in completing the second questionnaire. It is possible that participants will be more likely to accurately report their physical activity on the second questionnaire due to an increased knowledge and understanding of the questions gained from completing the first questionnaire. In addition, the questions asked on the first questionnaire may lead participants to be more aware of their physical activity over the intervening time period.
>
> *Describe the impact on your findings*
> This would result in lower agreement between the first and second questionnaires and produce an underestimation of the intraclass correlation coefficient.
>
> *Describe the methods to minimize the limitation*
> Therefore, in interpreting our findings, we will consider the observed reproducibility as a lower bound of the questionnaire's true reproducibility.

14.8.2 Threats to Observed Validity Scores

A common threat to observed validity scores is correlated error between the measurement tool and the comparison measure.

1. *Correlated error*
   Observations of high validity between your measurement tool and comparison measure may reflect correlated error. For example, if both your measurement tool and the comparison measure omit an item, they will be highly correlated, but they will both be similarly incorrect (invalid). Similarly, if both your measurement tool and the comparison measure include questions that are misinterpreted, they will also be likely highly correlated but again less than valid. Third, if both your measurement tool and the gold standard rely upon self-report, then both will be

similarly influenced by limitations of memory as well as social desirability bias (e.g., the tendency of respondents to report what they think they should be doing or what they feel would be the correct behavior but not what they are truly doing).

In other words, high validity scores may simply indicate that error in the questionnaire and the comparison methods are correlated. As noted above, given that neither method will be perfect, it is critical that the errors of both methods be as independent (uncorrelated) as possible. To the extent that errors in a comparison method are uncorrelated with error in the questionnaires, the correlation between the two tends to be underestimated. Alternatively, correlated errors will result in spuriously high estimates of validity.

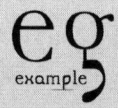

> **example**
>
> Recall the proposal above to conduct a reproducibility and validity study of a physical activity questionnaire. The questionnaire was administered at the beginning of the year. As a validation tool, four comparison measures (e.g., 7-day activity diaries) were then administered during each season to capture day-to-day and seasonal variation in activity levels. At the end of the year, the questionnaire was administered for a second time.
>
> *Identify the limitation*
> Diaries, however, are not a gold standard as they share several sources of errors with the questionnaires. While diaries, unlike questionnaires, are not subject to errors due to restrictions imposed by a fixed list of activities, memory, and interpretation of questions, both diaries and questionnaires likely elicit socially desirable responses. Also, if the diaries are not filled out properly (e.g., at the end of the day), they may involve memory as well as the questionnaires.
>
> *Describe the methods to minimize the limitation*
> However, diaries are judged to be superior to questionnaires and are considered an acceptable method to validate questionnaires.[1] Because errors associated with the questionnaires and diaries will be largely independent, our validity scores will likely be underestimated.

14.8.3 Threats to Generalizability

As with any research study, participants in reproducibility/validity studies tend to be convenience samples, that is, people who are available and volunteer to be in the study as opposed to a random sample of the study population. These volunteers may differ in important ways from those who do not volunteer. In turn, these differences may be responsible for your observed reproducibility and validity scores. For example, volunteers may be healthier or more likely to have higher levels of education than those who do not volunteer. As such, they may be more likely to accurately report their behavior or be more aware of their behaviors than the general population.

However, this *concern is minimized* if the measurement tool is actually intended for use in a healthy or college-educated population. In this situation, your findings for reproducibility and validity would be relevant for epidemiologic studies among this population.

In addition, the fact that people who participate in this study may be different from those who could not or would not participate does not necessarily mean that findings cannot be generalized. Generalizing depends on whether you think the *ability to self-report such information would be different* among participants as compared to those who did not participate.

If you have any concerns about generalizing, you can consider repeating your reproducibility/validity study among participants who share the characteristics of the population for whom the measurement tool is intended.

14.9 HOW TO INTERPRET FINDINGS FROM REPRODUCIBILITY/VALIDITY STUDIES

It is important to note that the range of acceptable reproducibility and validity measures for a questionnaire will tend to be lower than the acceptable range for a laboratory measure. For example, measures of agreement ranging from 0.5 to 0.7 are not unusual for behavioral questionnaires. Indeed, dietary and physical activity questionnaires with these ranges of reproducibility and validity have been found to be strong and consistent predictors of disease.

Various recommendations have been published for interpreting measures of reproducibility and validity. These recommendations vary slightly but in general are consistent with the following:

- <0 poor
- 0–0.20 slight
- 0.21–0.40 fair
- 0.41–0.60 moderate
- 0.61–0.80 substantial
- 0.81–1.00 almost perfect

Once you have conducted your reproducibility and validity study, you will need to consider these ranges in deciding whether you want to rely upon these measurement tools in your subsequent proposals.

It is important to note that there are no generally accepted thresholds below which agreement is considered too low. However, if you find that your reproducibility and validity are poor to slight, you may want to consider modifying your assessment tool for future use. In the case of a questionnaire, focus groups on the acceptability and interpretability of the questionnaire could be considered. On the other hand, as described above, there are other explanations for low reproducibility and validity (e.g., true changes in behavior, error in the reference method). All these factors need to be considered in deciding whether or not to accept your measurement tools. Therefore, interpret your findings with caution!

14.10 ISSUES OF SAMPLE SIZE AND POWER FOR A REPRODUCIBILITY AND VALIDITY STUDY

The number of subjects to be included in a reproducibility and validity study varies and depends upon

- The expected correlation between the measurement tool and the comparison measure
- The degree of desired precision

For example, if the goal is to observe a correlation between a dietary or physical activity questionnaire and a comparison measure of 0.5–0.7, it is generally recommended that the study population include 100–200 subjects. Often, power calculations are not included in proposals for reproducibility and validity studies as the goal of these studies is to generate findings that will be utilized for sample size calculations for future proposals.

However, if conducted, such calculations should not rely entirely upon significance testing, because whether or not a measure of agreement is statistically significant depends largely on the number of participants, typically a small number in such studies. In addition, power calculations for a correlation coefficient only indicate the ability of the correlation coefficient to differ from 0, which is not particularly informative.

Instead, it is possible to present the reviewer with a range of desired measures of agreement and the corresponding CIs that you will be able to detect at 80% power. That is, power the study to achieve a particular range of CIs for a desired measure of agreement.

> **eg** *example* The study was powered to achieve CIs of 0.66–0.90 for a sensitivity of 0.80.

14.11 SUMMARY

Evaluating the reproducibility and validity of your proposed measurement tools is critical. A variety of comparison methods are available and the study design should be tailored to your specific population. Interpretation of results should be informed by a comprehensive understanding of the possible reasons for over- or underestimates of your observed reproducibility and validity scores. Finally, because there is typically no gold standard comparison measure, interpretation of results of validity/reproducibility studies should be informed by an understanding of the sources of error associated with both the measurement tool and the comparison method.

14.12 EXAMPLE

A Proposal to Evaluate the Reproducibility and Validity of an Exercise Questionnaire for Use in the Elderly

I. *Study design*
Participants will complete the exercise questionnaire and then wear an actigraph as a validation tool for the following 7 days. At the end of the 7-day period, the exercise questionnaire will be repeated.

II. *Methods*
The actigraph detects vertical accelerations ranging in magnitude from 0.05 to 2.00 G with frequency response from 0.25 to 2.50 Hz. The above parameters will detect normal human movement while filtering out high-frequency movements such as vibrations. The filtered acceleration signal is digitized and the magnitude is summed over a user-specified time interval (epoch). At the end of each epoch, the activity count is stored in memory and the accumulator is reset to zero. A 1 min epoch will be used in this study.

The actigraph will be affixed with an adjustable belt on the right hip under clothing during the waking hours of the following seven days. While wearing the actigraph, participants will be given a form on which to note if they removed the actigraph during the day for longer than one hour to swim, shower, or nap.

Total energy expenditure will be calculated from both the questionnaire and the actigraph. In addition, data from the questionnaire and the actigraph will be classified by intensity: light, moderate, or vigorous.

III. *Statistical analysis*
The reproducibility between the two administrations of the exercise questionnaire will be described by intraclass correlation coefficients. We will calculate reproducibility for total energy expenditure, as well as according to activity intensity (i.e., light, moderate, and vigorous).

To evaluate the validity of the exercise questionnaire, we will calculate Spearman correlation coefficients between the exercise questionnaire and the actigraph values for total energy expenditure, as well as according to activity intensity (i.e., light, moderate, and vigorous).

IV. *Study limitations*
This study will be subject to several limitations. Wearing an activity monitor during the one-week interval between the administrations of the questionnaires may lead to a heightened awareness of activity among participants. In addition, although less likely, true changes in activity patterns may have occurred during the one-week interval. However, as the exercise questionnaire assesses usual activity, which is less likely to have changed over a one-week time period, we believe that the correlations will largely reflect the reproducibility characteristics of our questionnaire. Given these changes in awareness or true activity over the week, the correlations we observe will provide a lower limit on the questionnaire's actual reproducibility.

As our comparison measure of usual activity, we will utilize estimates of physical activity from an actigraph worn for a one-week period. A number of studies have been conducted to determine how many measurement days are needed to reliably estimate habitual physical activity. In these studies, the number of days has varied between 4 and 12 depending on the precision that is required, the accuracy of the reference method, and the intraindividual variation in activity. In light of these factors, we feel that seven days of actigraph use will be appropriately conservative.

The validity results will be impacted by errors in the actigraph data as well as in the exercise questionnaire measures. For example, when the actigraph is worn on the hip, error results from the inability of the actigraph to accurately measure activities involving upper body movement, pushing or carrying a load, stationary exercise (e.g., cycling), and weight lifting. In contrast, errors in the exercise questionnaire may result from subject inaccuracy in self-reporting physical activity. Given that neither method is perfect, it is critical that the errors inherent in each method be as independent as possible, as correlated errors will result in spuriously high validity coefficients. Therefore, because errors associated with the actigraph and exercise questionnaire are largely independent, our correlation coefficients will not likely be overstated.

Abstracts and Titles

15

An abstract can be considered the most critical component of a proposal. The skill of learning to write a concise, persuasive abstract will serve you well. Due to its short length, and ability to encapsulate the crux of the study rationale and methods, the abstract plays a powerful role in funding decisions. In the NIH grant review process, the abstract is termed the *project summary* and may be the only component of the proposal read by the entire review panel. As noted in Chapter 1, *Ten Top Tips for Successful Proposal Writing*, the bulk of your writing time should be spent refining your **abstract** and specific aims.

The overall goal of the abstract is to show how your proposed study will extend prior research in the area, briefly encapsulate the study methods (particularly any innovative methods), as well as provide the key public health and clinical significance of potential study findings. Keep in mind that your goal is to provide enough information for potential readers to make informed decisions on whether to read the rest of your proposal. The abstract is the *teaser* or *appetizer*. If it doesn't grab the reader's attention now, you may have permanently missed your window of opportunity.

Therefore, this chapter will provide strategies for abstract writing within the context of the strict word count or line limitations typical of most funding agencies. The chapter provides tips and strategies for how to write your abstract and, more importantly, what merits inclusion in your abstract. In addition, guidelines and tips for how to **title** your grant proposal will also be provided.

Finally, it is important to note here that this chapter **comes after** the chapters on writing the body of your proposal for a specific reason: abstracts should not be finalized until the remainder of the proposal has been written.

15.1 OUTLINE FOR PROPOSAL ABSTRACT

In a grant proposal, an abstract is usually the first scientific page of the proposal—coming immediately after the face page (which contains data on the applicant and their institution). In a dissertation proposal, an abstract is usually placed on a separate page following the title page.

Early-career faculty and graduate students may be most familiar with journal article abstracts, the summary of the report that is placed immediately below the title

TABLE 15.1 Proposal abstract outline

I. Background
II. Research aims
III. Highlights of the methodology
IV. Summary of the significance and innovation

TABLE 15.2 Journal article abstract outline

I. Background
II. Research aims
III. Highlights of the methodology
IV. Highlights of the results
V. Conclusions
VI. Summary of the significance and innovation

in a journal article. The key difference between an abstract for a journal article and an abstract for a proposal is that the former will include study findings. In contrast, the abstract for a proposal needs to convey the ***potential importance of* study findings**.

The following is a general outline for a proposal abstract, shown in Table 15.1.

In contrast, note in Table 15.2 that an abstract for a journal article includes highlights of the results and conclusions.

The following sections will break down each of the four subcomponents of the proposal abstract (Table 15.1) in more detail.

15.2 HOW TO GET STARTED WRITING AN ABSTRACT

Before setting pen to paper, it is important to step back and try the following tactic.

A *tactic* to try Consider the following exercise. Pretend that you standing at the edge of a diving board. Immediately after you jump, someone yells out, "What is so important about your new proposal?" You quickly yell out the key factors before you hit the water. In my experience, this tactic is most productive when conducted **out loud** with a colleague (but not actually on a diving board!). It does not matter if this colleague is an expert in the field. To be successful, a proposal needs to be understandable by anyone with a scientific background. After answering this overall question, have the colleague hold a timer set to 15 s and ask you the following questions relating to each item in Table 15.1. You get 15 s to respond to each question:

- What **background** motivates your study?
- What are your key **aims**?

- What are the key aspects of your **methodology**?
- What is the **significance and innovation** of your proposed study?
  - What are the **implications** of your potential findings?

I have used this verbal technique for years in my course on grant proposal writing. Students are always surprised how much easier it is to express themselves verbally when the identical questions, presented in writing, can cause them to freeze up or, even worse, use professional jargon.

15.3 WHEN TO FINALIZE THE ABSTRACT

It may be surprising to learn that the process of finalizing the abstract ideally comes after the process of writing the entire proposal. This is also true when writing a journal article. Indeed, the order of the chapters of this text was done purposefully to follow this recommendation.

The reason for this recommendation is efficiency. A well-written proposal will include within it the key sentences needed for an abstract. Remember back in Chapter 7 when I recommended bolding key sentences in the Background and Significance sections. Here, you are allowed to plagiarize from yourself! Simply start out by copying and pasting, perhaps with a modicum of tweaking, these key sentences into your abstract. Continue on through the proposal choosing key sentences from your methods section. This repetitive use of key sentences (i.e., both in the abstract and then again in the body of the proposal) actually makes it easier for the reviewer. It usually takes seeing these items at least twice, before the reviewer really *gets* the key aspects of your proposal (Table 15.3).

Excerpt the key sentences from your proposal that relate to each component of the abstract outline

It is important to note here that this process also serves a dual purpose. If you find that you are unable to find key sentences in the body of your proposal—this raises a red flag about your writing style. To improve the proposal, reread and review Chapter 5 *Scientific Writing*.

TABLE 15.3 Proposal abstract writing: Correspondence with body of the proposal and book chapter

ABSTRACT OUTLINE	PROPOSAL SECTION	CHAPTER #
I. Background	Background and Significance	Chapter 7
II. Research aims	Specific Aims/Hypotheses	Chapters 6 and 3
III. Highlights of the methodology	Study Design and Methods	Chapter 9
IV. Summary of significance and innovation	Background and Significance	Chapter 7

15.4 NIH REVIEW OF AN ABSTRACT

As discussed in more detail in Chapter 19, *Review Process*, NIH grant reviews are conducted by study sections—panels of anywhere from 20 to 30 members. Prior to this meeting, your grant application will have been read in its entirety by one primary reviewer and two to three secondary and tertiary reviewers. The remainder of the grant review panel will likely have never seen your application prior to this meeting.

Many study sections will start the grant review process by asking the entire grant review panel to take 2–3 min to silently read over the abstract and specific aims of the application under review. Others will not even allow this time before the discussion starts. Therefore, the majority of reviewers on the panel will only have time to read your abstract. The remainder of the discussion typically lasts 10–20 min—not enough time for these members to read the body of your proposal. This first impression of your application will likely be the first and primary exposure to your grant by the majority of the review panel.

Because every review panel member's vote counts equally on your application—regardless of whether they are a primary/secondary/tertiary reviewer or a committee member—it is vital that your abstract get all committee members excited about your application.

15.5 EXAMPLES OF FUNDED ABSTRACTS

An excellent resource in abstract writing is the NIH Reporter (http://projectreporter.nih.gov/reporter.cfm). This site provides the abstracts for active funded grants as well as grants over the past 10 years or so. These abstracts of successful applications can serve as examples in helping you to write your own abstract—in terms of both writing style and scope and depth.

You can limit your search of the NIH Reporter to key terms as well as particular grant mechanisms (e.g., early-career awards, smaller grant mechanisms, and larger grant mechanisms). The NIH Reporter, in addition to listing the abstract, will also provide the name of the review panel and the NIH institute that funded the proposal.

The abstracts that your search reveals can help you answer the questions:

"How did the writer convey the significance and innovation of the project? How many aims did the authors include? What was their sample size? How did they concisely summarize their study methods? How did they express the public health and clinical significance?"

For general familiarity with abstract writing style in your field, it is also advisable to read through the top journals in your area. For example, a perusal through the abstracts in *American Journal of Epidemiology* or *Preventive Medicine* would also provide excellent examples of concise abstract writing.

15.6 STRATEGIES FOR MEETING THE WORD COUNT/LINE LIMITATIONS

Current NIH guidelines limit abstracts (termed *project summaries*) to 30 lines with 0.5″ margins. Other funding agencies will have their own requirements. For a dissertation proposal, it will be important to check your graduate school requirements. Failure to comply with these rules can be a reason for the grant being rejected and/or not successfully submitted.

Often, early-career faculty and graduate students have difficulty fitting everything that they would **like** to say about their proposal within these strict word count or line limits. This difficulty is often due to insecurity or confusion as to which aspects of the proposal are most important to mention. By following the outline in Table 15.1 and the corresponding strategies below, you should be well on your way to fitting within these limits.

15.7 ABSTRACT: STEP BY STEP

15.7.1 Background Section

Table 15.4 below provides a detailed outline for the background section of the abstract. **A pitfall to avoid** It is important to note that while this background section is key, a common pitfall is to spend too much time on this section before getting to the aims and methods. Remember that you will have a chance to expand in detail on the background in the *Background and Significance* section of the proposal. Your goal here is to concisely justify the need for your study—touching on the major points in the outline below but then immediately moving on to the highlights of the methodology.

TABLE 15.4 Outline for the background section of the abstract

I. The background section
   a. Public health impact of outcome (disease)
   b. Physiology of exposure–outcome relationship
   c. Epidemiology of exposure–outcome relationship

15.7.1.1 Public health impact of outcome (disease)

Recall that Section a of the Background and Significance section of your proposal already specified the number or percentage of people affected by your outcome of interest. This is typically done by citing the prevalence and/or incidence rates of your outcome of interest. For example, depending upon your study outcome, these data can be found on such websites as the CDC and SEER Program or in published findings from large surveillance studies such as the *National Health and Nutrition Examination Survey*.

Another efficient way to locate such incidence/prevalence data can be found by carefully reading the introductions of journal articles that you included in your summary table (see Chapter 4, *Conducting the Literature Search*). A well-written introduction to a journal article will cite current rates and provide a corresponding citation.

Because you have already collected this information, the examples below are excerpted sentences from a proposal's background and significance section that would then be **inserted into the abstract**. You will note that abstracts typically **do not allow citations or references**.

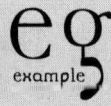

> *e.g. example* In the United States, 5% of women over age 60 years, 12% of those over 75 years, and as many as 28% of women over 85 years suffer from Alzheimer's disease.

> *e.g. example* Epidemiological evidence suggests that approximately 10%–12% of high school students experience clinically significant levels of depression. Similarly, thoughts about suicide, or suicide ideation, affect approximately 11% of adolescents in high schools.

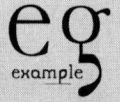

15.7.1.2 Physiology of exposure–outcome relationship

The abstract can also include a justification for the physiologic mechanism between your exposure and your outcome. You will have already written a section on physiology as part of your Background and Significance section. Here, you will want to excerpt the key sentence(s) from that subsection.

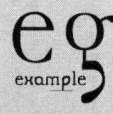

> **e.g.** *example*
>
> Imagine a proposal to conduct a study of prenatal physical activity and risk of low birth weight.
>
> Redistribution of uterine blood flow during physical activity poses a potential threat to fetal growth and development through increased risk of fetal hypoxia, hyperthermia, decreased carbohydrate availability, and preterm labor.

Remember that it is important to avoid focusing on simply the physiology of your outcome, or your exposure, in isolation. That is, in the example above, you can assume that the reviewer will be familiar with the basic mechanisms behind low birth weight. Instead, choose a sentence for the abstract that focuses on the physiologic mechanism for how your exposure (e.g., physical activity) could **impact** your outcome (e.g., low birth weight).

15.7.1.3 Epidemiology of exposure–outcome relationship

Next, the abstract should summarize the prior epidemiologic literature.

When you wrote this section for the Background and Significance section of your proposal, you opened with a paragraph that gave the reader an overview of the number and designs of the prior epidemiologic studies that evaluated your exposure–outcome association of interest. The goal of this overview was to quickly give the reader a synopsis of the state of the research in this area. For example, is this a well-studied area? Or are prior studies sparse?

Although already concise, this overview will likely be too long for the abstract but can be readily condensed as indicated in the example below.

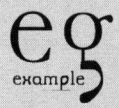

> **e.g.** *example*
>
> Imagine a proposal to conduct a study of physical activity and risk of breast cancer.
>
> **Original sentences in the Background and Significance**
>
> Prior studies of physical activity and breast cancer have been contradictory.[1–21] Fifteen of the 21 published studies observed decreased risk of breast cancer for women who were physically active compared with inactive women.[1–15] No overall association between physical activity and breast cancer was found in four studies.[16–19] Increased risk of breast cancer was associated with higher levels of physical activity in the Framingham cohort study[20] and the Turkish case–control study.[21]
>
> **Corresponding sentence for the Abstract**
>
> Prior studies of physical activity and breast cancer have been contradictory with 15 observing a decreased risk for active women, 4 failing to find an association, and 2 observing an increased risk.

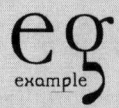

eg *example*
Refer back to our prior proposal to conduct a study of prenatal physical activity and low birth weight.

Original sentences in the Background and Significance Section
A total of 15 epidemiologic studies have evaluated the relationship between physical activity and birth weight.[1-15] These studies, however, have assessed women's occupational activities only,[1-5] recreational activities only,[6-11] or a combination of occupational and household activities.[12,13] Only two studies have measured total activity (recreational, occupational, and household).[14,15]

Corresponding sentence for the Abstract
Prior studies that evaluated the relationship between physical activity and birth weight have been limited by an assessment of occupational activities only, recreational activities only, or a combination of occupational and household activities. Only two studies have measured total activity (recreational, occupational, and household).

Or an even shorter sentence for the Abstract
The majority of prior studies that evaluated the relationship between physical activity and birth weight have failed to measure total activity (recreational, occupational, and household).

15.7.2 II. Research Aims

The abstract should convey the **overall goal** of the proposal and, if space permits, a concise version of your **specific aims**. Remember that you will have an entire page to devote to the specific aims and hypotheses later in the proposal. Therefore, they do not need to be included verbatim in their entirety here.

Below is an example that shows how to **condense** your Specific Aims page into a concise excerpt for inclusion in the Abstract.

eg *example*
Original Specific Aims in the Specific Aims Section
Specific Aim #1. Evaluate the impact of a 12-week individually targeted exercise intervention on risk of recurrent GDM among prenatal care patients with a history of GDM.
  Hypothesis #1. Compared to subjects in the comparison health and wellness intervention, women in the individually targeted exercise intervention will have a lower risk of recurrent GDM.
Specific Aim #2. Evaluate the impact of a 12-week individually targeted exercise intervention on biochemical factors associated with insulin resistance among prenatal care patients with a history of GDM.

> Hypothesis #2. Compared to subjects in the comparison health and wellness intervention, women in the individually targeted exercise intervention will have lower fasting concentrations of glucose, insulin, leptin, TNF-α, and CRP and higher concentrations of adiponectin.
> Specific Aim #3. Evaluate the impact of a 12-week individually targeted exercise intervention on the adoption and maintenance of physical activity during pregnancy among prenatal care patients with a history of GDM.
> Hypothesis #3. Compared to subjects in the comparison health and wellness intervention, women in the individually targeted exercise intervention will participate in more physical activity in mid and late pregnancy.
>
> **Condensed version for Abstract**
> We propose to test the hypothesis that an exercise intervention is an effective tool for preventing GDM among women with a history of GDM.
> The primary goals of the proposal are to investigate the effects of a motivationally tailored, individually targeted 12-week physical activity intervention on (1) the risk of recurrent GDM, (2) serum biomarkers associated with insulin resistance, and (3) the adoption and maintenance of exercise during pregnancy.

15.7.3 III. Highlights of the Methodology

The abstract should specify the study design, sample size, and the tools that you propose to use to measure your key exposure and outcome variables. If any of your methods are particularly innovative, you will want to note that here.

Key features of the methods to include in the abstract:

- Study design
- Sample size
- Assessment tools
- Any methodological innovations

A pitfall to avoid One common pitfall in abstract writing is the failure to mention your sample size. Abstracts that do not include this number can be misinterpreted as trying to *hide* a study limitation—that is, a small sample size.

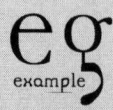

> **example** This example methodology section of an abstract omits several items that would be useful for the reviewer.
>
> **Original Version**
> The investigation will be a supplementary study to an existing dataset of 8000 older adults based in New Mexico. We will conduct tests of cognitive function. Baseline data from this testing will serve as the initiation of a study of predictors of cognitive decline. Second interviews will be given to the same adults after a 2-year interval and again at 4 years. Multivariable logistic regression will be used to model the association between diet and risk of cognitive decline controlling for confounding factors.

The above abstract excerpt could be improved by including

- The type of study design (e.g., prospective cohort study, case–control study, cross-sectional study)
- The name of the tool used to measure cognitive function and whether it has been validated
- The name of the existing database/study

Remember that you want to be kind to the reviewer. You do not want to leave it to them to deduce your study design. In addition, if a study is particularly well known (e.g., NHANES) and has generated many published findings, it definitely adds to the value of the abstract to mention it by name.

> **example** **Improved Version**
> The investigation will be a supplementary study to the **Lincoln Health Study, an existing cohort study** of 8000 older adults based in New Mexico. We will conduct tests of cognitive function **using an instrument validated for use in this population**. Baseline data from this testing will serve as the initiation of **a prospective cohort study** of predictors of cognitive decline. Second interviews will be given to the same adults after a 2-year interval and again at 4 years. Multivariable logistic regression will be used to model the association between diet and risk of cognitive decline controlling for confounding factors.

When choosing which highlights of the methodology to include in an abstract, elements that make your research **innovative** deserve more emphasis (e.g., if you will be using a novel measurement tool or study design feature).

A pitfall to avoid Many grant proposals involve the use of existing datasets (i.e., secondary data from cohorts that are already established). While use of these rich datasets can be viewed as a study advantage, it can be risky to emphasize **cost efficiency** as the reason for choosing to use such a dataset. Instead, it is always best to provide a scientific rationale for your proposed methods. Then, as a secondary advantage, you could mention efficiency, by stating that *the study capitalizes upon the existence of previously collected data*, which implies, but does not overtly state, the cost savings.

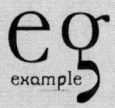

> **example**
>
> **Original Version**
> The Lincoln Health Study provides a highly cost-efficient setting in which to investigate these issues.
>
> **Improved Version**
> The proposed secondary study capitalizes upon the comprehensive data on diet collected by the Lincoln Health Study as well as objective measures of key potential confounding factors such as cigarette smoking and physical activity. Retention rates to date have been excellent.

15.7.4 IV. Summary of the Significance and Innovation

The proposal abstract, despite the lack of study findings, still must summarize the significance of the *potential* findings. The abstract needs to justify, in a nutshell, why it will be worthwhile to conduct the study before conducting the study, irrespective of study findings. When reading your abstract, reviewers will be asking, "Why would it be worthwhile to fund your study?"

Given that you have already drafted the section on significance and innovation as part of the Background and Significance section in Chapter 7, this section should be relatively easy to draft. Significance and innovation are both key drivers of the *overall impact* score on the NIH reviewer critique sheet. Don't rely upon the reviewer to figure it out for you—be kind to your reviewer!

The **key principle** in summarizing the significance and innovation of the proposal is to highlight the research gap that your proposal will be filling and how it extends the prior research in your area.

Remember the example research gaps originally presented in Table 15.5 of Chapter 7, *Background and Significance Section*, and repeated again below. These example research gaps can be succinctly summarized in an abstract. They can serve to answer the question, what is the demonstrated need for this new study? The more research gaps that you can point out that you will be filling, the better. In other words, at least one is necessary but more are value-added.

TABLE 15.5 Example research gaps

PRIOR LITERATURE IS…

Limited to particular study designs
Limited to particular methodology
Limited sample size
Conflicting findings
Limited control for confounding factors
Limited to particular study populations
Limited number of prior studies

Below are examples of sentences for the abstract that both summarize the prior epidemiologic literature and simultaneously highlight the research gap.

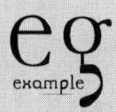

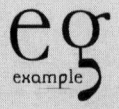

> *example*
>
> Imagine, again, a proposal to conduct a study of prenatal exercise and low birth weight.
>
> **Original sentences in the Background and Significance Section**
> In summary, the prior epidemiologic studies of prenatal exercise and low birth weight faced several limitations: (1) the majority involved small numbers of nonminority women who exercised regularly before pregnancy limiting the generalizability of results, (2) few assessed the validity of their measure of physical activity, and (3) many failed to account for confounding variables that can lead to misleading results (e.g., birth weights will appear lower if not adjusted for length of gestation).
>
> **Corresponding sentence for the Abstract**
> Prior studies of prenatal exercise and low birth weight were limited by small sample sizes, limited generalizability, and failure to use tools validated for pregnancy and to adjust for important confounding factors. In contrast, our proposal is innovative by evaluating this association in a large, well-characterized prospective cohort of minority women using validated tools to assess physical activity. The significance of the proposal is reflected in the high rates of low birth weight in this understudied population.

> *example*
>
> Prior studies of vitamin D and risk of breast cancer have been limited by cross-sectional study designs; therefore, our proposal to conduct a prospective cohort study of the association between vitamin D and breast cancer is innovative. The proposal is significant as findings of an association could inform future prenatal intervention programs that would help to reduce breast cancer.

> **e.g.** *example*
> Very little is known about ways to reduce Alzheimer's disease. Most prior investigations have been cross-sectional. In addition, while genetic aspects of Alzheimer's disease are increasingly being appreciated, virtually no studies have explored interactions between environmental and genetic factors. Therefore, the proposed study is innovative in prospectively evaluating genetic risk factors for Alzheimer's disease. The results of the proposed study are significant in that they will help to elucidate the etiology of Alzheimer's disease.

Even if you are writing a dissertation proposal abstract, the exercise of imagining that you are writing a grant proposal abstract makes the stakes higher—and can provide greater impetus to think about the potential implications of your findings.

As always, throughout this process, if you cannot think of any relevant significance and innovation, then it may be time to go back and rethink your aims and hypotheses. Remember that proposal writing is an iterative process, and it is always acceptable to go back and tweak or even entirely scrap your original aims.

15.8 HOW TO WRITE A TITLE FOR YOUR PROPOSAL

There are several strategies to consider in writing the title for your proposal. However, first and foremost is that the title should be **concise**, yet as informative as possible, while complying with the specific guidelines of the funding agency or your graduate school. For example, NIH and other Public Health Service (PHS) agencies limit the title character length to 81 characters, including the spaces between words and punctuation. Titles in excess of 81 characters are truncated.

Similarly, journal article titles will also have character limits. Finally, if you are a graduate student, it is best to use the dissertation proposal writing process as an opportunity to practice grant proposal writing. In that vein, follow the guidelines of the funding agency to which you plan on targeting your future grant applications—as long as their rules are consistent with those of your graduate school.

> **e.g.** *example*
> **Titles That Exceed Character Limits**
> The Measurement of Physical Activity in Free-Living Humans and the Effect of Seasonal and Short-Term Changes in Physical Activity on Cardiovascular Disease Risk Factors
> A Dietary Strategy to Reduce Breast Cancer Risk: Estrogen Metabolism and Brassica Vegetable Consumption

> **example**
>
> **First Improved Version**
> Seasonal Changes in Physical Activity and Cardiovascular Disease Risk Factors
> **Second Improved Version**
> A Dietary Strategy to Reduce Breast Cancer Risk

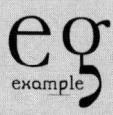

The revised versions are compliant with the 81 character limit while retaining the primary focus of the proposal (e.g., the key exposure and outcome variables).

The overall goal in crafting the title for an NIH grant proposal is to ensure that your proposal gets **routed to the correct review panel** (i.e., study section) within NIH. While you can request what you feel is the appropriate review panel in your cover letter, your title will help to further ensure that your suggestion is followed. This issue is discussed in more detail in Chapter 18, *Submission of the Grant Proposal*. In addition, the tips below not only help to correctly route your application but also reflect good practices in titling.

15.8.1 Tip #1: Use Agency-Friendly Keywords

Using terms in the title that correspond to the names of review panels at the granting agency will help ensure that officials direct your proposal to the correct review panel.

For grant proposals in epidemiology and preventive medicine, using the term *epidemiology of* will help the application go to an epidemiology review panel. It is one of the key ways to indicate that the study is population-based. In contrast, removing this term might lead the same application to be misdirected to more of a *bench science* review panel. Such groups may not be comfortable with the use of self-reported assessments or other techniques considered acceptable in large studies in preventive research.

Including study design terms in the title that are characteristic of grants in epidemiology or preventive medicine proposal will also be helpful such as *A Case–Control Study of…* or *A Prospective Study of…*.

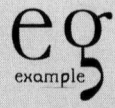

> **example**
>
> **Original Version**
> Stress and Gestational Diabetes
> **First Improved Version**
> The Epidemiology of Stress and Gestational Diabetes
> **Second Improved Version**
> A Prospective Cohort Study of Stress and Gestational Diabetes

15.8.2 Tip #2: Titles Should Include the Key Variables Being Evaluated

A proposal title should list your key **exposure** and **outcome** variables. If there are too many exposure and outcome variables to fit concisely in the title, then the corresponding umbrella terms should be used. For example, if your outcome variables include markers of cardiovascular disease such as HDL, LDL, and triglycerides, it is more efficient to simply use the umbrella term *cardiovascular disease risk factors*. Similarly, if your exposures involve lifestyle behaviors such as diet, exercise, and weight management, instead use the term *lifestyle behaviors*. Additional examples include *nutritional factors*, *risk-taking behaviors*, or other terms that summarize groups of variables.

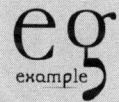

> *eg example*
> The Relationship between Blood Lead and Cardiovascular Risk Profile among Adult Women

This tip has a second benefit. If you find that you are having trouble coming up with a concise title, this could be an indicator that your topic is overly ambitious and that you are taking on a dissertation/proposal topic that is too broad.

15.8.3 Tip #3: The Title Should Not State the Expected Results of the Proposed Study

Stating the expected or hypothesized outcome of your study in your title is considered inappropriate for several reasons. First, this is the title for a proposal and not a completed study. Indeed, the proposal includes hypotheses to be tested. Secondly, even if prior studies have observed an association between your exposure and outcome, causality has likely not been established. The merits of your proposal rely upon your assertion that there is a research gap and that your association of interest is not fully known.

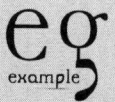

> *eg example*
> **Original Version**
> Emphasis on Patient Care Delivery and Collegial Interaction Lead to Successful Recruitment of Physicians in Health Maintenance Organizations
> **Improved Version**
> Critical Factors in Recruiting Health Maintenance Organization Physicians

> **Original Version**
> Chocolate Increases the Risk of Heart Disease
> **Improved Version**
> The Association between Chocolate and Heart Disease

15.8.4 Tip #4: Titles Should Mention the Study Design If a Strength

Including the study design in your title is important if the design is a particular strength of your proposal and a means by which you are extending the prior literature. In addition, if you are conducting a large prospective study, or a randomized clinical trial, or using data from a national survey—these would be considered strengths. On the other hand, conducting a cross-sectional study or a qualitative study may be appropriate as a study design but likely not worth highlighting in your title.

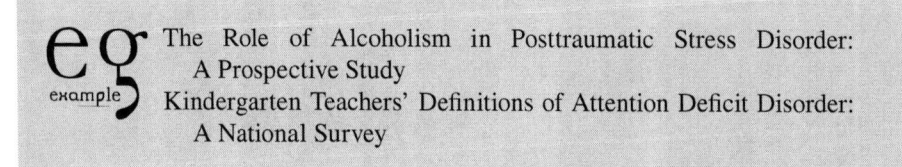

> The Role of Alcoholism in Posttraumatic Stress Disorder: A Prospective Study
> Kindergarten Teachers' Definitions of Attention Deficit Disorder: A National Survey

15.8.5 Tip #5: The Title Should Mention the Study Population When Important

Including the study population in a title is important when one of the key strengths of your proposal is the study population. In other words, if the means by which your proposal is extending the prior literature is by virtue of conducting the analysis in your study population, then mention this population in the title.

Another reason to mention the population is if you are conducting a large population-based study—for example, among the US population—or using data from a well-established cohort such as the NHS or the BRFSS. Finally, if your study population will be limited to a particular racial or ethnic group, to a particular age group, or to some other characteristic (e.g., overweight and obese; patients with diabetes; disabled people), the study population is also important to mention in the title.

Potential reasons to mention the study population in your title:

- A new study population
- A large national database
- An established cohort

- A specific racial/ethnic group
- A study population with a particular disease or disability
- A particular age group

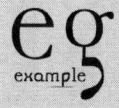

> **example**
> Age and Automobile Crash Risk in a Community Population of Older Persons
> Relationship of Drug Therapy with Mortality in the National Health Interview Survey
> The Association between Vitamin D and Depression in African-American Men

15.8.6 Tip #6: Titles Should Mention Any Other Unique Features of the Study

In addition to mentioning the study population and study design, titles can also mention any other unique features of the proposal—if you feel that they are study strengths. For example, if you will be conducting the first long-term follow-up study in your area, this would be important to point out in your title. Similarly, if you were using a novel measurement tool, this could also be mentioned in your title—if space allows. The bottom line is to be sure that the title (or at least the abstract) touches upon those aspects of your proposal that you believe will be pivotal in its funding success.

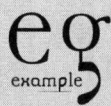

> **example**
> The Long-Term Effects of Tetracycline on Tooth Enamel Erosion
> Objective Measurement of Physical Activity and Risk of Respiratory Disease

15.8.7 Tip #7: A Title Should Be Consistent with the Overall Study Goal

This may seem like a straightforward tip, but caution should be taken to draw your title from your overall research goal and specific aims. It may be easy to get distracted by some of the above tips and emphasize the study methods to the exclusion of your overall exposure and outcome variables. In other words, be sure not to miss the forest for the trees.

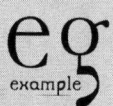

> **example**
> **Specific Aim:**
> The purpose of this study is to investigate whether those who experience sexual harassment have a higher rate of suicide ideation than those who do not experience sexual harassment.
> **Corresponding Title:**
> The Relationship between Sexual Harassment and Suicide Ideation

> **example**
> **Specific Aim:**
> To examine the association between alcohol consumption and cataract extraction in a prospective cohort of older adults.
> **Corresponding Title:**
> A Prospective Study of Alcohol Consumption and Cataract Extraction among Older Adults

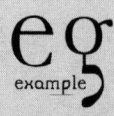

15.8.8 Stylistic Tip #1: Avoid Clever Titles

Dissertation proposals in the humanities often include a catchy phrase to capture the attention of the audience. It is best to avoid use of such subtitles for proposal titles in epidemiology and preventive medicine.

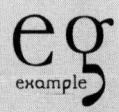

> **example**
> The Smoking Gun: The Association between Cigarette Use and Oral Cancer
> Doctors without Borders: Health Care Utilization Patterns and HIV Risk in Developing Countries

The use of clever titles may lead reviewers to take you less seriously. Such titles are more appropriate for a magazine or newspaper article, as opposed to a scientifically rigorous proposal. If your topic is timely and important, it will speak for itself without the need to be clever or provocative in the title.

15.8.9 Stylistic Tip #2: Avoid Writing Titles as Questions

While a title written in the format of a question might at first appear *sexy* or interesting, the use of a question as a title is considered more appropriate for a magazine or newspaper article. It is not a generally acceptable approach for a scientific proposal.

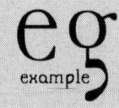

> **example**
> **Original Version**
> Does a Mediterranean Diet Reduce Risk of Heart Disease?
> **Improved Version**
> The Mediterranean Diet and Risk of Heart Disease

15.9 EXAMPLES

15.9.1 Example #1

A Proposal to Evaluate Stress and Risk of Hypertensive Disorders of Pregnancy

The following example presents the background and significance section of the proposal first and then the corresponding abstract. Presenting the sections in this order shows how key sentences can be excerpted from the Background and Significance section and cut and paste directly into the Abstract.

Background and Significance

Hypertensive disorders of pregnancy affect up to 8% of pregnancies and can result in poor outcomes for both mother and child.[1] Additionally, there is sparse data on the Latina population, a group at a twofold increased risk of preeclampsia relative to non-Latina white women.[2] This group is a growing segment of the US population[3] and has a higher birthrate than non-Latina white women.[4] There are few modifiable risk factors for hypertensive disorders of pregnancy.

Stress may increase risk of hypertensive disorders of pregnancy through a number of pathways, including neuroendocrinological mechanisms and through an inflammatory response to stress. Previous research has shown a link between adrenocorticotropin hormone and cortisol and both stress and hypertension.[5] CRP[6] and TNF-α,[7] markers of inflammation, are also elevated among women with high stress levels and are associated with increased blood pressure[8] and preeclampsia.[9]

Previous epidemiologic data suggest an association between psychosocial stress and hypertensive disorders. While limited in some respects, previous data suggest that high levels of job stressors, as well as depression, may result in a twofold increased risk of preeclampsia.[10–12] However, prior research has yielded conflicting results with one study showing no association between job stress and preeclampsia.[13]

Given the serious nature of hypertensive disorders of pregnancy and their sequelae, the proposed study will be significant in evaluating the association between general stress and this disease in a Latina population, an understudied high-risk group with high rates of stress. The proposal is innovative by using a validated measure of psychosocial stress in the underrepresented Latina population.

Abstract

Hypertensive disorders of pregnancy affect approximately 8% of pregnancies and can lead to serious medical complications for both mother and child. While Latinas are at twofold increased risk of preeclampsia relative to non-Latina white women, little research on hypertension in pregnancy has been conducted in this population. Prior studies suggest an increased risk of hypertensive disorders of pregnancy associated with high levels of work-related stress. However, to date, there are no data on psychosocial stress in early pregnancy and hypertensive disorders of pregnancy in any population. Therefore, our proposal is innovative by evaluating the association between perceived stress and hypertensive disorders of pregnancy using data from the Salud study, a prospective cohort study of 1231 women, and Salud II, an ongoing cohort of approximately 900 women. Psychosocial stress was measured in early pregnancy through the perceived stress scale. Hypertensive disorders of pregnancy were confirmed through obstetrician review of medical records. Data on potential confounders were obtained through interviews conducted during pregnancy and from medical records. We will use multivariate logistic regression to evaluate the association between early pregnancy stress and hypertensive disorders of pregnancy. Results of this study will be significant by providing needed information on a potentially modifiable risk factor for hypertensive disorders of pregnancy and inform future intervention studies.

15.9.2 Example #2: Needs Improvement

A Proposal to Acid-lowering Agent Use and Vitamin B12 Deficiency among Older Puerto Rican Adults

Abstract

Vitamin B12 deficiency affects approximately 6% of adults aged over 60 years and is associated with several chronic illnesses, including cardiovascular diseases, insulin resistance, and anemia. Puerto Ricans are the second largest Hispanic subgroup in the United States with the worst health outcomes; however, few studies of vitamin B12 status have been conducted among this population. Although prior studies suggested an increased risk of vitamin B12 deficiency among the elderly associated with acid-lowering agents (ALAs) use, to date, this relationship has not been examined among older Puerto Ricans. Therefore, we propose to evaluate the association between ALA use and vitamin B12 deficiency using data from the Providence Puerto Rican Health Study, a longitudinal prospective cohort of 1500 older Puerto Ricans from 2004. ALA use was self-reported by interview at the time of enrollment along with potential confounding factors. Vitamin B12 deficiency was defined as serum vitamin B12 concentration <200 pg/mL collected the subsequent day. Multivariable logistic regression will be used to evaluate the association between ALA use and vitamin B12 deficiency. Results of this study will attract more attention on older Puerto Ricans and inform further research in diverse population.

Comment:
- Try to always say your exposure prior to your outcome.
- The significance and innovation of the proposal need to be strengthened. Calling for additional research is too vague and could be said at the end of any abstract. Instead, this last sentence(s) needs to comment on the implications for public health and clinical practice.

15.9.3 Example #3: Needs Improvement

A Proposal to Examine the Impact of Dance Programs on Physical Activity Levels of African-American Girls

Abstract

African-American girls suffer disproportionately from obesity and type 2 diabetes mellitus (T2DM) compared to their age matched non-Hispanic white counterparts. One factor associated with the development of obesity and T2DM disparities in children is a decrease in their physical activity (PA) levels. Reductions in PA are more prevalent in African-American girls; therefore, effective PA interventions that result in behavior change and ultimately improvements in their PA levels are needed. For a PA intervention message to be effective among African-American girls, the program must resonate among them and they must enjoy participating in the intervention activity (e.g., Afrocentric dance). Afrocentric dance has a strong cultural and historical significance in the African-American community and can provide girls with sustained bouts of moderate-to-vigorous physical activity (MVPA). One study in African-American girls has shown that Afrocentric dance can result in improvements of self-reported measures of PA but not objectively measured PA; it is possible that the participation in the dance program did not have any impact on girls' home PA environment due to lack of parental participation. It has been speculated that one way to increase children's PA level is to increase parental PA level, as there is a strong positive correlation between parental and children PA levels. In the African-American culture, maternal health behaviors have a strong influence on children's health behaviors, making studies exploring methods to enhance maternal and child health behaviors critical. There are sparse data (mostly in Caucasian families) suggesting that parent–child interventions could have a beneficial impact on children's PA. In one of the few family-based interventions in African-American girls, Beech et al. examined the effects of a family-based behavioral intervention in the prevention of weight gain and found a 12% non-significant increase in girls' self-reported levels of MVPA, compared to the control group. The lack of significant differences could potentially be attributed to the lack of impact on girls' home PA environment. *Currently, there are no studies examining the effects of a daughter–mother Afrocentric dance program on the PA levels of African-American girls.* Therefore, we propose a two-phase study. Phase 1 is designed to develop and formalize the culturally tailored daughter–mother Afrocentric dance intervention curriculum. The second phase will examine the feasibility of a 12-week randomized control daughter–mother afterschool Afrocentric dance PA intervention and explore its impact on the PA levels of African-American girls.

Comment

- Too much space is dedicated to background. Instead, the abstract should more quickly shift to the proposed study methods.
- Similarly, too much space is dedicated to the psychobehavioral model underlying successful programs.
- Specific authors and specific studies should not be highlighted in the abstract unless they are the only evidence on the topic. Instead, the abstract should summarize the current state of the literature in the area.
- The background of the abstract points out that prior studies were limited by their lack of objective measures. However, the abstract does not state if the proposed studies will use objective measures.
- The sample size is not provided and other important details on the methods to be used in phase 1 and 2 are not included.
- The significance and innovation of the study are not emphasized. Study implications for public health and clinical practice are not provided.

Presenting Your Proposal Orally 16

Learning how to best present a proposal is a skill that will serve you well not only in graduate school but throughout your career. As a graduate student, you will likely be asked to present your proposal as part of a doctoral proposal defense. As an early-career faculty, you may be asked to present your grant proposal to fellow faculty, potential coinvestigators, and/or at a scientific meeting.

Care should be taken with proposal presentations, keeping in mind that in science, if one is to make an impact, you must persuade your colleagues of it. Presentations need to be understandable to the audience without relying on their having read the written proposal. To achieve this goal, slides should be clear and readable with figures, images, and tables playing a major role.

Therefore, this chapter provides strategies and tips for clearly conveying the importance and rationale for your proposal via an oral presentation. The chapter covers tips for how to present each component of the proposal—from the background and significance through the aims, methods, and study limitations.

16.1 HOW TO GET STARTED

In advising my graduate students on their proposal presentations, I always ask them to first step back and take a moment to think about presentations that they have seen in the past. I ask them to name 2 rules of thumb that they feel are important to follow and then to name 2 things to avoid at all costs. Without exception, the students highlight the need to speak slowly, use slides that are clear and not busy, and avoid being overly ambitious in the scope of the presentation. Students all comment negatively on presenters that simply read their slides.

16.2 GENERAL GUIDELINES

16.2.1 Guideline #1: Organize the Presentation Based on Your Proposal Outline

The titles of your slides should match your proposal subheadings. In this way, the audience can easily follow along and, at the same time, know where you are within the context of the proposal. This technique also ensures that you do not fail to include a particular section of your proposal (Table 16.1).

16.2.2 Guideline #2: How to Allocate Presentation Time

A common pitfall to avoid

The overall emphasis of a proposal presentation should be on the presentation of **study methods**. This should constitute the bulk of the presentation time. Instead, a common pitfall is to spend too much time on the prior literature. Students can get lost in presenting the prior literature and find that they run out of time before even getting to their own study methods. Instead, the review committee (or general audience) will be most interested in what you plan to do, the methods of your proposed work, and if it is feasible and reflects the state of the science.

Therefore, the presenter should start with a **brief literature review** and clear statement of the **significance of the study problem**. Remember, as noted in Chapter 7,

TABLE 16.1 Example presentation outline and corresponding slide titles

- Title slide (proposal title, investigators, institution)
- Background and significance
  - Highlight the significance
  - Snapshot of summary literature table
  - State the innovation—research gap
- Methods
  - Study design
  - Population
  - Exposure, outcome, covariate assessment
  - Data analysis
  - Power calculations
- Study limitations

TABLE 16.2 Time breakdown for a 25 min proposal presentation

TOPIC	TIME (MIN)
Background and significance and study goal	10
Methods and limitations	15
Total time	25

Background and Significance Section, that the goal of this section is to show how the proposed work is **innovative** by extending prior research in the area and filling a research gap. The presenter should then go on to describe the *methods and study limitations*—this is the primary focus of the presentation.

Table 16.2 provides the time breakdown for a 25 min proposal presentation but can be proportionally modified for proposals that are longer in length depending upon the guidelines of your institution. One advantage of limiting the proposal presentation time to 25 min is that, after the study has been conducted, you will have the space and time to include your study findings. In this way, your final doctoral defense will fall within 50 min—a common time limitation for doctoral defenses at most institutions.

In general, it is best to plan about 1–2 slides/min. Using this guideline, the above presentation would include approximately 25–40 slides. Some of these slides will be brief—such as the title slide—while others will have more detail.

16.2.3 Guideline #3: A Presentation Cannot Have Too Many Figures or Tables

As mentioned in Chapter 1, *Ten Top Tips for Successful Proposal Writing*, the more figures and tables in a grant application, the better. Similarly, a presentation can also never have too many figures or tables. Not only does the process of creating these figures and tables help you to crystallize your specific aims and study methods, they are also kinder to the audience. As compared to slides of dense text, tables and figures are easier for audience to digest and help them more quickly grasp your methods. They demonstrate to the audience that you have an excellent grasp of your proposal and high organizational skills.

Figures and tables can be used for almost every section of a presentation—just as they can be used in almost every section of a grant application. For example, in the Specific Aims Section, a figure can be included showing how the specific aims interrelate (see Chapter 6, *Specific Aims*, for example figures).

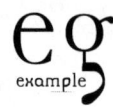

Example Specific Aims Slide

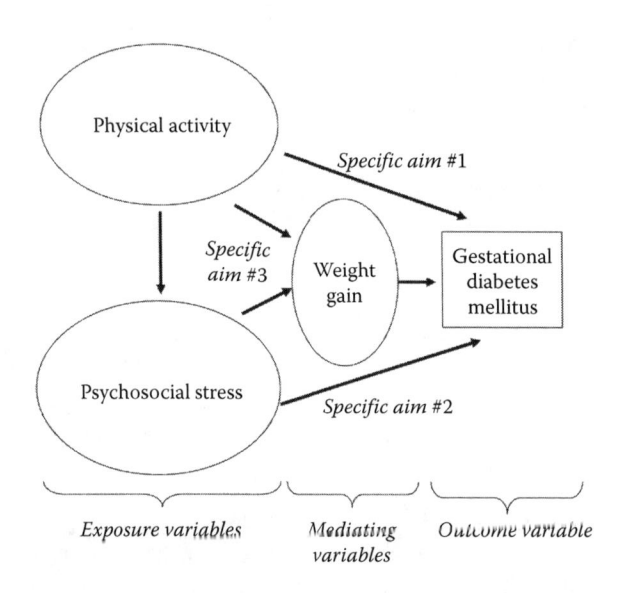

Figure: Conceptual model showing Physical activity and Psychosocial stress (Exposure variables) affecting Weight gain (Mediating variables), which affects Gestational diabetes mellitus (Outcome variable). Specific aim #1: Physical activity → Gestational diabetes mellitus. Specific aim #2: Psychosocial stress → Gestational diabetes mellitus. Specific aim #3: Physical activity → Psychosocial stress → Weight gain.

Another key figure to include is a figure of your anticipated results. Some reviewers feel that this latter figure is essential.

Example Anticipated Results Slide

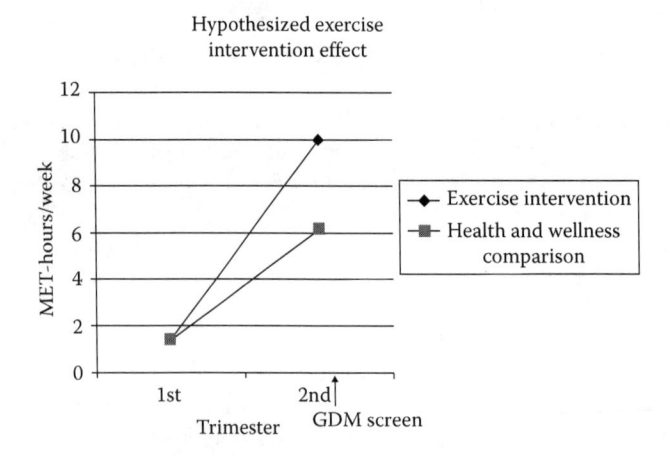

Figure: Hypothesized exercise intervention effect. Line graph with MET-hours/week on y-axis (0–12) and Trimester on x-axis (1st to 2nd/GDM screen). Exercise intervention rises from ~1.5 to 10; Health and wellness comparison rises from ~1.5 to ~6.

Other examples include study design figures, tables listing study variables, and statistical power displays. Images of assessment tools such as surveys or questionnaires are also recommended. Typically, an entire questionnaire will be too large to include on a slide—therefore, an image of an example question or a relevant section of the questionnaire would be ideal. The presentation can end with a timeline figure—showing each study activity and the quarters during which it will be conducted.

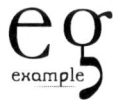

example | Example Study Design Slide

Study design

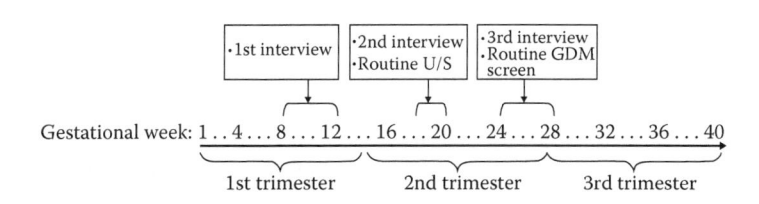

	•1st interview	•2nd interview •Routine U/S	•3rd interview •Routine GDM screen

Gestational week: 1 .. 4 ... 8 ... 12 ... 16 ... 20 ... 24 ... 28 ... 32 ... 36 ... 40

1st trimester   2nd trimester   3rd trimester

example | Example Questionnaire Excerpt

	Average use						
Type of food	Never	1 per month	2–3 per month	1 per week	2–4 per week	4–6 per week	1 per day
Fruit							
Apples	■	■	■	■	■	■	■
Pears	■	■	■	■	■	■	■
Bananas	■	■	■	■	■	■	■

Sections that can benefit from display as a figure or image:

- Specific aims figure
- Anticipated results
- Findings of prior literature
- Preliminary study findings
- Study design
- Study population
  - Recruitment
  - Exclusions
- Exposure/outcome assessment
  - Questionnaire excerpt
  - Scales
- Power and sample size
- Timeline

16.2.4 Guideline #4: How to Create User-Friendly Text Slides

Some text slides will always be necessary in a presentation. Your overall goal in creating text slides is to be brief and **save elaboration for your speech**. Remember that neither the slides nor your speech should be directly repetitive of each other. Instead, both should supplement and compliment the other and, surprisingly enough, neither the slides nor the speech should be able to stand alone.

In creating your slides, you will want to ask yourself if the audience is spending more time reading than listening. An audience cannot both read and listen to what you are saying. When faced with a dense slide, the audience will tune out what you are saying and focus on reading the slide or vice versa: they will only listen to what you are saying and ignore the slide entirely.

In this vein, avoid full sentences or paragraphs in slides. Use outline form such as bullets and short phrases. In general, slide software, such as PowerPoint, provides default slides with large font. A typical slide may have 9 lines of text, with approximately 30–50 words. Use no more than 3–4 points under one heading. After drafting your slides, review them for brevity. This process should be repeated several times, so that you distill your slides down to essential terms. **Make sure every word counts**.

The example below may look fairly brief but could be made more concise.

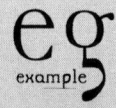

> **Original Slide**
> Our intervention approach was threefold:
>
> - We used a one-on-one strategy to target those that survived from breast cancer.
> - We used a media approach to target residents and college students at risk.
> - Finally, we used a helpline to provide support to friends and family.
>
> **Improved Version of Slide**
> Threefold intervention
>
> 1. One-on-one strategy → breast cancer survivors
> 2. Media approach → at-risk residents and college students
> 3. Helpline → friends and family

The authors of this slide were trying to convey that they had three strategies and that each strategy had a target group. However, these facts were not immediately apparent in the original slide given its structure. The improved version revises each bullet point to first state the approach and uses an arrow to point to the target group. Words that did not add to the meaning of the slide such as *we used*, *finally*, and *our* were removed. These changes resulted in a reduction in the total word count from 45 to 27, a 40% reduction.

Remember that all the deleted words can now be stated verbally by the presenter and the presenter will make the point that the arrow is pointing to the *target* group. This approach to slide making leads to a speech that adds to the slides, as opposed to repeating them. Neither the slide nor the speech can stand alone.

16.2.5 Guideline #5: Recommended Slide Aesthetics

As a general rule, try to avoid having more than 3–4 colors on a slide. Typically, slides have a dark background (such as navy), while posters at scientific presentations have a light background (such as white). The PowerPoint default of white or yellow text on blue background is easy to read. Often the bullet shapes (e.g., the dots, squares, or stars) appear in red with this format option.

Figures should be kept simple in terms of both design and color. Avoid using overly detailed figures. One rule of thumb is to use no more than 3 curves. Avoiding orange and yellow for figures is also recommended as those colors may be difficult for the audience to see.

For **complicated tables and figures**, I recommend that you parse these into multiple figures to illustrate different stages. Or start with a slide that contains a simple framework and build the additional components onto this slide using the *animation* feature of PowerPoint. In this way, the audience is not overwhelmed with information at one glance.

For example, below is a complex study design slide that is virtually unreadable. Instead, this slide could be separated into two sequential slides. This revised approach allows the audience to read the slide and goes through the design in a step-by-step process.

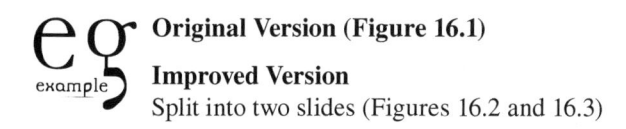

eg *example*
Original Version (Figure 16.1)
Improved Version
Split into two slides (Figures 16.2 and 16.3)

16.3 PRESENTING BACKGROUND AND SIGNIFICANCE

As noted in Chapter 7, the main goal of the background and significance section is to demonstrate that your proposal is significant and innovative by filling a research gap and thereby extending prior research in the area. Recall that, in the body of the proposal, you made this point via a summary literature review table (created as part of Chapter 4, *Conducting the Literature Search*). However, including this entire table in a slide would be too dense for the audience to digest.

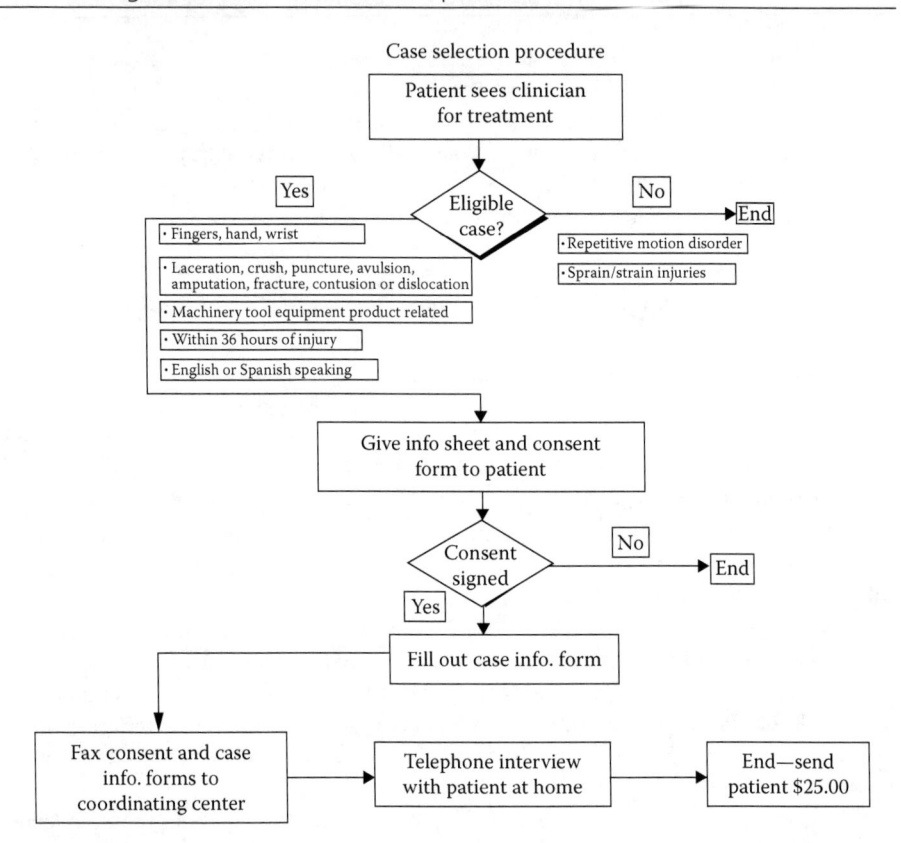

FIGURE 16.1 Example of an overly complex study design slide.

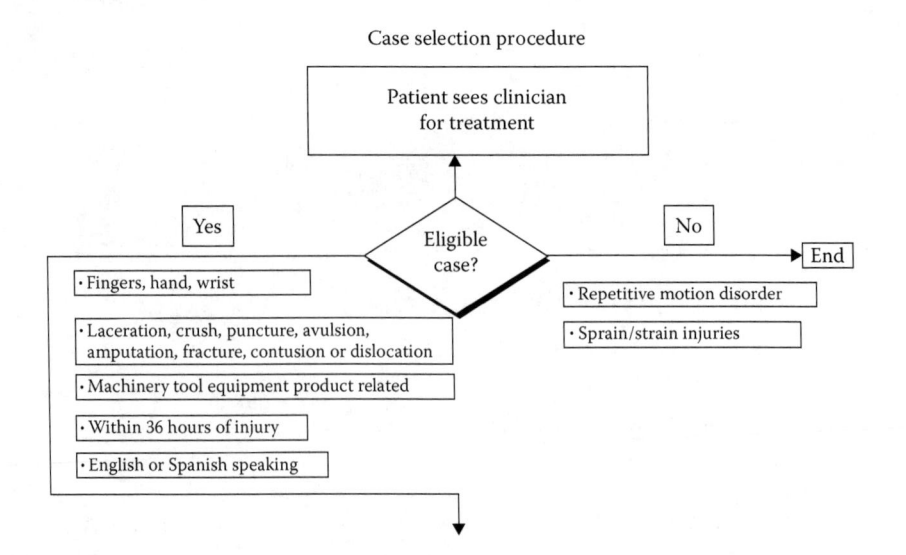

FIGURE 16.2 Improved study design slide #1.

16 • Presenting Your Proposal Orally 317

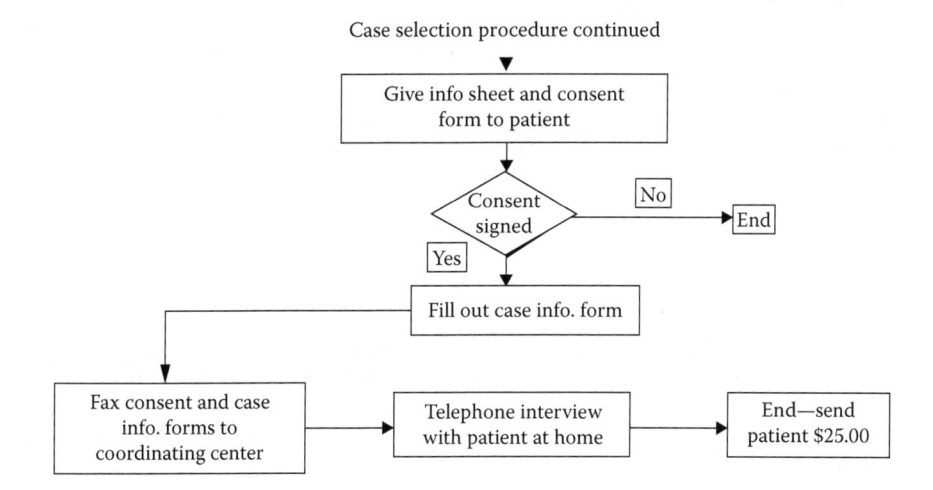

```
Case selection procedure continued
              │
              ▼
   ┌─────────────────────────┐
   │ Give info sheet and consent │
   │     form to patient         │
   └─────────────────────────┘
              │
              ▼
          ╱Consent╲   No
          ╲signed ╱ ──────▶ [End]
           ╲    ╱
            Yes
             │
             ▼
   ┌─────────────────────────┐
   │  Fill out case info. form   │
   └─────────────────────────┘
             │
             ▼
┌──────────────────┐   ┌──────────────────┐   ┌──────────────────┐
│ Fax consent and  │──▶│ Telephone interview │──▶│   End—send       │
│  case info. forms│   │  with patient at home│   │  patient $25.00  │
│ to coordinating  │   │                  │   │                  │
│     center       │   │                  │   │                  │
└──────────────────┘   └──────────────────┘   └──────────────────┘
```

FIGURE 16.3 Improved study design slide #2.

Instead, in a presentation setting, your goal is for the audience to be able to quickly note **trends** across the studies. Therefore, it is best to present an excerpt of the summary literature review table modified for the purposes of the presentation as follows.

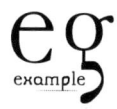

eg *example* A Summary Table of Fiber and Risk of Type 2 Diabetes (Figure 16.4)

This summary table slide presents a representative sampling of the studies from the authors original summary literature review table. The slide uses brief and consistent

Epidemiologic evidence fiber and type 2 diabetes

Author	Type Place	Diet	Outcome Method	Quintiles: Highest to Lowest	
Taylor 2000	Cohort U.S.	FFQ	Self-report	Total fiber 0.78 ↓	Cereal fiber ↓
Sheridan 2000	Cohort U.S.	FFQ	Self-report, glucose levels, meds	Total fiber 1.0 ↔	Cereal fiber ↓
Montoyo 2003	Cohort Finland	FFQ	Social insurance and med. records	Total fiber 0.51 ↓	Insoluble fiber ↓
Stein 2004	Cohort U.S.	FFQ	Self-report and supp. questionnaire	Total fiber 1.00 ↔	Cereal fiber ↓

FIGURE 16.4 Summary table of fiber and risk of type 2 diabetes.

terms across the methods section columns. No more than two to three words are used per cell box. Instead of dense numerical results, findings are primarily conveyed by the use of arrows—with an *up* arrow showing increased risk, a *flat* arrow showing null effects, and a *down* arrow indicating a protective effect. With this approach, the audience can quickly scan down the results column and see the general direction of previous findings. Note that you can always bring a hard copy of the complete table to the presentation as backup reference if there are specific questions about a particular study.

16.4 PRESENTING PRELIMINARY STUDIES OR FINDINGS FROM THE PRIOR LITERATURE

When presenting your preliminary results or the findings of prior studies, *figures are always preferable to tables; and both figures and tables are preferable to text.*

The example below is excerpted from the *preliminary studies* slide of a proposal to evaluate the association between coffee drinking and risk of melanoma. The author starts out presenting these preliminary findings via a text slide, then converts them into a table slide and finally into a figure slide.

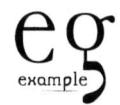

eg example — A Proposal to Evaluate Coffee Drinking and Melanoma Risk

- Option #1: Text version of slide
  "We investigated the association between coffee drinking (cups/day) and risk of melanoma in our pilot study. There was no increase in risk with increasing coffee consumption (p_{trend} = 0.20). As compared to those with no coffee consumption, the RR for melanoma among those with 1 cup/day of consumption was 0.79 (95% CI = 0.18–1.30); for 2 cups/day of consumption, the RR was 1.47 (95% CI = 0.55–1.56); for 3 cups/day of consumption, the RR was 3.03 (95% CI = 0.95–8.55); and for 4 or more cups/day, the RR was 1.30 (95% CI = 0.54–1.35). Lack of statistically significant findings may have been due, in part, to the small sample size, particularly among those with the highest level of coffee consumption."

- Option #2: Table version

COFFEE CONSUMPTION	RR	95% CI
None	1.0	Referent
1 cup/day	0.79	0.18–1.30
2 cups/day	1.47	0.55–1.56
3 cups/day	3.03	0.95–8.55
4+ cups/day	1.30	0.54–1.35

- Option #3: Figure version (Figure 16.5)

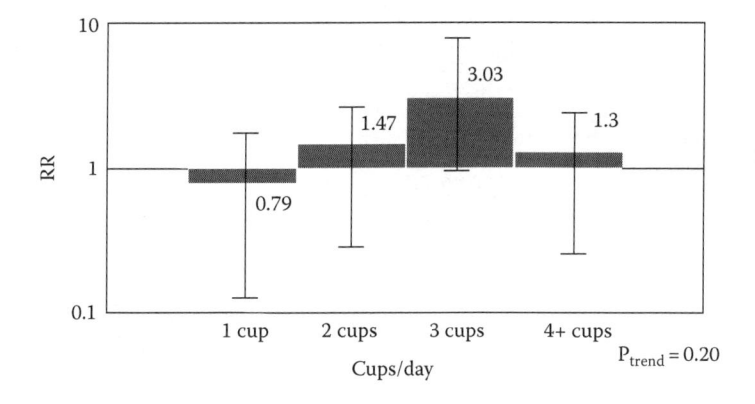

FIGURE 16.5 Coffee and melanoma risk.

As you can see, the figure version is the clearest way to show a potential trend to the reviewers. It saves the work for the reviewer of translating dense text or numerical findings to a visual image. In addition, the additional information regarding the reason for the lack of statistically significant findings can be stated orally. In this way, the speech complements the slide.

16.4.1 Keep Results Tables Simple

If your preliminary study findings or findings from prior literature do not readily translate themselves into figures, then present tables. However, tables should be kept simple in terms of both design and the amount of data included. Avoid dense slides filled with numbers or nonessential columns and rows.

A common pitfall to avoid In showing findings from the prior literature, it may be tempting to cut and paste a table directly from the published article. This is not kind to your audience and we've all heard speakers say the dreaded **I know you can't read this.** Such tables are stand alone, as per the requirements of the journal. As such, they contain complete titles with the name of the study, the study year and location, as well as tiny footnotes. They also likely contain additional data that do not relate to your study aims. Or they may contain columns and rows that, while relevant to your aims, would take too much time to go over (e.g., descriptive statistics or both raw numbers *and* percentages). All of these items will be hard for the audience to read and take up room on the slide. Remember that your primary goal is to tell the audience the main results of preliminary studies.

example The original example below is a table slide that is too dense (Figure 16.6).

Relative risks and 95% confidence intervals for work during overtime and exposure according to clinic; The Franklin study 2003–2008.

Exposure in Past Month

Risk Factor: Work during Overtime	Exposed in the Hazard Period[a]	Exposed in the Past Month[b]	Total # Hours Worked	Medium # Hours Overtime (% Total)	Relative Risk	95% CI
Clinic-Total (N = 1097)	41 (3.7%)	794 (72.4%)	193.3	21.5 (11.1%)	0.31	0.23–0.42
Clinic-OH & R (N = 458)	20 (4.4%)	325 (71.0%)	191.7	21.5 (11.2%)	0.41	0.26–0.64
Clinic-IHC (N = 370)	18 (4.9%)	273 (73.8%)	194.0	24.0 (12.4%)	0.38	0.23–0.61

[a] The number of subjects exposed only in the hazard periods; 10 min before injury.
[b] The number of subjects exposed (reporting worked overtime) anything in the past month.
Clinic hours OH & R: IHC:
   0800–1600   0800–1900
   0800–1630 (primarily)   0800–2000 (primarily)
   0800–1700
   0800–1800

FIGURE 16.6 Example of a dense table slide.

In the improved table below, the author was kind to their audience by creating a new streamlined version of their table. The improved version uses an abbreviated title and deletes table footnotes. The raw numbers and extraneous columns that were removed can be commented upon verbally. Reformatting the slide assures that the font and background is consistent with the style of the remainder of the author's presentation (Figure 16.7).

Overtime and hand injury

Total	Exposed in Hazard Period	Exposed in Past Month	Percent Overtime	RR and 95% CI
Total N = 1097	3.7%	72.4%	11.1%	0.31 (0.23–0.42)
OH & R Clinic N = 458	4.4%	71.0%	11.2%	0.41 (0.26–0.64)
IHC Clinic N = 370	4.9%	73.8%	12.4%	0.38 (0.23–0.61)

FIGURE 16.7 Improved table slide.

16.4.2 Presenting *Mock Tables* for a Dissertation Proposal

Recall the *mock tables* that you created as part of Chapter 10, *Data Analysis Plan*, for the preparation of a dissertation proposal. Because these tables are, by definition, empty of results, they cannot be converted into figures. However, including these tables, or a selection of them, will more clearly convey your data analysis plan to your audience than the use of text slides. They will help to assure your audience/doctoral committee that your analysis plan will address your study aims—and make your analysis plan more accessible.

To make such slides more user-friendly, it is fine to include a representative excerpt of each relevant table—for example, several rows by several columns—and discuss the rest of the table verbally. It may be difficult to fit all the rows or columns within one slide.

16.5 INCLUDE *BACKUP* SLIDES

You will likely find that you cannot fit all the information that you would like within the time limits of a presentation. *Backup* slides are not presented as part of your presentation but are placed after your *thank you* slide at the end of your presentation. You can use them if they respond directly or even indirectly to a particular question raised by the audience.

In fact, it is always most impressive to have a nicely created slide in response to an audience question as opposed to responding extemporaneously. Pulling out one of these backup slides is so impressive that some graduate students have their peers ask them a predetermined question that directly corresponds to one of these slides!

However, on a more serious note, anticipating what types of questions you may be asked and the process of developing backup slides in response to those questions is an excellent exercise—making you more prepared for the presentation and hopefully less nervous.

Examples of *backup* slides

- More images of the proposed physiologic mechanism
- More statistics/charts/graphs on the prevalence of your exposure
- Additional details on prior studies that examined your association of interest
- Slides responding to anticipated concerns about potential biases
- Alternative approaches that you considered
- Slides demonstrating additional design or analysis techniques to minimize potential biases

16.6 GUIDELINES FOR YOUR SPEECH

16.6.1 Guideline #1: Consider How Your Words Will Supplement Your Slides

The most important item to remember in developing the speech that corresponds to your visual presentation is to **avoid reading from a script** and to **avoid reading your slides verbatim**. This is important for several reasons.

Speaking without notes, although more challenging, is always more impressive to the audience—it is highly effective in assuring them that you have a solid grasp of your proposed research area. Start by writing out your entire speech word for word—the speaker notes section of the PowerPoint can be very helpful for this purpose. After your first draft, have your advisor/mentor look over these notes. Check that your speech is consistent with your slides and flows smoothly.

One area that is often problematic for presenters is the **transition from slide to slide**. We've all been to presentations where the presenter appears surprised by the next slide that appears. This suggests that the speaker is not familiar with their talk and has not adequately prepared. Therefore, nail down and focus on **transition phrases**.

A caveat If the thought of speaking without notes makes you nervous, it is possible in PowerPoint to have your notes appear in a side bar on your laptop screen as you progress through your talk. This way, in an emergency, these notes will be there for you to refer to. Sometimes, knowing that your notes are there even if you do not use them is sufficient to calm any nerves!

16.6.2 Guideline #2: How to Discuss Tables/Figures

There is a real art to verbally presenting tables and figures to your audience. This is an important aspect of your proposal that, if done well, can demonstrate your grasp of the research area. Ironically, as with scientific writing, the more simply and clearly that you discuss a table/figure, the more impressive you seem. Remember that while you are very familiar with your slides, the audience is not! The act of presenting tables and figures in a step-by-step fashion gives them the chance to acclimate to each slide.

How to present a table or figure

- Step #1: Read the title of the slide.
- Step #2: Read the title of the x- and y-axes.
- Step #3: Define an example data point.
- Step #4: Discuss the main finding.

First, read the title of the slide. This gives the audience a chance to orient themselves to your slide. Then read the title of the x- and y-axes. At this point, it is now best to physically point to an example data point in the center of the table/figure and give the meaning of this data point.

Lastly, and most importantly, discuss the **main message** that the table or figure conveys. This will also likely involve pointing directly to the data points of interest.

Tell the audience what you feel is the **take-home message** of the table or figure. This would be the finding(s) that directly shows support for your primary hypotheses.

In your speech, avoid repeating each value that appears in the tables/figures. Remember that the reader can see all of these data. Instead, limit yourself to **highlighting, at most, 2–3 main findings per table**.

Also, in your speech, be sure to point to out the *magnitude of your findings* (e.g., mean differences, RRs) with their accompanying measures of variation (e.g., standard deviations, confidence intervals) and not just their statistical significance.

> **eg** *Example Speech Corresponding to Slide* (Figure 16.8)
> example
> This slide shows "alcohol consumption by hospital and trimester." The y-axis shows the estimated percent of the study population who consumed alcohol. The x-axis shows time period: that is, prepregnancy and then the first, second, and third trimesters. Public hospitals are indicated in dark shading and private hospitals in light shading. So, for example, approximately 30% of the prenatal care patients in public hospitals consumed alcohol in their first trimester. Overall, the slide shows that, alcohol consumption decreased over pregnancy with lower rates in public as compared to private hospitals. Alcohol consumption appeared to increase slightly in the third trimester in private hospitals.

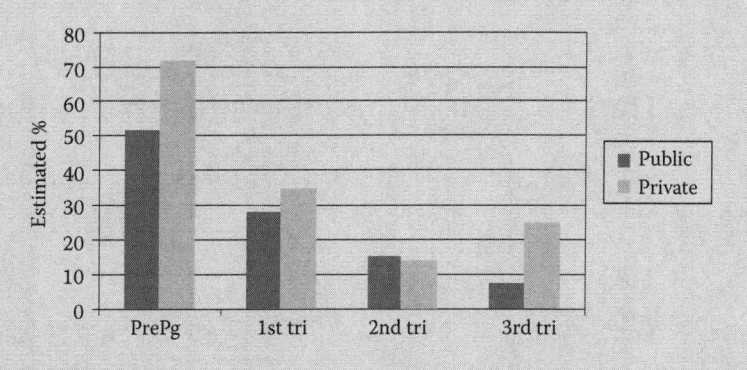

FIGURE 16.8 Alcohol consumption by hospital and trimester.

Common pitfalls to avoid In contrast to this step-by-step approach, we have all seen presenters skip directly to Step #4 (i.e., the main findings). The audience can barely keep up and just ends up taking the presenter's word for the main findings. Another common pitfall in a presentation is when the presenter points at their slide from a distance with their hand/finger. The audience is then forced to visualize an imaginary line leaving the presenter's finger, crossing the trajectory to the screen, and then landing somewhere on the screen. It is rarely clear to the audience where exactly the presenter is pointing! Instead, it is important to **get physical with your slides**—either by reaching out and physically touching the relevant data point on the screen (in a small room setting), using a laser pointer, or the mouse. This is particularly important for Steps #3 and #4 in the table above.

16.6.3 Importance of Rehearsing Your Speech

The importance of rehearsing out loud several times cannot be emphasized enough. In my experience, the audience can always tell which presenters have rehearsed their talk and which have not. Rehearse to yourself first but do so **out loud**. Check the amount of time spent on each topic. Allow 1–2 min/slide. Remember to focus on transition phrases between slides so that awkward pauses do not occur.

If you find that there are slides that you cannot easily describe verbally, this should raise a **red flag**. Difficulty in describing a slide may reflect lack of knowledge or confusion about the area on your part. In this case, doing some additional background research may be warranted. Difficulty in describing a slide may also be due to a problem in the slide itself. Consider revising your slide or separating a complicated slide into several sequential slides so that your speech can more clearly convey your thoughts.

After rehearsing to yourself out loud, it is now time to rehearse in front of some colleagues. I find that a total of *3 out-loud* rehearsals are essential in order to achieve a smooth presentation.

16.6.4 Cultivating a Relationship with the Audience

The goal of your speech is to cultivate a relationship with the audience. At all costs, avoid facing the screen behind you and talking to it. This is tempting, particularly if you are nervous, but will detract from your presentation. Instead, have your laptop in front of you so that you can glance down at the slide. Then, it is okay to turn briefly to point to a section of the screen.

While presenting, look at the audience as much as possible. At the same time, avoid fixating your gaze upon one individual! We've all been in talks where the presenter seems to look more in one direction or at one person. Often, from the presenter's point of view, this person is the one who is looking most interested and nodding. However, instead, it's important not to leave anyone, or any side of the room, out of your gaze.

16.6.5 Tip #1: Don't Undercut Your Message

Comments such as "I know this is a boring topic" or "I'm not good at presenting" or "I wrote this on the plane" are all ways that speakers can undercut their message. Do not undercut your reason for being there: "I don't know why they invited me." All of these comments result in reducing the audience's confidence in you as a speaker.

16.6.6 Tip #2: Try Not to Talk Too Quickly

This is one of the most important aspects of presenting. Typically, speaking quickly is due to nervousness. If you have followed my recommendation for rehearsing your talk at least three times out loud, you will gain confidence in your talk and this will help to ensure that you speak at a measured pace.

Relax, knowing that audiences need to orient themselves to your slides first and remembering that you are much more familiar with your slides than they are. Give the audience time before you start talking and read the titles of your slides first.

16.6.7 Tip #3: Try Not to Spend Too Much Time on Each Slide

It is disconcerting to be halfway through your talk and receive the 1 min warning. In addition, the audience will get bored with anything on screen for longer than 5 min. Instead, for a complicated concept, consider using several slides to make your point. Or, for concepts that build upon each other, consider having items enter the slide through special animation so that you can build upon a more simple slide. In this way, you will not lose the audience's interest.

16.7 CONSIDER HOW THE PRESENTATION WILL BE EVALUATED

It is useful to know how your presentation will be evaluated. If you are a graduate student, try to obtain this information from your committee. In practicing your talk in front of colleagues, consider giving them a critique form for direct, confidential written feedback. An example form is included at the end of this chapter.

In the course I teach, each student presents their proposal at the end of the semester. During the presentation, the rest of the class completes the critique form and hands it directly to the presenter without my seeing it. In this way, students can receive informal and anonymous feedback from each other. Seeing patterns in the comments and suggestions can also help to persuade the presenter of items that need to be conveyed more clearly.

Presentations are typically rated on a number of factors.

Has the presenter provided a clear and concise overview of the:

- Background and significance
- Research hypothesis
- Mechanism (physiologic or behavioral)
- Prior epidemiologic research
- Innovation and research gap
- Study design
- Exposure assessment
- Outcome assessment
- Strengths and weaknesses

16.8 PROPOSAL PRESENTATION CRITIQUE

Name of speaker:_____

Please circle the number corresponding to your response.

1. Did the speaker convey the background and significance of the topic?
   7----------6----------5----------4----------3----------2----------1
   well presented,   inadequate
   understandable   and/or not logical

   Comment:

2. Did the speaker convey the innovation of the proposal and the research gap it will be filling?
   7----------6----------5----------4----------3----------2----------1
   well presented,   inadequate
   understandable   information provided

   Comment:

3. Study methods:
   7----------6----------5----------4----------3----------2----------1
   well presented,   inadequate
   understandable   information provided

   Comment:

4. Data analysis plan and statistical power:
   7----------6----------5----------4----------3----------2----------1
   well presented,   inadequate
   understandable   information provided

   Comment:

5. Tables and figures:
   7----------6----------5----------4----------3----------2----------1
   Yes,   confusing and/or
   Very clear   too complicated

   Comment:

6. Limitations section:
   7----------6----------5----------4----------3----------2----------1
   Yes,   no, did not address
   Addressed well   and/or too confusing

   Comment:

7. Response to audience questions:
   7----------6----------5----------4----------3----------2----------1
   Very clearly,   with confusion and/or
   and thoughtfully   missed the point

   Comment:

8. The pace of the presentation was
   7----------6----------5----------4----------3----------2----------1
   too fast   too slow

   Comment:

9. *Other comments*: (This is the most important.) Please counsel the speaker on any aspects of his/her presentation that you felt could have been delivered better. What suggestions do you have?

PART THREE

Grantsmanship

Choosing the Right Funding Source 17

Welcome to Part Three of this book, *Grantsmanship*. In this third and final part of the book, I will walk you through choosing the right funding source for your grant proposal (Chapter 17), submitting your proposal to a granting agency (Chapter 18), and the grant review (Chapter 19) and resubmission process (Chapter 20).

This chapter is divided into three parts—Part I: "Developing Your Grant-Funding Plan" provides strategic advice for launching your grantsmanship career in collaboration with a mentor. Part II: "Choosing the Appropriate Funding Mechanism for Your Early Grants" goes over considerations in choosing the right funding source. Part III goes on to provide "Step-by-Step Advice for Finding the Right Funding Source at NIH." Navigating the NIH grant system can be overwhelming; however, NIH is the most typical funding source for epidemiology and preventive medicine, particularly for larger awards—the ultimate career goal. Indeed, the NIH Office of Extramural Research is the largest funder of biomedical research in the world, and NIH funds research in just about every area that's remotely related to human health and disease.

17.1 PART I: DEVELOPING YOUR GRANT-FUNDING PLAN

17.1.1 Step #1: Locate a Mentor for Grantsmanship

A key factor in developing your grantsmanship plan is the advice of your mentor(s). If you do not currently have a mentor, speak to your department chair and ask if she or he can provide you with one. If not, it is usually considered acceptable to seek out your own mentor. Indeed, many early-career faculty will assemble a *mentorship team,* each member of which can provide guidance in a different aspect of their career (e.g., a teaching mentor, a research mentor, and a work–life balance mentor).

Consider both on-site and off-site faculty as potential mentors. In particular, if the work of your departmental colleagues does not relate to your primary area of inter-est, then seeking external mentors is particularly important. Luckily, in these days of electronic communication, Skype, and other electronic media, it has become increasingly easy to communicate with colleagues at other institutions electronically.

17.1.1.1 How to identify a mentor

Regardless of their location, a useful technique in identifying mentors is via the use of web-based resources such as Community Of Science (COS) (http://pivot.cos.com/) and NIH Reporter (http://projectreporter.nih.gov/reporter.cfm). Searching on your research topics of interest on the COS website will provide you with a list of faculty with similar interests. You can then use the NIH Reporter site to view the grant track record of these faculty. Be sure to select not only *active grants* but also the faculty member's history of grants obtained over the past 10+ years.

Ideally, your mentor should have the grant track record that you yourself also hope to achieve. Specifically, a mentor should have been successful in securing and maintaining funding—including large R01-type grants, even if she or he is in a different field. A mentor like this will be invaluable in advising you on grantsmanship.

17.1.2 Step #2: Develop Your Overall Grantsmanship Goal

Once you have identified a mentor or mentorship team, it is best to sit down together to create your overall grantsmanship plan. Indeed, it is critical that postdoctoral fellows and early-career faculty have an overall larger vision for their research. Each small grant—be it a seed grant, a predoctoral fellowship, or an early-career award—should be viewed as providing preliminary data for one or two of the specific aims of your ultimate larger grant. Typically, large grants are funded by the NIH R01 mechanism.

Therefore, early on in the process, it is critical to try to envision your ultimate large project. For example, let's assume that a typical R01 contains three to five specific aims. Once you are able to envision these aims, your next steps become clear: Step by step, you start *biting off* small chunks of this larger grant through writing small grants designed to support **one or two** of these ultimate aims. These small grants should not be designed to provide the definitive answer to these aims but instead to show that the aims are feasible and/or provide preliminary data in their support. These small grants will be limited by smaller sample sizes and budgets but will be able to demonstrate proof of principal—that you can *pull it off*.

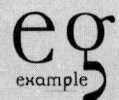

---

e.g. *example*

Overall Grantsmanship Goal/Research Theme:

To obtain an R01 grant to conduct a large prospective study of vitamin D intake and risk of depression.

Specific Aims of the R01

Aim #1: To evaluate the association between self-reported vitamin D and risk of depression

Aim #2: To evaluate the association between a biomarker of vitamin D and risk of depression

Aim #3: To evaluate whether the impact of vitamin D on depression risk is stronger among those with gene x as compared to those without the gene

Small grant proposal to support aim #1: A reproducibility and validity study of the proposed vitamin D questionnaire against an objective measure. *This small grant would support the validity of your measurement tool for your exposure of interest.*

Small grant proposal to support aims #1, #2, and #3: A reproducibility and validity study of the proposed depression questionnaire against a clinical diagnosis of depression. *This small grant would support the validity of your measurement tool for your outcome of interest.*

Small grant proposal to support aim #3: Evaluate the influence of gene x on the association between vitamin D and depression using an existing available dataset. *While this small grant would not be conducted in your population of interest, findings from this project could support your proposed association between vitamin D, gene x, and depression.*

Small grant proposal to support aims #1, #2, and #3: A pilot/feasibility study of recruiting a prospective cohort study at the proposed study site. *This small grant would generate recruitment and retention rates and provide measures of the variability of your exposure and outcome of interest in the study population. These findings would support the power and sample size calculations for the larger grant.*

17.1.2.1 Plan for a steady trajectory of grants from small to large

Start out by capitalizing on funding mechanisms designed to support small projects targeted to early-career faculty or postdoctoral fellows. Below is an example schematic demonstrating the progression from a small internal seed grant to modest NIH grants (e.g., Career Awards) and then culminating in the receipt of an NIH R01 (Figure 17.1).

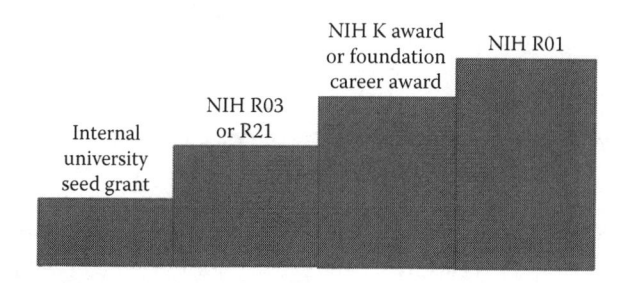

FIGURE 17.1 Example trajectory of grants from small to large.

These early grants typically have the advantage of not requiring pilot data or are specifically designed to support pilot/feasibility studies and are therefore an excellent way to start.

Note that the **order of the smaller steps is flexible**. For example, you might consider submitting an application to NIH for a Career Development Award (K award) prior to a R21 or R03 due to any requirements for submission of a Career Award within 5 years of your postdoctoral degree. Then, you might consider applying for an R21 or R03 second.

17.1.2.2 Avoid classic pitfall #1: Don't skip straight to large funding mechanisms

Early-career faculty want to be successful and, as such, are often tempted by the wish to immediately make a big impact and *land a big grant*. Others are under pressure from their institutions and department chairs to immediately apply for a large grant (e.g., an NIH R01) without a track record of smaller grant funding. In my experience as an NIH review panel member, this approach is almost certainly destined to fail.

The majority of review panels consider a large grant to be the culmination of a growing body of work. They want to see evidence of this stairway to success, and it's your job to demonstrate that you have been on this stairway. You do this by showing your successful procurement and management of previous smaller grants, as well as the translation of these grants into publications. A desirable grant-funding history starts from small seed grants progressing to larger and larger awards in a cumulative fashion. While it is always tempting to skip to the last page of a novel to see what happens, one needs to earn one's way there.

Smaller grants provide critical evidence to reviewers that you can successfully

- Write grant applications
- Manage the logistics of grant projects
- Translate these grants into publications

There are certainly some exceptions to this rule. For example, you may be an early-career faculty member within a research team that already has a track record in your area. If so, you gain the advantage of including any preliminary data they may have in your application. This will give you a head start. However, as described in Chapter 19, *Review Process*, one of the key criteria upon which a grant is scored is the expertise of the PI as a PI. Regardless of your investigative team, if you are the PI, the reviewers will be looking for *your* track record in managing such a large grant. It is unlikely you will be able to provide this assurance of feasibility at an early stage in your career.

One way to minimize this concern is by including a senior team member as co-PI on your proposal. This is described in more detail in Chapter 18, *Submission of the Grant Proposal*.

17.1.3 Plan for More Than One Potential Funding Pipeline

Given today's difficult grant-funding climate, the only way to ensure grant success is to have several proposals in the pipeline and/or under review **at the same time**. For example, you could take the "Small Grant Proposal to Support Aim #1" described above and submit it for an internal seed grant at the same time that you submit the "Small Grant Proposal to Support Aim #1, #2, and #3" to NIH as an R03. Because all these initiatives fit within your overall grantsmanship goal, in the wonderful event that all are funded, they can all serve as pilot data for your larger R01-type grant.

Consider multiple funding options for the same application Another strategic approach is to consider multiple funding options for the *same* application. In this vein, I always advise my mentees to take the same or similar grant application and submit it to multiple potential funders. For example, the **Small Grant Proposal to Support Aim #1**, *A reproducibility and validity study of the proposed vitamin D questionnaire against an objective measure*, could be submitted for (1) an internal seed grant as well as to (2) a small foundation and (3) to NIH for a smaller grant mechanism. On the highly unusual chance that you obtain funding for this grant from more than one source, you will simply be faced with the luxury of declining one of these sources. Most often, the grant submission requirements differ between these funding agencies, such that you will already have made modifications between each version of the proposal. The **key** here is that you are being efficient by taking the same small grant topic and shaping it to apply to several granting mechanisms.

17.1.4 Serve as a Coinvestigator on Established Teams

Developing your own independent line of research funding is of high priority. Indeed, one criterion for tenure and promotion at many research institutes is movement away from the area of your dissertation work and development of independence in terms of your own research aims.

However, given today's difficult grant-funding climate, another way to ensure grant success is to also serve as a **coinvestigator** on a grant led by one of your more senior colleagues while launching your own **independent** research track.

The advantages of serving as a coinvestigator on ongoing or new proposals should not be underestimated. These grants will require a somewhat reduced effort on your part (in comparison to being a PI). In addition, because these ongoing projects may have been underway before you joined, you can also anticipate an earlier payoff in terms of published manuscripts.

Joining an established research project also provides you with the opportunity to apply for supplementary funding that builds upon the established methods and successes of these ongoing grants. Research supplements are described in detail in Part III.

In this vein, consider projects that align with the interests of your senior colleagues with the caveat that the proposed project should not be too far afield from your expertise. Remember that this collaborative work only needs to serve as one of the several streams of your research track.

17.1.5 Avoid Classic Pitfall #2: Do Not Propose Overly Ambitious Specific Aims

An *ambitious* grant proposal by a new investigator is one of the most common reasons for an application to receive a poor score or to be streamlined. (For a definition of the term *streamline* often known as *triage*, see Chapter 19, *Review Process*.) Instead, it is much more impressive to exercise restraint and have focused aims in your early grant proposals.

Recommendation for a feasible topic for a first grant

As mentioned in Chapter 14, *Reproducibility and Validity Studies* or *Pilot Feasibility Studies* make excellent choices as the topics of early grant proposals. Due to their fairly small size and delineated methods, they are quite feasible for early stage investigators. Furthermore, their critical role in the development of a larger project makes them particularly appealing for reviewers—as it is clear that they are a critical first step toward answering a larger etiologic question.

For example, it is perfectly appropriate for a proposal for a small pilot study to state that its ultimate objective is to support the submission of a larger award. The specific aims can conclude by saying, *Findings from this study will yield critical evidence to support the subsequent submission of an R01 application.* Reviewers like to see this evidence of a carefully thought out plan for the future. It demonstrates that the findings from the proposal will have future utility.

In this vein, avoid asking too big of a question or including too many specific aims. If you truly find you cannot delete any aims, consider listing some as *exploratory aims*. Exploratory aims should be limited in number, and while they may require a data analysis plan, they do not typically require power calculations. However, caution should be taken with this approach. Reviewers will carefully examine your application to detect if you are labeling a key aim as *exploratory* as a way to hide poor power.

17.1.6 Avoid Classic Pitfall #3: Do Not Embed Pilot or Validity Studies within a Larger Proposal

Avoid interdependent aims

It is important to acknowledge here that in earlier more economically advantaged times, it was considered acceptable for a large R01 grant to include pilot studies as one or more of its specific aims. However, in the current economic climate, reviewers do not look favorably upon this practice. They naturally ask, "What if the pilot study finds that the methods are not successful? How would the investigator accomplish the subsequent aims of the project?" For example, imagine if aim 1 proposes to conduct a validation study of the questionnaire to be used in aims 2 and 3. If aim 1 subsequently fails to find that the questionnaire is valid, then how can the remainder of the project proceed? These are termed interdependent aims, and reviewers often consider such aims to be a fatal flaw of a proposal.

17.2 PART II: CHOOSING THE APPROPRIATE FUNDING MECHANISM FOR YOUR EARLY GRANTS

17.2.1 Focus on Grants Targeted to Early-Career Faculty and Postdoctoral Fellows

Funding is more difficult to obtain than it ever has been before. However, graduate students and early-career faculty have certain advantages that they can capitalize upon. **Doctoral and postdoctoral training grants or fellowships** as well as **early-career awards** provide the highest chances for success. A primary advantage of these mechanisms is that they typically do not require significant preliminary data. Instead, funding decisions for these awards rely most heavily on your promise and potential as a candidate. This potential is indicated by three items: (1) your education to date, (2) the mentors with which you have surrounded yourself, and (3) the public health importance of your topic.

A key advantage of these funding mechanisms is that, unlike larger grant awards, you will be competing in a smaller pool of investigators, all of whom will be at a comparable stage in their career as yourself. This advantage should not be minimized, as it avoids the risk of competing against senior investigators who already have established track records. As one senior investigator once advised me, "Avoid competing against the 'big boys & girls' as long as you can!" This advantage that you now have will quickly be over after several years pass by, and you find yourself no longer eligible for these early-career investigator awards.

Therefore, if you are a **graduate student**, seek out grant mechanisms designed for graduate students. If you are an **early-career faculty** member, look for grants designed for early-career faculty members.

17.2.2 Internal University Funding

Internal awards vary by institution but may include seed grants and faculty research grants. Take advantage of these opportunities as these grants are typically designed for early-career faculty, and therefore the institution will be motivated to award these to you. In these applications, highlight that the proposed work is critical to the ultimate submission of a larger grant to show your clarity of purpose and the key role that this smaller grant will play. Typically, such awards are small in size.

17.2.3 Foundation Grants

Many foundations have grants targeted for career development. Foundation websites are the best place to start.

Examples are as follows:

- The American Diabetes Association offers the Junior Faculty Award and the Career Development Award.
- The March of Dimes offers the Basil O'Connor Starter Scholar Research Awards.
- The American Heart Association offers the Mentored Clinical & Population Research Award and Scientist Development Grant.

These grants can total as much as $150,000–$200,000 in direct costs per year and provide support for anywhere from 2 to 5 years, but these specifics vary widely by foundation.

17.2.4 Resources for Selecting the Right Funding Source

Universities have resources to help you find grants relevant to your interest area and level. For both graduate students and early-career faculty, your university's office of research will help you identify **funding databases** and **funding sources** and subscribe to **funding alerts**.

Selected examples include:

The Foundation Center offers free *Funding Watch* newsletters in health funding. They are only available to registered users, but registration is free.

Grant Forward features more than 10,000 research funding opportunities from US federal agencies and private foundations. It includes in-depth and up-to-date indexing and abstracting of critical grant information; subject search access; limited submission management; customizable alert service; and an expertise profile service, private foundation sources, and research fellowships.

Grants.gov is a centralized, searchable clearinghouse for over 900 grant programs from the 26 federal grantmaking agencies. Several e-mail alert features are available so that you can receive notifications of new grant opportunity postings.

IRIS funding alerts allow you to create a search profile that will alert you to upcoming funding opportunities in your areas of interest.

NIH Guide for Grants and Contracts (http://grants1.nih.gov/grants/guide/index.html *and* www.http://grants.gov) provides weekly funding alert e-mail notifications of research priorities and open solicitations from NIH to subscribers.

NIH Reporter allows you to search a repository of NIH-funded research projects and access publications and patents resulting from NIH funding. You can limit your search to particular key terms and to particular funding mechanisms.

National Science Foundation (NSF) is an independent federal agency that funds approximately 20% of all federally supported basic research at U.S. colleges and universities. The NSF provides funding alert e-mail notifications.

17.2.5 Look at Who and What They Funded before You

Funding agencies will often make publically available a list of prior grant awardees. These lists may include the grant title, recipient name, amount awarded, and institution. If the granting agency does not provide a list of past grant recipients, your own institution's office of grants and contracts may have a list of investigators on your campus who have obtained these same grants. Look over this list and see if you or your mentors know any of these investigators.

This is useful for several reasons. First, it shows the interest of the funding agency in funding research in **epidemiology and preventive medicine**. Some funding agencies simply don't have the interest or track record in funding population-based research and instead limit their funding to laboratory studies (*bench science*). Second, it is reasonable to consider asking successful fundees to share their successful applications with you, particularly if you, or your mentors, recognize any names on the fundee list or see that they are from your institution. Reassure these successfully funded investigators that you are simply seeking a model for the appropriate scope and depth of the research plan, not the actual content of their aims. When framed in this manner, people are typically willing to share.

17.2.6 Look at Who Serves as Reviewers

In addition to posting prior grant awardees on their website, funding agencies may also post a list of prior and current grant reviewers and their affiliations. Go through this list and review the expertise of these investigators. Ask yourself if their expertise overlaps with your study aims and methodology.

For example, are any of these investigators population health researchers? Are any from similar departments/divisions to yours? It would be a high-risk proposition to write a proposal for a foundation that does not include reviewers with expertise in epidemiology or preventive medicine on their review panels.

17.3 PART III: STEP-BY-STEP ADVICE FOR FINDING THE RIGHT FUNDING SOURCE AT NIH

Due to the complex nature of NIH, this section of the chapter focuses on recommended sources of grants for early-career faculty, postdoctoral fellows, and doctoral students at NIH.

Below, I provide a step-by-step approach for finding the right funding mechanism at NIH (Table 17.1).

17.3.1 Step #1: Determine Which NIH Institute's Mission Encompasses Your Topic

Once you have identified a mentor, created your overall grantsmanship goal, and bitten off a chewable section of that larger goal into a first feasible grant proposal, the next step is to view the NIH institute websites.

NIH is made up of **27 institutes and centers**, each with a specific research agenda, often focusing on particular diseases or body systems (Table 17.2).

Alternatively, you can also start by searching the NIH Guide for Grants and Contracts (http://grants1.nih.gov/grants/guide/index.html and www.http://grants.gov) for your scientific area of interest, and this search will generate a list of institutes that support these interest areas.

17.3.2 Step #2: Choose a Funding Mechanism Sponsored by Your Selected NIH Institute

Now that you have selected the NIH institute that encompasses your topic, go to the institute's website and see which funding mechanisms they offer and who/what it is designed to support. For example, does the institute fund Career Development Awards (K series), and if so, which ones? Do they fund Research Awards (R Series such as R03s and R21s)? Not all NIH institutes offer every funding mechanism. In addition, even for the same funding mechanism, each institute may have different emphases and program requirements. Therefore, it is perfectly appropriate to contact the relevant institute staff member early in the process to determine whether your planned research and/or training falls within their mission for that type of award.

The funding mechanisms listed in Table 17.3 are examples of funding mechanisms particularly suited to early-career faculty and doctoral students.

TABLE 17.1 Step by step: Finding the right funding mechanism at NIH

Step 1: Determine which NIH institute's mission encompasses your topic.
Step 2: Choose a funding mechanism sponsored by your selected NIH institute.
Step 3: Choose the corresponding funding opportunity announcement (FOA) (PA or RFA number).

TABLE 17.2 NIH institutes

National Cancer Institute (NCI)	National Eye Institute (NEI)
National Heart, Lung, and Blood Institute (NHLBI)	National Human Genome Research Institute (NHGRI)
National Institute on Aging (NIA)	National Institute on Alcohol Abuse and Alcoholism (NIAAA)
National Institute of Allergy and Infectious Diseases (NIAID)	National Institute of Arthritis and Musculoskeletal and Skin Diseases (NIAMS)
National Institute of Child Health and Human Development (NICHD)	
National Institute of Diabetes and Digestive and Kidney Diseases (NIDDK)	National Institute on Deafness and Other Communication Disorders (NIDCD)
National Institute of Environmental Health Sciences (NIEHS)	National Institute of Dental and Craniofacial Research (NIDCR)
National Institute on Minority Health and Health Disparities (NIMHD)	National Institute on Drug Abuse (NIDA)
	National Institute of Mental Health (NIMH)
National Institute of Nursing Research (NINR)	National Institute of Neurological Disorders and Stroke (NINDS)

TABLE 17.3 Selected examples of funding mechanisms suitable for early grants

	DOCTORAL STUDENTS	POSTDOCTORAL FELLOWS	EARLY-CAREER FACULTY
Mentored/Training Awards			
Doctoral and Postdoctoral Fellowships (F series)			
F30, F31	X		
F32		X	
Training Grants (T series)	X	X	X
Career Development Awards (K series)			
K08, K12, K22, K99/R00		X	
K01, K07, K18, K23, K25			X
LRP		X	X
Research supplements	X	X	X
Independent Awards			
Research Awards (R series)			
R03, R15, R21		X	X

17.3.2.1 Doctoral and postdoctoral fellowships (F series) "Ruth L. Kirschstein Individual National Research Service Award" (NRSA)

Doctoral and Postdoctoral Fellowships (F series) are named for Dr. Ruth L. Kirschstein, an accomplished scientist in polio vaccine development, who became the first female director of an NIH institute. She was a champion of research training and a strong advocate for the inclusion of underrepresented individuals in the scientific workforce.

These fellowship awards require a proposed **research and training plan**, which will be conducted under the supervision of a **mentor (sponsor)**. The sponsor and any cosponsors are also expected to have a successful track record of mentoring and provide an assessment of the applicant's qualifications and potential for a research career.

Note that you can identify more than one mentor (i.e., a mentoring team) to ensure that you receive expert advice in all aspects of the research and training program. In such cases, one individual must be identified as the principal sponsor who will coordinate the applicant's research training program. Your sponsor should have a key role in helping you to prepare the application (Figure 17.2).

For Doctoral Students

F30 Individual Predoctoral MD/PhD and Other Dual Doctoral Degree Fellows
This award provides support to doctoral candidates enrolled in a formally combined MD/PhD program to perform a research project in clinical or basic sciences.

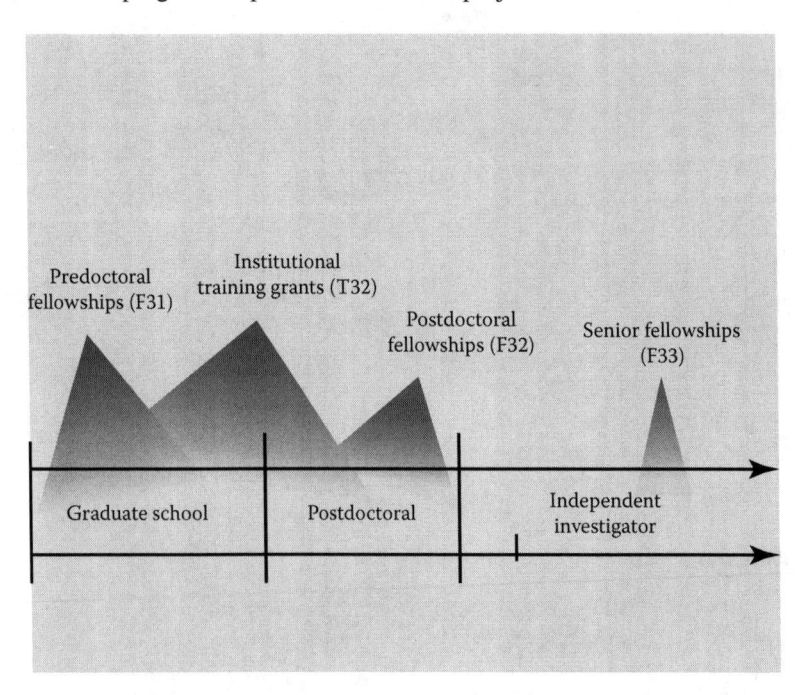

FIGURE 17.2 Training grants and fellowships for researchers.

This fellowship is awarded to applicants with the potential to become productive, independent, highly trained physician-scientists and other clinician-scientists, including patient-oriented researchers in their scientific mission areas.

F31 Individual Predoctoral Fellows
This award provides support for promising doctoral candidates to perform dissertation research and receive training in scientific health-related fields relevant to the missions of the participating NIH institutes.

F31 Individual Predoctoral Fellowships to Promote Diversity in Health-Related Research
This award is identical to the F31 but provides support for promising doctoral candidates who are from underrepresented racial and ethnic groups, individuals with disabilities, and individuals from disadvantaged backgrounds.

For Postdoctoral Fellows

F32 Individual Postdoctoral Fellows
This award provides support for promising postdoctoral fellows to perform a research project within the broad scope of biomedical, behavioral, or clinical research.

17.3.2.2 Training grants (T series) "Ruth L. Kirschstein Individual National Research Service Award"

Training Grants (T series) are also named for Dr. Ruth L. Kirschstein. Training grants are **awarded to universities under the direction of a senior faculty member** who serves as the training project director (PD)/PI. Therefore, you would not apply directly to NIH yourself for a training grant. Ask your chair or mentor if this type of program is available at your institution. Then, you would follow **internal university guidelines** to apply to be a fellow in this program (Figure 17.2).

For Doctoral Students and Postdoctoral Fellows

T32 Institutional Research Training Grants are awarded to support predoctoral and postdoctoral research training to help ensure that a diverse and highly trained workforce is available to assume leadership roles related to the nation's biomedical, behavioral, and clinical research agenda. The training grants tend to require a proposed **research and training plan**, which will be conducted under the supervision of a **mentor or preceptor**. Often, the next step for a T32 fellow is to apply for a K award.

17.3.2.3 Career development awards (K series)

Most career development awards are designed for applicants who have completed their academic or clinical training and who have accepted (or have recently started) a faculty position. Note that some career development awards (e.g., K99) require that applicants have no more than 5 years of postdoctoral research training at the time of application. It is important to note that you will not be eligible for a career development award if you have already received a large NIH R01 grant (as PI) but that you are still eligible if you have been awarded an NIH small grant (R03), exploratory/developmental grant (R21), or dissertation award (R36). Therefore, these eligibility limitations make a K award an excellent choice for an early-career faculty member.

Proposals for K awards require a proposed **research project** and a **career development training plan** to be conducted under the supervision of a *mentor (sponsor)*. As with other mentored awards, the mentor, co-mentor, or mentoring team should be recognized as accomplished investigators in the proposed research area and have a track record of success in training and placing independent investigators. The sponsor and any cosponsors are also expected to provide an assessment of the applicant's qualifications and potential for a research career and a plan for mentoring and monitoring the candidate's research, publications, and progression toward independence.

In addition, the proposals also require a description of the candidate's background, career goals and objectives, and training in the responsible conduct of research.

For Postdoctoral Fellows

K08 Mentored Clinical Scientist Research Career Development Award
This award provides support and *protected time* to individuals with a clinical doctoral degree for an intensive, supervised research career development experience in the fields of biomedical and behavioral research, including translational research.

K12 Mentored Clinical Scientist Developmental Program Award
This is an award to universities, and interested candidates should ask the chair of their department if such an award exists.

K22 Career Transition Award
This award provides support for a postdoctoral fellow in transition to a faculty position during the early years of a new faculty position.

K99/R00 Pathway to Independence Award
This award is designed to facilitate the transition from a mentored postdoctoral research position to a stable independent research position. The K99/R00 award consists of two phases. The initial mentored phase (K99) provides support for career development and the conduct of a research project by a postdoctoral candidate with no more than 5 years of postdoctoral research training. The second phase (R00) provides support to continue the research as an independent scientist at the institution to which the individual has been recruited for a tenure-track full-time assistant professor position (or equivalent). The goal is for the individual to continue to work toward establishing his or her own independent research program and prepare an application for regular research grant support (R01).

For Early-Career Faculty

K01 The Mentored Research Scientist Development Award
This award supports new faculty members who need additional supervised research experience because they have had a career hiatus or they are moving to a substantially new area of research. For example, if your doctoral work was in nutrition, but you would like to shift your focus to mental health, you should consider a K01.

K07 Academic Award
This award is used to recruit research faculty into areas where there is a growing need for research and instructional capabilities.

K18 and K25 Career Enhancement Awards
These awards are used to support individuals interested in stem cell research or quantitative methods.

K23 Mentored Patient-Oriented Research Career Development Award
This award provides support for individuals with a clinical doctoral degree interested in pursuing a career in patient-oriented research.

17.3.2.4 Loan repayment programs

Loan repayment programs (LRPs) are designed to attract health professionals to pursue careers in biomedical, behavioral, social, and clinical research. The program offers up to $35,000 per year to repay student loans of scientists, physicians, dentists, and other doctoral-level health professionals. The program requires that you commit at least 2 years to conducting qualified research. Loan repayment benefits are in addition to your institutional salary. The application requires a description of your current or proposed **research and training** plan as well as a statement from the **mentor(s)**.

For Postdoctoral Fellows and Early-Career Faculty

There are five LRPs—each with a different focus:

1. LRP-CR (clinical research)
2. LRP-PR (pediatric research)
3. LRP-HDR (health disparities research)
4. LRP-CIR (contraception and infertility research)
5. LRP-IDB (clinical research for individuals from disadvantaged backgrounds)

17.3.2.5 Research supplements

This program provides administrative supplements to existing NIH research grants for the purpose of supporting full-time or part-time research by individuals meeting the eligibility criteria described below. Therefore, if your mentor is a PI of an active research grant with 2 years or more remaining on that active grant, they may be eligible to submit an administrative supplement to the grant to support you and your research project. Note that while the mentor will be listed as the PI on this supplement, you will be listed as the *candidate*. These supplemental funds are targeted toward attracting targeted populations within the research workforce in the United States and internationally and providing reentry opportunities to the research workforce.

There are a variety of different types of supplements. Examples are as follows:

For Postdoctoral Fellows and Early-Career Faculty

Supplements to Promote Diversity in Health-Related Research
These supplements are designed to improve the diversity of the research workforce by supporting and recruiting students, postdoctoral fellows, and eligible investigators from groups that have been shown to be underrepresented in health-related research.

Supplements to Promote Reentry into Biomedical Research
These supplements are designed to support individuals with high potential to reenter an active research career after an interruption for family responsibilities or other qualifying circumstances. The purpose of these supplements is to encourage such individuals to reenter research careers within the missions of all the program areas of NIH.

17.3.2.6 Research awards (R series)

The smaller Research Awards such as R21s and R03s are **not mentored** and are designed to support your **independent research**. While they typically provide smaller budgets than an R01, they are well suited to early-career faculty as they do not require preliminary data. In addition, receipt of these awards does not remove your NIH new investigator advantage as described below. However, it is important to note that these awards are not offered by all NIH institutes.

For Postdoctoral Fellows and Early-Career Faculty

R03 NIH Small Grant Program
This award provides support for small research projects that can be carried out in a short period of time (i.e., 2 years) with limited resources. Such projects include pilot or feasibility studies, collection of preliminary data, secondary analysis of existing data, small research projects, or development of new research technology. Direct costs are generally quite limited (e.g., up to $50,000 per year). Note that this funding mechanism is not utilized by all the NIH institutes.

R15 NIH Academic Research Enhancement Award (AREA)
This award is designed to stimulate research in educational institutions that have not been major recipients of NIH support. They are intended to support small-scale research projects proposed by faculty members from these eligible institutions, to expose students to meritorious research projects, and to strengthen the research environment of the applicant institution. Check with your institution's office of grants and contracts regarding your eligibility for an R15. The majority of NIH institutes utilize this award.

R21 NIH Exploratory/Developmental Research Grant Award
This award is designed to support exploratory studies during the early and conceptual stages of project development. Exploratory studies are defined as novel studies that break new ground or extend previous discoveries toward new directions or applications. High-risk/high-reward studies that may lead to a breakthrough in a particular area or result in novel techniques, agents, methodologies, models, or applications that will impact biomedical, behavioral, or clinical research are an excellent fit for R21s. Direct costs (e.g., $275,000 over 2 years) are typically higher than an R03. Note that this funding mechanism is not utilized by all the NIH institutes.

Choosing between an R03 and an R21 R03s are smaller in budget, but don't have the high impact requirement of an R21. However, given the current funding environment, one could argue that all grant proposals have to be high impact to be competitive. This doesn't mean that as an epidemiologist or preventive medicine specialist, you have to propose to create a new methodology for an R21 proposal. Instead, high impact could be defined as the investigation of a novel hypothesis or use of better methods to evaluate an existing hypothesis for which prior findings have been conflicting. For example, proposals to conduct the first prospective study in an area, the first study to use a better assay to evaluate a particular biomarker, or the first study to evaluate an association among a high-risk group could all be interpreted as high impact. All this being said, projects of limited cost or scope that use widely accepted approaches and methods are likely better suited for the R03 small grant mechanism.

17.3.2.7 New investigator advantages

Once you reach the step of applying for an NIH R01 award, you will have several advantages as an early-career faculty member.

NIH defines **new investigators** as PIs who have **not** received a substantial NIH independent research award such as an R01. In other words, you will remain a *new investigator* even after you receive early stage or small research grants (e.g., an R03 or R21) or Training Grants/Fellowships (e.g., T and F series awards), infrastructure (e.g., R15 awards), or Career Development Awards (e.g., K series awards).

NIH defines Early Stage Investigators (*ESIs*) as new investigators who are within 10 years of completing their terminal research degree or within 10 years of completing their medical residency at the time they apply for R01 grants. Applications from ESIs, like those from all new investigators, are given special consideration during peer review and at the time of funding. Peer reviewers are instructed to focus more on the proposed approach than on the track record and to expect less preliminary data than might be provided by an established investigator.

Check your specific NIH institute of interest for their policies for new investigators and/or ESIs. These **special considerations** may include funding priority and ensured years of support. For example, some NIH institutes have separate paylines (e.g., more generous) for awards to ESI applicants and/or monitor their new investigator pool to make sure that a certain percent has ESI status.

17.3.3 Step #3: Choose the Corresponding Funding Opportunity Announcement Number

Once you have followed the steps above, then you will need to choose the corresponding funding opportunity number. There are three types of funding opportunity announcements (FOAs) as described in Figure 17.3. Most simply, the type of FOA that you list on your submission cover/face page will dictate the specific submission instructions that you will follow (as described in Chapter 18). The FOA will also have implications for your probability of receiving funding as described below.

```
                    ┌─────────────────────────┐
                    │ Types of funding        │
                    │ opportunity             │
                    │ announcements (FOA)     │
                    └─────────────────────────┘
              ↙              ↓               ↘
  ┌──────────────┐  ┌──────────────────┐  ┌──────────────────┐
  │ Parent       │  │ Insitute-specific│  │ Request for      │
  │ announcements│  │ program          │  │ applications     │
  │              │  │ announcements(PAs)│ │ (RFA)            │
  └──────────────┘  └──────────────────┘  └──────────────────┘
```

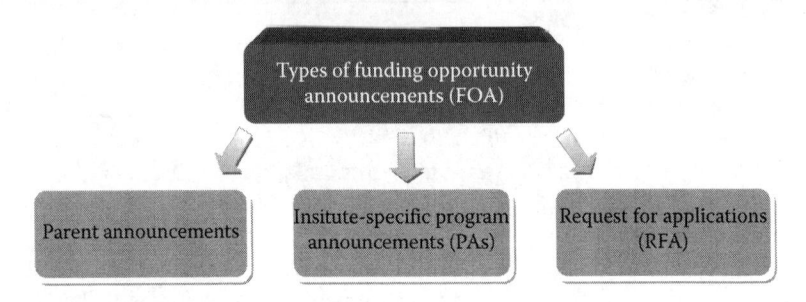

FIGURE 17.3   Types of FOAs.

Parent announcements simply refer to general investigator-initiated, unsolicited research. More simply stated, this means that if you, as the PI, propose a grant on any topic within the breadth of the NIH mission, it will likely fit under a general parent announcement. In other words, the individual grant project designs reflect the ideas and creativity of the investigator. For example, the R03 and R21 grants described above are general parent announcements. Submission dates are standard (approximately three times per year), and the funding payline is determined by the NIH institute of choice. **Advantages** of parent announcements are your flexibility in topic.

Institute-specific *PAs* are similar to parent announcements but are generated by the specific NIH institute themselves and reflect the institute's broad research interests or a reminder of a scientific need. Again, if you, as the PI, have a grant proposal on any topic within the breadth of that particular institute, it will likely fit under a PA. PAs use standard receipt dates (approximately three times per year). All **training grants** are in the form of PAs. **Advantages** of PAs are that the institute may have flexibility in funding **above the payline**. This is a key advantage that should not be overlooked—and if at all possible, you should see if your grant topic relates to one of the PAs.

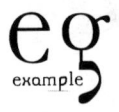

e.g. example   For example, the National Institute on Aging (NIA) offers the parent R03. In addition, they offer a **specific** R03, which is focused on Acute Kidney Injury in Older Adults (R03). If your R03 topic happened to be focused on kidney injury in older adults, then applying for this specific PA would be preferable. Instead, if your R03 topic focused on risk factors for aging muscles, then you would apply through the parent R03 announcement.

Request for Applications (RFAs) are formal statements inviting applications on a well-defined area with specific objectives. They have specific, one-time application receipt dates and plan to fund a limited prespecified number of awards. RFAs use a special review panel that is convened on a one-time basis. There are several **disadvantages** of RFAs:

- Revising and resubmitting your proposal are typically not possible as there is only one review.
- The review panel has not worked together before, which may make the review process more unpredictable.
- The topic is not investigator initiated.

How to choose between a parent announcement and PA and RFA

I always advise my mentees to prioritize their overall research/grantsmanship vision over and above these time-specific PAs and RFAs. Certainly if you find a PA that fits closely with your overall research vision, it is preferable to apply under that announcement even if it might require some modest *tweaks* to your application. However, I would not suggest that you substantively alter your research vision in response to a specific PA or RFA. As you will see in Chapter 18, *Submission of the Grant Proposal*, your application is scored by a study section at NIH which is **independent** from the NIH institutes. As long as you receive a strong scientific score from this study section, you will have a high chance of success. Response to a specific PA simply gives you an extra boost, as it gives the NIH institute more flexibility in their payline for what scores are funded.

17.3.3.1 Read the FOA carefully!

Finally, be sure to read the FOA carefully for specific eligibility requirements as well as any special review criteria or application instructions before writing your application. **Then take a second look at the FOA!**

17.4 EXAMPLES OF CHOOSING THE RIGHT FUNDING SOURCES

17.4.1 Example #1: A Postdoctoral Researcher Transitioning to Early-Career Faculty

Using our example provided early in the chapter, below is a reminder of the overall grantsmanship goal of a postdoctoral researcher (Table 17.4).

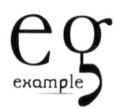

eg example

Overall Grantsmanship Goal/Research Theme:
To obtain an R01 grant to conduct a large prospective study of vitamin D intake and risk of depression.

Specific Aims of the R01
"Aim #1: To evaluate the association between self-reported vitamin D and risk of depression"
"Aim #2: To evaluate the association between a biomarker of vitamin D and risk of depression"
"Aim #3: To evaluate whether the impact of vitamin D on depression risk is stronger among those with gene x as compared to those without the gene"

TABLE 17.4 Grantsmanship timeline example for a postdoctoral researcher

TIME	FUNDING MECHANISM	TOPIC
Postdoctoral Fellow		
Year 01	F32 Individual Postdoctoral Fellow through NIMH	Small Grant Proposal to Support Aim #1: A reproducibility and validity study of the proposed vitamin D questionnaire against an objective measure.
Year 02	K99/R00 Pathway to Independence Award (NIMH)	Small Grant Proposal to Support Aims #1, #2, and #3: A pilot/feasibility study of recruiting a prospective cohort study at the proposed study site.
Assistant Professor		
Year 01	Internal Faculty Research Grant	Small Grant Proposal to Support Aim #3: Evaluate the influence of gene x on the association between vitamin D and depression using an existing dataset.
Year 01	Continuation of K99/R00 through NIMH	
Year 02	American Society for Nutrition—starter scholar[a]	Small Grant Proposal to Support Aims #1, #2, and #3: A reproducibility and validity study of the proposed depression questionnaire against a clinical diagnosis of depression.
Year 02	R03 NIH Small Research Grant Program at NIMH	Small Grant Proposal to Support Aims #1, #2, and #3: A reproducibility and validity study of the proposed depression questionnaire against a clinical diagnosis of depression (Note in case American Society for Nutrition grant not awarded).
Year 03	Resubmission and/or conduct of above grants	
Year 04	R01 at NIMH	Proposal to conduct a large prospective study of vitamin D intake and risk of depression.

[a] Hypothetical foundation grant.

17.4.2 Example #2: An Early-Career Faculty Member

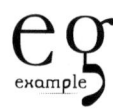

Overall Grantsmanship Goal/Research Theme:
To obtain an R01 grant to conduct a randomized trial of exercise in the prevention of obesity in early childhood (Table 17.5).
Specific Aims of the R01
"Aim #1: To evaluate the impact of the 6-month exercise intervention on BMI"
"Aim #2: To evaluate the impact of the 6-month exercise intervention on markers of insulin resistance"
"Aim #3: To evaluate the impact of the 6-month exercise intervention on levels of cardiovascular risk factors"
"Aim #4: To evaluate the efficacy of the 6-month exercise intervention on measures of compliance (i.e., exercise and diet)"

TABLE 17.5 Grantsmanship timeline example for an early-career faculty member

TIME	FUNDING MECHANISM	TOPIC
Assistant Professor		
Year 01	Internal Faculty Research Grant	*Small Grant Proposal to Develop the Intervention*: Conduct focus groups among at-risk children.
Year 01	American Diabetes Association Junior Faculty Award	*Small Grant Proposal to Support Aim #4*: To evaluate the efficacy of the exercise intervention on measures of compliance.
Year 02	R21 NIH Small Research Grant Program NIDDK[a]	*Small Grant Proposal to Support Aims #1, 2, 3, and 4*: A pilot feasibility study of the proposed intervention among a sample of at-risk children.
Year 03	Resubmission and/or conduct of above grants	
Year 04	R01 from NIDDK[a]	Proposal to conduct a randomized trial of exercise in the prevention of obesity in early childhood.

[a] In response to a specific PA from NIDDK for "Home and Family Based Approaches for the Prevention or Management of Overweight or Obesity in Early Childhood (R21) and (R01)."

Submission of the Grant Proposal

18

This chapter picks up where Chapter 17, *Choosing the Right Funding Source*, left off by walking you step by step through the actual submission of your grant proposal to a funding agency. As noted in the prior chapter, throughout this last section of the book, I use NIH submission criteria as the primary example because NIH is the most typical funding source for epidemiology and preventive medicine, particularly for larger awards.

The submission of a grant includes not only the research proposal itself but also such forms as the biosketch, budget, facilities, and protection of human subjects, and it can even include the coordination of subcontracts with off-site coinvestigators. Part I of the chapter, "Getting Started," begins with suggested first steps and techniques to obtain both internal and external review of your grant proposal. Part II of the chapter provides "Strategic Tips for Each Component of the Grant Submission." Finally, Part III of the chapter provides a "Timeline for the Grant Submission Process." Chapter 19 follows up with the *Review Process*.

A note: This chapter does not review the submission of Training Grants (T series) Ruth L. Kirschstein NRSA applications. These awards are granted to your university under the direction of a senior investigator who provides the administrative and scientific leadership for the implementation of the program. Ask your department chair or mentor if your institution has such a training grant. You would then apply internally at your institution.

18.1 HOW TO VIEW THE SUBMISSION PROCESS OVERALL

A colleague of mine once described the grant submission process as a race. You arrive at the finish line completely exhausted but still holding aloft your completed grant application with your last remaining iota of strength. However, there are ways to get help in this race.

If your institution provides you with the services of a **preaward grants manager** or an **office of grants and contracts**, it will be important for you to meet with these personnel early in the process and determine how they can assist you with the submission. Often, such personnel can complete many of the nonscientific forms required for the submission described later in the chapter.

In addition, if you are an early-career faculty, try to involve **graduate students** (e.g., research assistants or other mentees) in the submission process. This will provide the students with exposure to grantsmanship and the nuts and bolts of the submission process—critical for their own careers.

18.2 PART I: GETTING STARTED

18.2.1 How Far Ahead to Start the Grant Preparation Process

Back in the days when NIH pay lines were higher and 3 submissions of the same grant proposal were allowed, some investigators used the first of these submissions as a way of *testing the waters*. The first review would indicate if the reviewers *liked* the topic and put the onus on the reviewer to identify the proposal's limitations. The investigator would then correct and/or address any concerns for the second submission, knowing full well that they had a third submission to address any final issues.

This approach was a saving grace for those procrastinators who like to wait till the deadline nears or those spontaneous investigators who decided to respond to a PA or RFA at the last minute.

However, this old approach is no longer feasible given the drastic reduction in funding pay lines and the current limitation of two submissions for the same grant proposal. In this current economic climate, investigators not only need to perfect the application down to the finest detail before submitting but need to choose among their ideas and only submit their **best work**. The onus is now on the investigator to find their own study limitations and to present alternative strategies.

In light of these concerns, I always recommend the following:

Start the grant proposal writing process 4 months in advance of the due date. This provides time:

- To adequately review the prior literature such that the research gap can be identified
- To revise your specific aims if you find you have insufficient power
- To obtain advance feedback from your coinvestigators and mentors
- To incorporate the comments of your coinvestigators and mentors
- To consider alternatives and limitations
- To complete final fine-tuning and editing

A 4-month timeline allows for an adequate review of the prior literature such that the research gap can be identified and key studies can be cited. Most importantly, this timeline allows for iterative versions of the specific aims such that you can incorporate your colleagues' comments and then have time for rereview and revisions. There is nothing more insulting to a coinvestigator than to ask for their comments at the last minute—it implies either that they do not have competing responsibilities or that you will not be incorporating their comments—as there would clearly not be sufficient time.

An early stab at your power and sample size calculations avoids the last-minute panic of discovering that you have insufficient power given your budget. Instead, it allows for a consideration of alternatives and limitations. The 4-month timeline also allows for a final evaluation to see if submission should be delayed to the next cycle to allow for the conduct of small pilot studies or the accumulation of more preliminary data to support the proposed aims.

Lastly, the timeline comfortably incorporates time for a final fine-tuning such that reviewers don't become frustrated with inconsistent table references/titling and other typographical errors, omissions, or lack of adequate citations. These small errors can significantly reduce a reviewer's enthusiasm.

See the end of this chapter for a detailed *example timeline for submission of an NIH grant*.

18.2.2 Begin to Assemble the Research Team Early

18.2.2.1 How to choose collaborators

Investigate opportunities for collaborating with more experienced, well-known grantees or a known laboratory. Keeping your proposed topic in mind, determine the expertise needed to strengthen your research study team (e.g., individuals, collaborating organizations, and/or their accompanying resources). Collaborators can fill gaps in your own expertise and can assure reviewers of the competence of your proposed team. In addition, NIH looks favorably upon interdisciplinary collaborations as they can lead to a more novel proposal with greater impact. You will find that many NIH PAs and RFPs emphasize the importance of interdisciplinary teams.

For grant writing in epidemiology and preventive medicine, reviewers often look for a doctoral-level epidemiologist and/or statistician on the research team. Failure to include such a *card-carrying* coinvestigator (unless you are one yourself) is a common reason for a lower score. Enlist an epidemiologist and/or statistician early in the grant-writing process right after the research question is elucidated. Collaborate closely with them on the methods, data analysis, and power/sample size sections. Be open to concerns they may have.

A common pitfall to avoid Avoid the common pitfall of scrambling to add an epidemiologist or statistician to the research team **after** the first round of reviews—just to patch problems found by reviewers. Similarly, unless you are a clinician already, enlist at least one clinician who is an expert in the particular outcome of interest. Also enlist at least one coinvestigator who is an expert in the main exposures of interest, even if the dataset is already built.

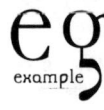

eg *example* Imagine that you are planning to submit a grant proposal designed to prospectively identify genetic and environmental risk factors for prostate cancer. Your research team should ideally include (1) an **oncologist** who has a track record of publications on prostate cancer, (2) an **epidemiologist** who has designed and led studies on prostate cancer or a related cancer, and (3) a **statistician** with expertise in genetic analyses, ideally in the cancer field.

On the other hand, reviewers will carefully watch for the inclusion of too many collaborators—with no clear ties to your aims!

18.2.2.2 Establish working relationships with coinvestigators before submission

Coinvestigators should not appear in name only Your grant application will need to demonstrate that you have established working relationships with these investigators. If you are early in your career, you may be concerned that you cannot establish such relationships in time, given the pressure you may be under to submit grants. However, the following will provide reassurance to the reviewers of such a relationship:

- Coauthored publications (or submitted publications under review)
- Copresentations
- An established mentoring relationship (e.g., as part of a training grant)
- Other grant applications on which you are both investigators or consultants

How will you demonstrate this established relationship? You cannot rely upon the reviewers to connect the dots between you and your coinvestigators. Instead, you want to make it easy for the reviewers by clearly integrating this prior collaboration into several components of the grant application. These include

- The preliminary studies section (see Chapter 8)
- Biosketches (Section A, *Personal Statement*) for yourself and your coinvestigators
- Letters of support
- The budget justification section

See Part II for relevant strategies for each of these individual sections.

18.2.2.3 Consider a multiple principal investigator model

If your work includes interdisciplinary efforts and collaboration where a team science approach could be more effective, then you may want to consider the NIH option of a multiple-PI model. This approach can be particularly helpful when you are an early-career faculty but are proposing to conduct a project that might be considered ambitious by some reviewers. For example, let's say you have a track record of publications on prostate cancer using secondary data sources. However, the proposal involves the de novo recruitment and follow-up of a relatively large sample of participants—a new area for you. In this case, you may consider a second PI with a track record of expertise in conducting large prospective follow-up studies.

The format, peer review, and administration of applications submitted under the multiple-PI model have some significant differences from the traditional single-PI model that will need to be taken into consideration as you plan. Therefore, if you are considering a multiple-PI model, you will want to contact the relevant NIH program official (listed on the relevant FOA) early in the grant preparation process to discuss whether this model would be appropriate for that mechanism.

18.2.3 Spend Half Your Time on the Specific Aims and Project Summary (Abstract)

As noted in Chapter 1, *Ten Top Tips for Proposal Writing*, the specific aims should be the first item that you write when you *set pen to paper,* prior to writing a literature review or methodology section. Indeed, writers of successful grant applications typically report that 50% of their time is spent on revising and rewriting their specific aims (Figure 18.1). Once a draft is ready, send it to your mentor and coinvestigators with the goal of kicking off an **iterative process of rewriting, revising, and rereviewing**.

After drafting your aims, the **second step** in this process is to calculate your statistical power to achieve these aims. This will help you to answer the question, "Will your sample size provide you with sufficient power to detect a difference between groups, if there truly is a difference?" If you are basing your grant upon a preexisting dataset, your sample size will typically be fixed, and the question of whether or not you have adequate power can be answered quickly. A negative answer, while disappointing, can quickly and efficiently result in a change in study aims.

If instead you are proposing to launch a new study and recruit participants, you can choose the sample size that you need to achieve sufficient power. However, in this case, progressing to Step #3 of calculating the budget will be critical. A common pitfall of new investigators is to be too ambitious in this regard—proposing a larger sample size than they have the budget and experience to handle.

Steps
✎ Draft aims
🖳 Calculate power
📖 Calculate budget

FIGURE 18.1 The first three steps in proposal writing.

Evaluate if your budget can afford your required sample size. Such costs include the number of assays, interviewer time for recruitment and follow-up, as well as the cost of participant incentives. Also, ask yourself whether your study site can feasibly provide that number of participants. For example, does the hospital actually see that number of patients per day/week/year? Are that many patients likely to be eligible *and* agree to participate? Such questions of feasibility can be answered by your own preliminary work, by that of your coinvestigators, or by other investigators at your proposed study site. Alternatively, if you are proposing a pilot grant, you can clearly state that the goal of your pilot is to assess recruitment and eligibility rates to calculate power for a larger grant submission.

Now, in light of everything you have learned from Steps 1, 2, and 3 and incorporating your mentors' and colleagues' feedback, go back and refine the aims and start the process over again. Once you have settled on the aims, you will find that writing the rest of the application will flow easily and fit within the rest of your time frame.

18.2.4 Allow Time for External Review Prior to Submission

In addition to asking your coinvestigators to read your grant application, the use of other external reviewers will substantially increase your odds of success. The **bottom line** being that the more comments you can obtain prior to submission, the fewer comments you are likely to receive from the actual grant review panel. Given that the majority of granting agencies provide only one opportunity for resubmission, this is critical. It is difficult to be able to improve from a poor score on a first submission to a fundable score on a second submission.

Your mentor should be able to assist you in identifying and recruiting the following types of external reviewers. Some departments will compensate outside scientists to review your grant proposal.

There are two types of external reviewers to consider:

1. Outside scientists with expertise in your proposed topic area
2. A grant-writing consultant and/or a colleague with a general scientific background but not necessarily in your proposed topic area

Recall that, depending on the review panel, some of your assigned grant reviewers may not have expertise in your area of interest. This is why a well-written application should be readable and understandable by anyone with scientific knowledge. Even a generalist reviewer will be able to assess (1) whether your goals are clearly stated, (2) whether your proposal clearly justifies what is new and how it extends prior work in the field, (3) what is innovative about your proposal, as well as (4) the overall impact of your potential findings on public health and clinical practice. In recent years, the last point has become an even more critical factor in funding decisions. With the recent revision in the NIH grant review process, reviewers now prioritize the overall impact. This aspect alone is often the most critical in the assigned score for an application.

The same person cannot write a proposal *and* review it for clarity

Regardless of how carefully you reread your grant, and no matter how conscientious you are, simply by virtue of your familiarity with the material, you will not be able to review your grant for final clarity. Therefore, many departments will provide funding for a grant-writing consultant. By encouraging you to convey the study aims and methods as clearly as possible, the best grant-writing consultants will help you to further refine your specific aims and convey the potential impact of your findings.

18.2.5 External Review: *Chalk-Talk Forums*

Another useful way to get constructive feedback on your grant proposal is to participate in a *chalk-talk forum* or similarly named forum. These consist of informal seminars in your department where investigators discuss their research ideas or draft specific aims early in the process—prior to writing a full proposal. If your department does not currently offer such a forum, suggest that they start one.

Example description of a Chalk-talk forum:

Chalk-talk forums will bring the department faculty together on a monthly basis to discuss research proposals generated by early-career faculty. Each session provides the opportunity for two early-career faculty in different divisions to present their proposed research. To maximize the utility of the session, the early-career faculty will submit a "press release" one week prior to the chalk-talk forum outlining their specific aims and corresponding public health significance. Mentors will be encouraged to assist their faculty mentee in crafting their press release.

18.2.6 External Review: Mock NIH Study Sections

Probably the most useful, albeit the most time-intensive, way to get constructive feedback on your grant proposal is to participate in a *mock NIH study section*. Mock study sections simulate real NIH review panels (termed *study sections*) by following the NIH grant proposal review process as closely as possible. It is generally acknowledged that a local *mock study section* review almost doubles your chances of funding. It provides the faculty member with substantive feedback enabling them to identify the key strengths and weaknesses of their proposal prior to formal submission. If your department or college does not currently provide such a review panel, encourage them to start one.

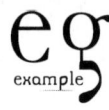

> **Example procedures for conducting a mock study section:**
>
> Early-career faculty will submit a proposal for review using the NIH submission guidelines. The review panel will be made up of senior faculty who have served on NIH study sections, are familiar with the area of study, and have a track record of mentorship. Each proposal will be reviewed by three section members. Faculty will receive the written reviews of their proposals and the NIH scoring system will be applied (1–9).

To provide even greater mentorship, a mock NIH study section can be modified in two key ways from a true NIH study section. For example, early-career investigators can be invited to **attend the session** and participate as silent observers. While it may be stressful to watch the reviewers discuss your proposal, you will gain firsthand experience of the dynamics of study section deliberations—and the proposal review process begins to become demystified. You will learn to look at proposals through the eyes of a reviewer. This is one of the most valuable ways to learn how to write fundable grants.

A second modification to a true NIH study section is to have a short **debriefing period** after the session, which allows the early-career faculty to ask questions and talk directly with their reviewers. This differs substantively from a true study section in which you will only receive written comments from the reviewers.

NIH posts videos of mock study sections on their website. These are invaluable to watch.

18.3 PART II: STRATEGIC TIPS FOR EACH COMPONENT OF THE GRANT SUBMISSION

The following table highlights the **key required components** for most NIH submissions (Table 18.1). This section follows with a description of each of these components along with strategies for completion.

The NIH grant application instructions are described in great detail in a document titled "SF424 (R&R) Application Guide for NIH and Other PHS Agencies" found on the NIH website. Be sure to check the NIH Guide for Grants and Contracts (http://grants1.nih.gov/grants/guide/index.html) to see if there have been changes in policy recently that may affect how you write the application. For example, an abstract that exceeds the allowable length can be flagged as an error upon submission and require a corrective action before the application will be accepted.

Note that this table is divided into three sections. Section I includes the **scientific component** of the submission. In an ideal world, this would be the only section that you,

TABLE 18.1 Components for NIH grant submissions

I. Scientific component
   a. Title
   b. Project summary (i.e., abstract) (30 lines of text)
   c. Specific aims (1 page)
   d. Project narrative (2–3 sentences on relevance to public health)
   e. Research strategy (6–12 pages depending on type of grant)
   f. Training information for fellowships (F series)
   g. Candidate information for career development awards (K series)
   h. Bibliography and references cited
   i. Human subjects protection component; responsible conduct of research
   j. Inclusion of women, minorities, and children; targeted/planned enrollment
II. Nonscientific forms
   a. Cover letter
   b. Facilities and other resources
   c. Equipment
   d. Biosketch (4 pages)
   e. Budget and budget justification
   f. Resource sharing plan
   g. Appendices
   h. Other forms (e.g., face page, select agents)
III. Items needed from coinvestigators
   a. Letters of support
   b. Biosketches for all key personnel (4 pages per person)
   c. For off-site coinvestigators: consortium/contractual arrangements, scope of work, facilities, budget, biosketches, and letters of support

as the PI, need to complete. Section II includes the **nonscientific forms**. Even if you do have a grants manager to handle these forms, it is best that you look them over for consistency with the scientific component. Finally, section III includes the forms that you will need from your collaborators. Again, you will want to review these forms for consistency with the remainder of the application.

18.3.1 Section I: Scientific Component

18.3.1.1 I.a. Title

The NIH guidelines ask for a short descriptive title limited to 81 characters, including the spaces between words and punctuation. Titles in excess of 81 characters are truncated. Only use standard characters in the title—letters and numbers and underscores (_) are all allowable.

Chapter 15, *Abstracts and Titles*, provides detailed strategies for creating your title, which are consistent with these NIH guidelines. Several key tips from that chapter are highlighted below.

Your title will help to direct your proposal to the correct review panel

Be accurate and use agency-friendly keywords to help officials direct your proposal to the appropriate study section. For grant proposals in epidemiology and preventive medicine, using the term *epidemiology of* in the title will help the application go to an epidemiology review panel. Including study design terms that are characteristic of grants in epidemiology or preventive medicine will also be helpful, such as *A Case–Control Study of...* or *A Prospective Study of...* Mention your disease outcome of interest in your title as well.

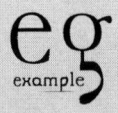

> **Original Version**
> "Stress and Gestational Diabetes"
> **First Improved Version**
> "The Epidemiology of Stress and Gestational Diabetes"
> **Second Improved Version**
> "A Prospective Study of Stress and Gestational Diabetes"

18.3.1.2 I.b. Project summary (abstract)

NIH guidelines require that the proposal abstract, termed *project summary*, be no longer than 30 lines of text and follow the required font and margin specifications.

Use an Arial, Helvetica, Palatino Linotype, or Georgia typeface, a black font color, and a font size of 11 points or larger. Type density, including characters and spaces, must be no more than 15 characters per inch. Type may be no more than six lines per inch.

The **project summary** is meant to serve as a self-contained succinct and accurate description of the proposed work when separated from the application. It should be informative to others working in the same or related fields and insofar as possible understandable to a scientifically or technically literate lay reader.

Briefly, the project summary should contain

- Overall goal
- Specific aims
- Research design and methods for achieving the stated aims
- The health relatedness of the project (i.e., relevance to the mission of the NIH institute sponsoring your funding mechanism)

Chapter 15, *Abstracts and Titles*, provides detailed strategies for creating your abstract, which are consistent with these NIH project summary guidelines.

18.3.1.3 I.c. Specific aims

The NIH guidelines limit the specific aims to one page. This page should state concisely the goals of the proposed research and summarize the expected outcome(s), including the impact that the results of the proposed research will exert on the research field(s) involved.

Chapter 6, *Specific Aims*, provides detailed strategies for creating your specific aims page, which are consistent with these NIH guidelines.

For grant proposals in epidemiology and preventive medicine, it is expected that specific aims be **hypotheses-driven**. In other words, each specific aim should be accompanied by corresponding hypotheses.

It is also helpful to search the NIH Reporter (http://projectreporter.nih.gov/reporter.cfm) for abstracts of both active and prior funded NIH awards in your field.

18.3.1.4 I.d. Project narrative

The NIH guidelines require that you write a project narrative that consists of two to three sentences on the *relevance* of your proposed project to public health. In this section, it is important to be succinct and use plain language that can be understood by a general lay audience.

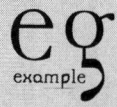

> **e.g. example**
>
> **Project narrative for a proposal to conduct a randomized lifestyle intervention in Hispanic women:**
>
> Hispanic women are the fastest-growing minority group in the United States and are more likely to begin their pregnancies overweight or obese as compared to non-Hispanic white women. This randomized controlled trial of a culturally and linguistically modified, individually tailored lifestyle intervention in Hispanic women aims to reduce excessive gestational weight gain, postpartum weight retention, and subsequent obesity using a high-reach, low-cost strategy, which has great potential for adoption on a larger scale and reducing health disparities in the United States.

18.3.1.5 I.e. Research strategy

The NIH guidelines require that the research strategy be 6 pages or 12 pages depending on the funding mechanism. For example, the research strategy for an R21 or R03 application is limited to 6 pages and for an R01 is limited to 12 pages.

The research strategy should explain the (i) significance, (ii) innovation, and (iii) approach as defined below:

(i) *Significance (see Chapter 7, Background and Significance Section)*
   – Explain the importance of the problem or critical barrier to progress in the field that the proposed project addresses.

- Explain how the proposed project will improve scientific knowledge, technical capability, and/or clinical practice in one or more broad fields.
- Describe how the concepts, methods, technologies, treatments, services, or preventative interventions that drive this field will be changed if the proposed aims are achieved.

(ii) *Innovation (see Chapter 7, Background and Significance Section)*
- Explain how the application challenges and seeks to shift current research or clinical practice paradigms.
- Describe any novel theoretical concepts, approaches or methodologies, instrumentation, or interventions to be developed or used and any advantage over existing methodologies, instrumentation, or interventions.
- Explain any refinements, improvements, or new applications of theoretical concepts, approaches or methodologies, instrumentation, or interventions.

(iii) *Approach (see Chapters 8 through 13)*
- Describe the overall strategy, methodology, and analyses to be used to accomplish the specific aims of the project. Include how the data will be collected, analyzed, and interpreted.
- Discuss potential problems, alternative strategies, and benchmarks for success anticipated to achieve the aims.
- Preliminary Studies (see Chapter 8): Preliminary studies, data, and/or experience pertinent to this application, if required by the funding mechanism, should be included in the research strategy.

Tips for the research strategy section

Tip #1: Include preliminary studies in the approach section Even though R21s and R03s do not require preliminary studies, if you **or your research team** have conducted relevant preliminary studies, definitely include them! It is common to forget that your coinvestigators are part of your research team—as such, their preliminary studies should be included as relevant. Using the terms *our lab has found that…* will strengthen the confidence of the reviewers in the ability of your team (not just you) to pull off the study.

Tip #2: Demonstrate established relationships with your coinvestigators in the preliminary studies section Insert a brief section at the beginning of the preliminary studies section reminding your reviewers of the expertise of your research team in all aspects of the proposal.

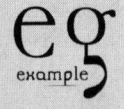

> *example:* Substantial preliminary work demonstrates the experience of the research team in all aspects of the proposed study: physical activity measurement (Drs. Jones, Thompson, and Levine), physical activity interventions (Drs. McGovern and Smith), racial/ethnic issues surrounding physical activity (Drs. Jones and Smith), gestational diabetes (Drs. Branson and Smith), obstetrics (Dr. Goldman), and statistical analysis of physical activity data (Dr. Francis).

Tip #3: Strive for consistency in tone and content It is common for particular sections of the research strategy (e.g., the data analysis section) to be written by one of your coinvestigators—such as a statistician. Read over and edit this section so that the writing style and content is consistent with the rest of the research strategy. Avoid the pitfall of simply cutting and pasting sections written by coinvestigators into your research strategy without checking for errors.

Tip #4: How to deal with the strict page limitations Chapter 5, *Scientific Writing*, provides detailed strategies for scientific writing style, which will help you comply with these strict NIH page limitations. Several key tips from that chapter are highlighted below:

- Use active voice.
- Use figures and tables.
- Be sure that every word is necessary.
- Proofread!

Remember that it takes longer to write a shorter research application. Only by reading and rereading your application will you have adequate time to make sure that every word counts.

Pitfalls to avoid In an attempt to save space, some investigators resort to the heavy use of **abbreviations**. These can become distracting for the reviewer. Try to use only those abbreviations that are well accepted in your field (e.g., PCR is commonly accepted for the polymerase chain reaction). Creating your own abbreviations should be avoided. Another space-saving approach to avoid is to circumvent the **strict formatting requirements** (e.g., font size, margin size, and line spacing details). These requirements are designed to ensure equity across applicants in terms of proposal length. They are also designed to make the review easier on the reviewers—such that the proposal is readable and not densely packed. It is critical to follow these guidelines to the letter as failure to comply can be rationale for the grant not to be reviewed. A final pitfall to avoid is to place some **research methods** in the **Appendix** or in the **Protection of Human Subjects sections**. Remember that NIH reviewers are not required to read the Appendix. If reviewers sense that you are trying to circumvent the page length guidelines with these strategies, this can lead to an unhappy reviewer and a low score.

18.3.1.6 I.f. Training information for doctoral and postdoctoral fellowships (F series)

The NIH guidelines for fellowships (F series) Ruth L. Kirschstein NRSA can be found in a separate guide: the *SF424 (R & R) Individual Fellowship Application Guide*.

Before applying for a fellowship, be sure to carefully *review the NIH FOA* for your F series grant of interest—noting especially the eligibility requirements, requirements for a mentor, review criteria, and any special application instructions. These factors may all vary according to the specific NIH institute that is sponsoring your selected F award and may change over time.

The NIH F Kiosk website (http://grants1.nih.gov/training/F_files_nrsa.htm) is an excellent source for the most recent funding announcements for fellowship funding opportunities as well as the relevant NIH personnel to contact with questions. It is best to contact this person well in advance of the submission deadline to confirm all these items.

The fellowship application requires a proposed **research and training plan** that will be conducted under the supervision of a **mentor (sponsor)**. The sponsor is expected to have a successful track record of mentoring and provide an assessment of the applicant's qualifications and potential for a research career. As noted in Chapter 17, *Choosing the Right Funding Source*, you can identify more than one mentor (i.e., a mentoring team) to ensure that you receive expert advice in all aspects of the research and training program. In such cases, one individual must be identified as the principal sponsor who will coordinate your research training program. Your sponsor should have a key role in helping you to prepare the application.

The fellowship applications are, in general, similar to a regular research awards (R series), with the addition of the sections noted below. Note that a portion of the application is completed solely by your sponsor. The forms below cannot exceed 25 pages in total:

- Sponsor and cosponsor information (6 pages)
  - Research support available
  - Sponsor's/cosponsor's previous fellows/trainees
  - Training plan, environment, research facilities
  - Number of fellows/trainees to be supervised during the fellowship
  - Applicant's qualifications and potential for a research career
- Research training plan
  - Specific aims (1 page)
  - Research strategy (6 pages)—following same guidelines as R series
- Respective contributions (1 page)
  - A description of the collaborative process between you and your sponsor in the development, review, and editing of the research training plan
- Selection of sponsor and institution (1 page)
  - An explanation for why the sponsor and institution were selected to accomplish the research training goals
- Goals for fellowship training and career (1 page)
- Activities planned under this award (1 page)
- Doctoral dissertation and research experience (2 pages)
- Letters of reference

The abstract (project summary) for a fellowship award, in addition to describing the proposed research, should describe the research training program design and methods for achieving the stated career goals.

Tips for fellowship awards

Tip #1: The **ideal fellowship application** is submitted by a candidate with high career potential and includes a research plan that is well balanced between originality and feasibility. Remember that the F programs are training awards and not research awards.

Major considerations in the review are your potential for a productive career, your need for the proposed training, and the degree to which the research training proposal, the sponsor, and the environment will satisfy those needs.

Tip #2: Therefore, it is essential that the fellowship application *be internally consistent and well coordinated*. For example, the research strategy should be **well suited to the stage** of your career development. In addition, the sponsor's description of your research training plan should be coordinated with your research strategy. Training in career skills, grant writing, and presentation skills are also looked upon as strengths of a fellowship application.

Tip #3: Choice of sponsor (mentor): As with all mentored grants, the sponsor(s) should have a successful track record of mentoring. Highly overcommitted mentors (e.g., with too many mentees) or off-site mentors may raise a red flag for reviewers. The mentors should demonstrate that their prior mentees have been successful through a table of prior mentees including their current positions and grant funding. For grants in epidemiology and preventive medicine, reviewers may also look for a statistical mentor on the team.

Tip #4: As with other funding mechanisms, it is particularly helpful to view examples of successfully funded fellowship applications by your colleagues. Searching on **NIH Reporter** for the abstracts of funded fellowship applications can give you a good sense of their depth and scope.

18.3.1.7 I.g. Candidate information for career development awards (K series)

The NIH guidelines for career development awards (K series) Ruth L. Kirschstein NRSA can be found in the supplemental instructions to the SF424 (R & R).

Before applying for a K award, be sure to carefully *review the NIH FOA* for your K award of interest—noting especially the eligibility requirements, requirements for a mentor, review criteria, and any special application instructions. These factors may all vary according to the specific NIH institute that is sponsoring your selected K award and may change over time.

The NIH K Kiosk website (http://grants.nih.gov/training/careerdevelopmentawards.htm) is an excellent source for the most recent funding announcements for career awards as well as the relevant NIH personnel to contact with questions. It is best to contact this person well in advance of the submission deadline to confirm all these items.

The NIH guidelines for career development awards (K series) are similar to regular research awards (R series). However, in addition to a research plan, the application also requires a **career development training plan** that will be conducted under the supervision of a **mentor (sponsor)**. As with other mentored awards, the mentors should be recognized as accomplished investigators in the proposed research area and have a track record of success in training and placing independent investigators. The sponsor is also expected to provide an assessment of your qualifications and potential for a research career and a plan for mentoring and monitoring your research, publications, and progression toward independence.

In addition, the proposals also require a description of the candidate's background, career goals, and objectives:

- Candidate information
  - Candidate's background
  - Career goals and objectives
  - Career development/training activities during award period
- Statement of support (mentors)
- Environment and institutional commitment to the candidate
- Letters of reference
- The research plan

In total, including the research plan, all of these components are limited to 12 pages.

Tips for career awards

Tip #1: The research plan for career awards: Follow the same guidelines covered above in the *research strategy* section for R series applications (and outlined in detail in Chapters 8 through 13). For career awards, however, it is important to *relate the research to your scientific career goals*. Describe how the research, coupled with the other planned career development activities, will provide the experience necessary to launch and conduct your **independent research career**. It is also important to explain the relationship between your proposed research and your mentor's ongoing research program.

Tip #2: The research plan is a major component of the career award application; however, note that it needs to fit, along with all the candidate information, within the 12-page limit. Therefore, it is understood that research plans for career award applications do not require the extensive detail usually incorporated into regular research applications. However, the plan still needs to be fundamentally sound. In addition, although candidates for mentored K awards are expected to write the research plan, it is expected that the mentor will play a major role in reviewing and shaping the draft. In fact, upon finding errors/inconsistencies in research plans for K awards, NIH review panels tend to hold the mentor responsible and become concerned about the quality of your proposed mentorship.

Tip #3: Choice of sponsor (mentor): As with all mentored grants, the sponsor(s) should have a successful track record of mentoring. Highly overcommitted mentors (e.g., with too many mentees) or off-site mentors may raise a red flag for reviewers. The mentors should demonstrate that their prior mentees have been successful through a table of prior mentees including their current positions and grant funding. For grants in epidemiology and preventive medicine, reviewers may also look for a statistical mentor on the team.

Tip #4: Accessing the *NIH Reporter* online to view the abstracts of successfully funded career awards will help you get a sense of the ideal scope of the research plan for a career award. You will want to ensure that your research plan is not overly ambitious and that it is achievable within the requested time period. On the other hand, proposals for routine collection of data or for small pilot studies are not usually considered sufficient as the sole component of the research plan for a career award. Your mentor should be able to help you with this.

Tip #5: Note that your mentor/co-mentor(s) statement of support cannot be counted toward the *three required letters of reference*. The reference letters are critically important and should address your competence and potential to develop into an independent investigator.

18.3.1.8 I.h. Bibliography and references cited

The NIH guidelines require a bibliography of all references cited in the research plan component. Any standard scholarly format for citations is acceptable, but the references should be limited to relevant and current literature. While there is not a page limitation for the bibliography, it is important to be concise and to select only those references pertinent to the proposed research.

When you are citing articles that fall under the public access policy, were authored or coauthored by yourself, and arose from NIH support, provide *the NIH Manuscript Submission reference number* (e.g., NIHMS97531) or the *PubMed Central (PMC) reference number* (e.g., PMCID234567) for each article. If the PMCID is not yet available because the journal submits articles directly to PMC on behalf of their authors, indicate *PMC Journal—In Process*. A list of these journals is posted at http://publicaccess.nih.gov/submit_process_journals.htm.

Citations that are not covered by the public access policy but are publicly available in a free online format may include URLs or PubMed ID (PMID) numbers along with the full reference (note that copies of publicly available publications are not accepted as Appendix material).

18.3.1.9 I.i. Human subjects protection/ responsible conduct of research

For research that involves human subjects and is not considered *exempt* (described below), you will need to write a justification for the involvement of human subjects and your proposed protections from research risk according to the following five criteria:

1. Risk to subjects
2. Adequacy of protection against risks
3. Potential benefits to the subjects and others
4. Importance of the knowledge to be gained
5. Data and safety monitoring for clinical trials

Exempt research involves human subjects but meets one or more of six criteria for exempt status listed in the NIH guidelines. For such research, you will need to write (1) the justification for the exemption, (2) human subjects' involvement and characteristics, and (3) sources of materials. One example of an *exempt* criterion met by proposals in epidemiology and preventive medicine is:

Research involving the collection or study of existing data, documents, records, pathological specimens, or diagnostic specimens, if these sources are publicly available or if the information is recorded by the investigator in such a manner that subjects cannot be identified, directly or through identifiers linked to the subjects.

For example, a proposal involving the use of a secondary dataset that is deidentified may qualify. However, it is always wise to contact relevant NIH personnel first and, when in doubt, to include the complete section on protection of human subjects.

A potential pitfall to avoid Simply noting that you already have Institutional Review Board (IRB) approval from your own institution for the proposed project is not sufficient for this section. Reviewers consider carefully issues in conducting research on humans in their overall *score* of your application.

Instruction in the Responsible Conduct of Research
A description of the plan for instruction in the responsible conduct of research is required for all mentored/training grant applications (T series, F series, and K series).

18.3.1.10 I.j. Inclusion of women, minorities, and children; Targeted/planned enrollment

When the proposed project involves clinical research, it must include plans for the inclusion of minorities and members of both genders, as well as the inclusion of children. This does not mean that your proposal must include such groups but that there needs to be a scientific rationale for their lack of inclusion. This can be straightforward. For example, a proposal to evaluate risk of Alzheimer's disease would likely not include children as they are not at risk for this disease.

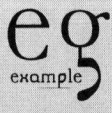

> *eg example* Imagine a proposal to conduct a lifestyle intervention in high-risk pregnant Hispanic women to prevent postpartum weight retention and risk of diabetes.
>
> **Inclusion of Women and Minorities**
> The population under study includes 300 pregnant and postpartum women between the ages 18 and 45 years at Taylor Hospital. The study is designed to test a lifestyle intervention to control gestational weight gain and positively influence maternal metabolic profile; therefore, all subjects are women.
>
> All women are Hispanic. Hispanic women are the fastest-growing minority group in the United States and have the highest rates of sedentary behavior as well as elevated rates of prepregnancy overweight and obesity. Hispanics have, overall, been underrepresented in prior research.
>
> **Inclusion of Children**
> Mothers between the ages of 18 and 21 will be included. Mothers younger than 18 will not be included as modifiable determinants of gestational weight gain may differ substantively among pregnant women under age 18 therefore precluding direct applicability of hypotheses to this age group. Their offspring from birth to age 1 will also be included.

If you answer "yes" to the question "Are human subjects involved?" on the R & R Other Project Information form and the research does not fall under an exemption, you will need to complete the targeted/planned enrollment table (found in an NIH guidelines) for each protocol.

18.3.2 Section II: Nonscientific Forms

18.3.2.1 II.a. Cover letter

I strongly recommend that you request in a cover letter, which accompanies your application, the assignment of your application to a specific NIH study section (i.e., review panel) and NIH institute. You may request a secondary institute as well.

NIH receives thousands of applications per cycle. A cover letter accompanying your application will assist NIH staff in correctly assigning your grant application. This cover letter can be uploaded electronically with the rest of the grant application.

The NIH website includes a description of each study section, their overall goals/objectives, and a list of the types of applications that they review. Quote key points from this description in your cover letter to support your request. A similar approach should be used when specifying the institute. The NIH Reporter can also be useful in identifying a study section. Search on grants with similar topics and funding mechanisms, and the search output, in addition to listing the abstract, will also provide the name of the review panel and the NIH institute.

One caveat in terms of requesting an institute is if your application is in response to a PA or RFP. In this case, the institute sponsoring these funding mechanisms will be prespecified. However, if multiple institutes are listed, you may still specify which institute is your primary choice.

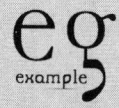

> **Example Cover Letter**
> Center for Scientific Review
> National Institutes of Health
> Suite 1040
> 6701 Rockledge Drive MSC 7710
> Bethesda, MD
>
> Dear People:
> The attached application entitled "Randomized Lifestyle Intervention in Overweight and Obese Pregnant Hispanic Women" would be most suitable for review by the **Health Disparities and Equity Promotion (HDEP) Study Section** for the following reasons:
>
>> The primary aim of HDEP is to address, reduce, or eliminate health disparities and improve equitable conditions related to health risks faced by minorities and/or ethnic groups, poor, urban, low literacy, and immigrant populations.

> The appropriate institutes are in order of relevance:
>
> 1. **NIDDK Division of Diabetes, Endocrinology, and Metabolic Diseases** as the primary focus of the proposal is on diabetes mellitus as well as physical activity and nutrition
> 2. **NINR** as the proposal promotes healthy lifestyles among at-risk and underserved populations, with an emphasis on health disparities
>
> Thank you for your consideration.

Note that requested assignments are not guaranteed. However, if your application was inadvertently assigned to what you feel is an inappropriate review panel or institute, contact the scientific research administrator (SRA) assigned to the application to clarify the fit of your application and to request reassignment if appropriate.

18.3.2.2 II.b. Facilities and other resources

Describe the facilities to be used (e.g., laboratory, animal, computer, office, clinical). Indicate their capacities, relative proximity, and extent of availability to the project. Describe only those resources that are directly applicable to your proposed project.

It is important to describe how the scientific environment in which the research will be done contributes to the probability of success. Discuss ways in which the proposed studies will benefit from unique features of the scientific environment or subject populations or will employ useful collaborative arrangements.

If you are an early stage investigator, also describe the institutional investment in your success (e.g., resources for classes, travel, training; collegial support such as career enrichment programs, assistance, and guidance in the supervision of trainees; availability of organized peer groups; logistical support such as administrative management and oversight and best practices training; and financial support such as protected time for research with salary support).

If there are multiple performance sites, describe the resources available at each site. Read over all the facilities statements (e.g., those sent to you by any off-site coinvestigators) and be sure that the writing style is consistent.

18.3.2.3 II.c. Equipment

List the major items of equipment already available for your project and, if appropriate, identify location and pertinent capabilities.

18.3.2.4 II.d. Biosketch

The NIH provides a template for your biosketch; you will need to complete sections A, B, C, and D as described below. Note that the biosketch cannot exceed 4 pages.

  A. *Personal statement*: Approximately 1 paragraph regarding why your experience and qualifications make you particularly well suited for your role in the project.
  B. *Positions and honors*: List in chronological order previous positions, concluding with your present position. List any honors. Include present membership on any federal government public advisory committee.
  C. *Selected peer-reviewed publications*: NIH limits the list of selected peer-reviewed publications or manuscripts in press to no more than 15. Do not include manuscripts submitted or in preparation. It is best to choose those publications that are most relevant to the topic of the proposed research to demonstrate your expertise, or growing expertise, in the proposed area. The reviewers will be looking for the connection between your publications and your topic.
  D. *Research support*: List both ongoing and completed (during the last three years) research projects (federal or nonfederal support). Begin with the projects that are most relevant to the research proposed. Briefly indicate the overall goals of the projects and your responsibilities on the project.

Demonstrate relationships with your coinvestigators in the biosketch

The biosketch can be used to demonstrate your established/ongoing relationships with your coinvestigators, a critical factor in the review. First, in the **personal statement** (Section A), describe your ongoing relationships with your coinvestigators. Second, include **publications** (Section C), if available, that include your coinvestigators as coauthors. Lastly, be sure to highlight any **research support** (Section D) that also includes your coinvestigators.

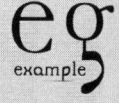

> **Example Personal Statement (Section A) on an NIH Biosketch**
>
> I am an assistant professor of epidemiology in the Division of Epidemiology at the Jones School of Public Health. I am a reproductive epidemiologist with a focus on physical activity during pregnancy. The proposed project will build upon a history of collaboration among our investigative team in conducting culturally modified, motivationally targeted, individually tailored interventions among Hispanic women. I led the development and evaluation of the feasibility of the proposed lifestyle intervention in collaboration with Dr. Branson and Dr. Smith (coinvestigators on the proposed study) in our pilot study, "Estudio Vida" (ASPH/CDC Sxxx). My research experience has lent me an appreciation of both the importance and difficulties associated with study design, measurement, quality data management, and analyses that will be instrumental in conducting the proposed study.

A potential pitfall to avoid Coinvestigators may send you versions of their biosketches from other grant applications. Therefore, check over their *personal statement* and make sure that their role is consistent with (1) the role that you delineated in the methods section, and (2) the budget justification section, where you also delineated each coinvestigators' role. Carefully review their selected list of 15 publications. Cross-check this against a complete list of their publications (e.g., using PubMed or a complete version of their CV if available) and check that they included those publications that most directly relate to your study aims, on which you are a coauthor, and/or those that demonstrate the seniority of the coinvestigator (e.g., on which the coinvestigator is the first or senior author, or those in top-ranked journals). For example, it would almost never make sense to leave out a *New England Journal of Medicine* paper.

18.3.2.5 II.e. Budget and budget justification

Engage the assistance of a grants manager or your office of grants and contracts to assist you with the budget and the budget justification section—a narrative in which you justify all your proposed costs, including personnel costs. Start this process early so that you can sketch out a draft budget.

Before such a meeting, be sure to calculate your power and sample size so that you have an approximate sense of the number of participants or samples that you will be analyzing. Think about the broad cost areas that you will include in the budget. Typical cost areas for grants in epidemiology and preventive medicine include

- Personnel
    - Professional (e.g., yourself and your coinvestigators)
    - Staff (e.g., research assistants, health interviewers, health educators, laboratory personnel, data analysts)
    - Consultants
- Materials and supplies (e.g., computer supplies, objective monitors)
- Other direct costs (e.g., computer lab charges, laboratory assays, travel, express mail, participant incentives)

For early small research grants (e.g., R21s and R03s), **modular budget guidelines** will be applicable. Modular budgets are for research grant applications requesting $250,000 or less per year in direct costs. These budgets are simplified and do not require detailed categorical information. However, one caveat is that your institution may still require you to submit a detailed internal budget.

Tips for the budget justification

Tip #1: Demonstrate established relationships with your coinvestigators in the budget section. The budget justification section is an excellent place to describe the means by which you will communicate with your coinvestigators. Recall that your coinvestigators do not have to be at your institution as long as you have a clear plan for communication.

Any long-distance relationship can be further bolstered by indicating that it has worked successfully in the past.

> **Example Personnel Section of a Budget Justification demonstrating established relationships:**
>
> Dr. Jones Ph.D., **PI** (2.70 academic months and 0.90 summer months, years 1–5) assistant professor of epidemiology in the Division of Epidemiology at the School of Public Health. Dr. Jones will be responsible for the scientific conduct of the study and oversee all aspects of the project. These will include patient recruitment and follow-up, patient interviews, patient interventions, laboratory analysis, medical record review, data analysis and interpretation, and manuscript preparation. As in our pilot study, Dr. Jones will oversee quality control procedures ensuring that stage of change and social cognitive constructs are consistently represented in both the physical activity and dietary interventions. Dr. Jones will meet face to face with (1) the project manager weekly, (2) the statistician monthly, (3) the coinvestigators at the recruitment sites monthly (Dr. Branson, Dr. Jones, and Dr. Smith), and (4) the intervention team via teleconference monthly (Dr. Smith, Dr. Francis, and Dr. Goldman). All the coinvestigators and consultants will meet quarterly via telephone conference call as well as yearly in a face-to-face meeting.
>
> Dr. Branson, Ph.D., **coinvestigator** (0.45 academic months and 0.15 summer months in years 1–5) is an associate professor of kinesiology at the School of Public Health whose research focuses on understanding how exercise, diet, and/or pharmacological agents interact to mediate insulin resistance and the risk for type 2 diabetes. Dr. Branson will provide expertise in the assessment and interpretation of the biomarker measures. He will participate, along with the other study investigators, in discussions of study design and in conducting analyses and disseminating study findings.

Tip #2: Ensure consistency between the budget justification section and the remainder of the proposal. Care should be taken that your budget justification section is consistent with your methods section. Inconsistencies can be viewed as a serious flaw in an application.

Tip #3: Check for consistency in the delineated roles of your coinvestigators between the research methods section, the biosketch personal statements, the budget justification, and the letters of collaboration. Any tasks mentioned in the facilities section (in relation to how the facilities are conducive to accomplishing the tasks of the grant) should also be cross-checked against these other forms.

18.3.2.6 II.f. Resource sharing plan

NIH considers the sharing of unique research resources developed through NIH-sponsored research an important means to further the advancement of research. These include plans for (1) data sharing, (2) sharing model organisms and (3) genome wide association studies. The data sharing plan is unlikely to be relevant to early-career faculty or postdoctoral fellows as it is typically only required of very large projects. Specifically, investigators seeking $500,000 or more in direct costs in any year are expected to include a brief 1-paragraph description of how final research data will be shared or explain why data sharing is not possible.

On the other hand, note that some specific FOAs may require that all applications include this information regardless of the dollar level. Therefore, it is important to read the specific FOA carefully.

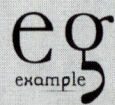

> **Example Resource Sharing Plan**
>
> Research resources generated with funds from this grant will be freely distributed, as available, to qualified academic investigators for noncommercial research. Our institution will adhere to the NIH Grants Policy on Sharing of Unique Research Resources including the "Sharing of Biomedical Research Resources: Principles and Guidelines for Recipients of NIH Grants and Contracts." Should any intellectual property arise that requires a patent, we would ensure that the technology remains widely available to the research community in accordance with the NIH Principles and Guidelines document.

> **Example General Data-Sharing Plan**
>
> Final data will be shared primarily through the vehicle of peer-reviewed publication. Raw data will be considered for sharing under the following rules. Raw datasets to be released for sharing will not contain identifiers. Data and associated documentation will be made available to users only under a signed and properly executed data-sharing agreement that provides for specific criteria under which the data will be used, including but not limited to (1) a commitment to using the data only for research purposes and not to identify any individual participant, (2) a commitment to securing the data using appropriate computer technology, and (3) a commitment to destroying or returning the data after analyses are completed.

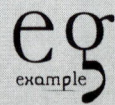

18.3.2.7 II.g. Appendices and supplemental materials

Read over the NIH guidelines for Appendix materials carefully and be sure to comply with them. A common pitfall is to try to use the Appendix as a way to circumvent the strict page limitations of the research strategy section. Reviewers are sensitive to this strategy and are not required to read appendices, although most try to do so.

Materials Allowed in the Appendix:

- Publications
    - You may submit up to three of the following types of publications. Any exceptions will be noted in specific FOAs.
        » Manuscripts and/or abstracts accepted for publication but not yet published
        » Published manuscripts and/or abstracts *only* when a free, online, publicly available journal link is not available
        » Patents directly relevant to the project
- Others
    - Surveys, questionnaires, data collection instruments, clinical protocols, and informed consent documents as necessary

18.3.2.8 II.h. Other pages

There are a number of other administrative pages required for an NIH grant submission. Try to enlist a grants manager or office of grants and contracts to assist you in their completion. For example, the first page of the grant (**cover component**) asks for such contact information for you and your university, the type of grant you are applying for, start and end dates, and other procedural information. Other pages include **Performance Sites pages** and **Other Project Information, Select Agents** (i.e., hazardous biological agents and toxins) pages. See the SF424 guide for details.

18.3.3 Section III: Items Needed from Others

18.3.3.1 III.a. Letters of support

If you have coinvestigators and consultants on your project, the grant application should contain a signed letter from each collaborator to the applicant that lists the contribution he or she intends to make and his or her enthusiasm for the work. These letters are often crucial information for the reviewers. Consultants, will also need to state their rate for consulting services.

Demonstrate established relationships with your coinvestigators in this section

As a doctoral student or early-career investigator, you will often find yourself in the position of soliciting collaborations with more senior faculty. Given their busy schedules, if they are willing to serve on your grant application, it is considered a courtesy for you to draft their letter of collaboration. They can certainly edit it as they see fit, but taking that first step of drafting the letter ensures timely receipt of this form and that the correct title and grant number (if a resubmission) will be referenced.

Recommended items to include in a letter of collaboration include:

- The title of the application
- The grant number (if a resubmission)
- The importance of the topic of the grant proposal
- The role that the investigator will be playing

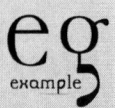

> *example*
>
> [on letterhead]
> Dear x [your name]:
> I very much look forward to building on our previous work in connection with your proposed study, "Study Title." This proposal builds on our previous work [can insert grant numbers and titles here] and has the potential to advance our understanding of modifiable risk factors for gestational diabetes. It will provide an invaluable opportunity to comprehensively assess the frequency, intensity, and duration of physical activity during pregnancy: the first step toward critically examining the relationship between activity during pregnancy and gestational diabetes.
> As we have discussed, I will be responsible, along with the other study investigators, for the analysis and dissemination of findings related to physical activity as well as weight gain and body fat distribution. I very much look forward to working with you on this important research.
> Sincerely,
> Dr. Smith
> Coinvestigator

18.3.3.2 III.b. Biosketches

Described in the relevant section above.

18.3.3.3 III.c. Consortium/contractual arrangements

If some of your coinvestigators are **off-site** at other institutions, your institution's office of grants and contracts will communicate with theirs to complete the required forms. Such forms include:

- Consortium/contractual arrangements
- Scope of work
- Subcontractor budget and budget justification
- Facilities

Work with your coinvestigators to draft the scope of work and budget justification pages.

18.4 PART III: TIMELINE FOR SUBMISSION OF AN NIH GRANT

Creating a timeline for the grant submission process is an excellent tool. Table 18.2 includes a suggested timeline for the submission of an NIH grant that can be modified depending on the requirements of your granting agency or the type of grant.

I highly recommend requesting any items needed from your coinvestigators or mentors early in the process. Unlike the rest of the application (e.g., the scientific component), these are the sections that you are relying primarily upon others to complete in a timely fashion. Examples of such items include mentor letters and letters of recommendation (if a training/mentored grant), coinvestigator biosketches, and letters of collaboration.

Similarly, if your coinvestigators are located at other institutions, you will need their consortium/contractual arrangements, scope of work, facilities, and budget signed off by their institution's office of grants and contracts. Given that you need all these materials in hand before submitting the grant to your own grants and contracts office for review, it is key to start the subcontract process early. Remember to factor in time for your own review of these external forms.

Anticipate being rejected In your timeline, anticipate having your first submission rejected. Even the most famous scientists have had their grant proposals rejected. Reviewers like to make their mark on your application. By having you revise and resubmit, they can see how responsive you are to their concerns and suggestions. Therefore, Chapter 20 focuses on *Resubmission of the Grant Proposal*.

TABLE 18.2 Timeline for submission of an NIH grant application

4 Months to submission deadline
  Identify the funding agency (see Chapter 17)
  Confirm eligibility and requirements with funding agency program officer
  Write specific aims (see Chapter 6)
  Calculate power (see Chapter 11)
  Meet with grants manager to draft budget and review timeline and responsibilities
  Send specific aims/power to coinvestigators/mentor to get feedback

3 Months to submission deadline
  Request relevant forms from coinvestigators
  Initiate any internal processing forms
  Complete research strategy (see Chapters 7 through 13)
  Write project summary/abstract (see Chapter 15)

2 Months to submission deadline
  Seek internal and external review of research strategy
  Meet with grants manager to finalize budget and budget justification
  Work on remainder of scientific forms (see Table 18.1, section I)
  Work on nonscientific forms (see Table 18.1, section II)
  Work on bibliography
  Write project narrative
  Update your biosketch
  Send final draft to coinvestigators

1 Month to submission deadline
  Incorporate comments from coinvestigators and internal/external reviewers
  Review all nonscientific forms submitted by coinvestigators
  Meet with grants manager to incorporate any final changes to budget
  Final update to biosketch (include any last-minute publications)

1 Week to submission deadline
  Submit application to office of grants and contracts
  Office of grants and contracts submits the grant to NIH

After submission
  Start collecting pilot data in anticipation of a rejection
  Resubmission (see Chapter 20)

Review Process   19

Now that you have passed the hurdle of submitting your grant proposal, this chapter moves on to describe the grant review process. Part I describes the review criteria for research, career, and fellowship awards; the review panel; ways to maximize your chances for a successful review; and potential reasons for rejection. Part II provides tips for how to proceed after the review including how to interpret your summary statement as well as issues that influence the potential funding of your award. Given today's economic challenges and the corresponding low NIH paylines, it is important to anticipate that your first submission will not be funded. Therefore, Chapter 20 follows up with *Resubmission of the Grant Proposal*.

19.1 PART I: REVIEW PROCESS

19.1.1 Scientific Review Group (*Study Section*)

After you (the *applicant*) complete your grant proposal according to the grant application instructions, your institution's office of grants and contracts submits the application to NIH (Figure 19.1). You will then be able to log onto the NIH website (Electronic Research Administration (**eRA**) **Commons** [https://commons.era.nih.gov/]) and see that it has been assigned to both of the following:

1. A Scientific Review Officer (SRO) of a specific Scientific Review Group (*study section*) at the Center for Scientific Review (CSR)
2. A program official(s) at a primary NIH institute and possibly one or more secondary NIH institutes

The first stage of the review is performed by the study section. The study section evaluates the application in terms of its **scientific and technical merit only**. In fact, the use of the term *funding* at this stage is forbidden and considered a *four-letter word*!

It is important to note that the study sections are based at the CSR within the NIH Office of the Director. It is a common **misconception** to believe that your grant is first

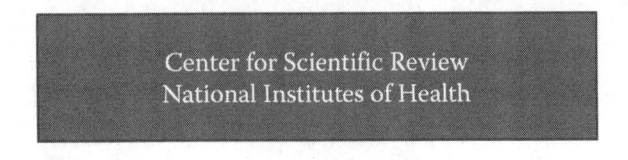

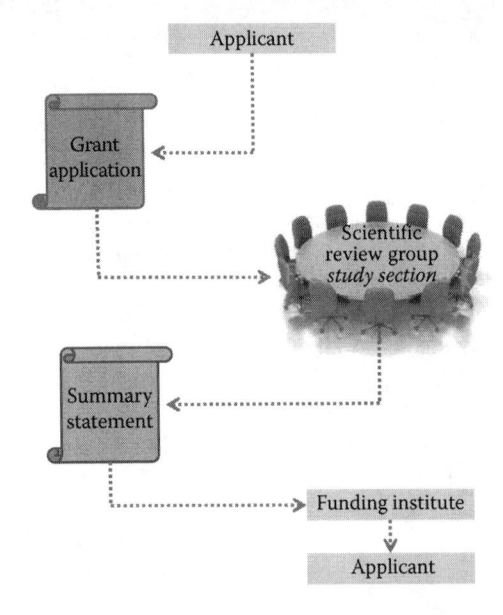

FIGURE 19.1 Where does my application go once I submit it?

reviewed by the relevant NIH institute which would ultimately award your grant if it were funded. Instead, science trumps NIH institute priorities during the **initial** stage of peer review. Indeed, a study section usually reviews applications assigned to several NIH institutes. It is not until **after** this first stage of peer view that your application makes its way to the institute (Figure 19.1).

A complete list of study sections can be found on the NIH CSR website http://www.csr.nih.gov/committees/rosterindex.asp.

The three types of study sections that are most relevant for early-career faculty are listed in Table 19.1.

19.1.2 Role of the Scientific Review Officer

Each study section is led by an SRO. The SRO is an extramural staff scientist responsible for ensuring that each application receives an objective and fair initial peer review and that all applicable laws, regulations, and policies are followed.

Once you have submitted your application, the SRO is your NIH point of contact until the study section meets. Make sure to avoid communicating directly with study

TABLE 19.1 Types of NIH scientific review groups (*study sections*)

TYPES OF STUDY SECTIONS	
Regular standing study sections	These study sections review most of the investigator-initiated research awards including R01, R03, R21, and Career Development Awards (K series) among others. They are typically made up of 20–30 members.
Fellowship study sections	These study sections review Fellowship (F series) applications including F30, F31, F32, and F33s.
Special emphasis panels	These *one-time* meetings are composed of temporary members only who are selected for their expertise regarding the applications under consideration. They are usually used to review specific RFAs.

section members about your application. Direct all questions only to the SRO in charge of the study section. Failure to observe this policy strictly will create a serious breach of confidentiality and conflict of interest in the peer review process.

SRO's Roles and Responsibilities

- Recruits qualified reviewers based on scientific and technical qualifications
- Assigns applications to specific reviewers
- Documents and manages conflicts of interest
- Ensures that proper review criteria are used during the review
- Prepares summary statements of the review, which are made available to you after the review is completed

19.1.3 Study Section Reviewers

Study section reviewers are either permanent or temporary members of their study section. They are scientists who are chosen as members due to their:

- Appropriate expertise for that review panel
- Authority in their scientific field
- Dedication to high-quality, fair, and objective reviews
- Ability to work collegially in a group setting
- Experience in research grant review

The **study section chair** is a member who also serves as a moderator of the discussion.

The names of the specific SRO, study section chair, reviewers, and their institutional affiliations and titles are all posted on the NIH CSR website (www.csr.nih.gov/).

19.1.4 How the Study Section Members Review Your Grant Application

The SRO assigns each application from two to three reviewers—a primary, secondary, and perhaps tertiary reviewer (sometimes termed *discussant*).

Prior to the study section meeting, each reviewer/discussant reads their assigned applications and completes a critique form. The critique form asks for bullet points regarding **strengths and weaknesses** as well as **preliminary scores** in each of the five specific review criteria (described later in the chapter) and in terms of the application's overall impact.

Scores are on a 9-point rating scale (1 = exceptional; 9 = poor) (Figure 19.2). These preliminary scores are used to determine which applications will be discussed by the entire panel of reviewers at the study section meeting (see Section 19.1.8).

19.1.5 Review Criteria for Research Grants (R Series)

There are five specific review criteria for Research Grants as well as consideration of the overall impact of the application (Table 19.2). Additional criteria that also influence the application's overall impact include protection of human subjects. Lastly, there are several items, such as the budget, which reviewers comment upon, but are not considered in their review of the overall impact.

19.1.5.1 Overall impact

The overall impact reflects the reviewer's assessment of the project's ability to exert a sustained, powerful influence on the research field. However, it is important to note that an application does not need to be strong in all five individual review criteria to still be

Impact	Score	Descriptor	Additional Guidance on Strengths/Weaknesses
High	1	Exceptional	Exceptionally strong with essentially no weaknesses
	2	Outstanding	Extremely strong with negligible weaknesses
	3	Excellent	Very strong with only some minor weaknesses
Medium	4	Very good	Strong but with numerous minor weaknesses
	5	Good	Strong but with at least one moderate weakness
	6	Satisfactory	Some strengths but also some moderate weaknesses
Low	7	Fair	Some strengths but with at least one major weakness
	8	Marginal	A few strengths and a few major weaknesses
	9	Poor	Very few strengths and numerous major weaknesses

Minor weakness: An easily addressable weakness that does not substantially lessen impact
Moderate weakness: A weakness that lessens impact
Major weakness: A weakness that severely limits impact

FIGURE 19.2 NIH 9-point rating scale.

TABLE 19.2 Review criteria for research awards (R series)

Scored review criteria
Overall impact
1. Significance
2. Investigators
3. Innovation
4. Approach
5. Environment

Additional scored review criteria
Protection of human subjects
Inclusion of women, minorities, and children

Nonscored criteria: Additional review considerations
Budget and period support
Resource sharing plans

---

judged likely to have a major scientific impact. In other words, the overall impact score is not an average of the scores for each of the five individual review criteria.

19.1.5.2 1. Significance

The subsection on **significance** on the NIH critique form asks reviewers to consider the following questions:

- Does the project address an important problem or a critical barrier to progress in the field?
- If the aims of the project are achieved, how will scientific knowledge, technical capability, and/or clinical practice be improved?
- How will successful completion of the aims change the concepts, methods, technologies, treatments, services, or preventative interventions that drive this field?

19.1.5.3 2. Investigator(s)

The subsection on **investigators** on the NIH critique form asks reviewers to consider the following questions:

- Are the PIs, collaborators, and other researchers well suited to the project?
- If the applicant is an ESI or a new investigator, do they have appropriate experience and training?
- If the applicant is an established investigator, have they demonstrated an ongoing record of accomplishments that have advanced their field?
- If the project is collaborative or multi-PI, do the investigators have complementary and integrated expertise? Are their leadership approach, governance, and organizational structure appropriate for the project?

See Chapter 18, *Submission of the Grant Proposal*, for tips on choosing your investigative team.

19.1.5.4 3. Innovation

The subsection on **innovation** on the NIH critique form asks reviewers to consider the following questions:

- Does the application challenge and seek to shift current research or clinical practice paradigms by utilizing novel theoretical concepts, approaches or methodologies, instrumentation, or interventions?
- Is a refinement, improvement, or new application of theoretical concepts, approaches or methodologies, instrumentation, or interventions proposed?

19.1.5.5 4. Approach

The subsection on approach on the NIH critique form asks reviewers to consider the following questions:

- Are the overall strategy, methodology, and analyses well-reasoned and appropriate to accomplish the specific aims of the project?
- Are potential problems, alternative strategies, and benchmarks for success presented?
- If the project involves clinical research, are the plans for (1) protection of human subjects from research risks and (2) inclusion of minorities and members of both sexes/genders, as well as the inclusion of children, justified in terms of the scientific goals and research strategy proposed?

See Chapters 8 through 13 for tips on writing the approach (Methods) section.

19.1.5.6 5. Environment

The subsection on **environment** on the NIH critique form asks reviewers to consider the following questions:

- Will the scientific environment in which the work will be done contribute to the probability of success?
- Are the institutional support, equipment, and other physical resources available to the investigators adequate for the project proposed?
- Will the project benefit from unique features of the scientific environment, subject populations, or collaborative arrangements?

See Chapter 18, *Submission of the Grant Proposal*, for tips on writing the environment section.

19.1.6 Review Criteria for Career Development Awards (K Series)

The review criteria for the Career Development Awards (K Series) differ from the review criteria for Research Awards (R series). In general, the primary focus of the review for career awards is on the candidate and the career development plan, with less emphasis on the research plan although it is still important. There are a variety of career awards depending upon your training and stage of career (as described in Chapter 17, *Choosing the Right Funding Source*), and the review criteria differ slightly across these awards. Therefore, it is important to consult the specific program announcement to which you are applying (http://grants.nih.gov/training/careerdevelopmentawards.htm).

In general, however, the review criteria for career awards can be summarized in Table 19.3.

19.1.6.1 Overall impact for a career award

The overall impact reflects the reviewer's assessment of the likelihood for the candidate to maintain a strong research program, taking into consideration the individual review criteria.

See Chapter 18, *Submission of the Grant Proposal*, for tips on writing a career award and choosing an appropriate mentor.

TABLE 19.3 Review criteria for career development awards (K series)

Scored review criteria
Overall impact
  1. Candidate
  2. Career development plan/career goals and objectives
  3. Research plan
  4. Mentor(s), co-mentor(s), consultant(s), collaborator(s)
  5. Environmental and institutional commitment to the candidate

Additional scored review criteria
Protection of human subjects
Inclusion of women, minorities, and children

Nonscored criteria: Additional review considerations
Training in the responsible conduct of research
Budget and period support
Resource sharing plans

19.1.6.2 1. Candidate

The subsection on **candidate** on the NIH critique form asks reviewers to consider the following questions:

- Does the candidate have the potential to develop as an independent and productive researcher? Is the candidate's academic, clinical (if relevant), and research record of high quality?
- Is there evidence of the candidate's commitment to meeting the program objectives to become an independent investigator?
- Do the letters of reference from at least three well-established scientists address the candidate's potential for becoming an independent investigator or that the program will meet the candidate's career goals?
- Is there likelihood that the award will contribute substantially to the academic and research career development of the candidate?

19.1.6.3 2. Career development plan/ career goals and objectives

The subsection on **career development plan/career goals and objectives** on the NIH critique form asks reviewers to consider the following questions:

- What is the likelihood that the plan will contribute substantially to the scientific development of the candidate leading to scientific independence?
- Are the content, scope, phasing, and duration of the career development plan appropriate when considered in the context of prior training/research experience and the stated training and research objectives for achieving research independence?
- Are there adequate plans for monitoring and evaluating the candidate's research and career development progress?

19.1.6.4 3. Research plan

The subsection on **research plan** on the NIH critique form asks reviewers to consider the following questions:

- Are the proposed research question, design, and methodology of significant scientific and technical merit?
- Is the research plan relevant to the candidate's research career objectives?
- Is the research plan appropriate to the stage of research development and as a vehicle for developing the research skills described in the career development plan?

19.1.6.5 4. Mentor(s), co-mentor(s), consultant(s), and collaborator(s)

The subsection on **mentors** on the NIH critique form asks reviewers to consider the following questions:

- Are the mentor's research qualifications in the area of the proposed research appropriate?
- Is there adequate description of the quality and extent of the mentor's proposed role in providing guidance and advice to the candidate? Are there adequate plans for monitoring and evaluating the career development awardee's progress toward independence?
- Is there evidence of the mentor's, consultant's, collaborator's previous experience in fostering the development of independent investigators? Is there evidence of previous research productivity and peer-reviewed support?

As you can see, the above points focus largely on the mentor's **expertise** and track record, as well as their strong **track record in training** future independent researchers. In this vein, as recommended in Chapter 17, it is important to identify a mentor not only with an NIH track record but who has the time to commit to mentoring you.

19.1.6.6 5. Environment and institutional commitment to the candidate

The subsection on **environment and institutional commitment** on the NIH critique form asks reviewers to consider the following questions:

- Is the commitment from the sponsoring institution to provide protected time for the candidate to conduct the research program adequate?
- Is the institutional commitment to the career development of the candidate appropriately strong?
- Is the environment for scientific and professional development of the candidate of high quality?

19.1.7 Review Criteria for Fellowship Awards (F Series)

In general, the review criteria for Fellowship awards can be summarized in Table 19.4.

19.1.7.1 Overall impact/merit for a fellowship award

The subsection on **overall impact** on the NIH critique form asks reviewers to consider:

- The likelihood that the fellowship will enhance the candidate's potential for, and commitment to, a productive independent scientific research career in a health-related field.

TABLE 19.4 Review criteria for fellowship awards (F series)

Scored review criteria
Overall impact
1. Fellowship applicant
2. Sponsors, collaborators, and consultants
3. Research training plan
4. Training potential
5. Institutional environment and commitment to training

Additional scored review criteria
Protection of human subjects
Inclusion of women, minorities, and children

Nonscored criteria: Additional review considerations
Training in the responsible conduct of research
Budget and period support
Resource sharing plans

19.1.7.2 1. Fellowship applicant

The subsection on **fellowship applicant** on the NIH critique form asks reviewers to consider the following questions:

- Are the fellow's academic record and research experience of high quality?
- Does the fellow have the potential to develop as an independent and productive researcher in biomedical, behavioral, or clinical science?

19.1.7.3 2. Sponsors, collaborators, and consultants

The subsection on **sponsors, collaborators, and consultants** on the NIH critique form asks reviewers to consider the following questions:

- Are the sponsor(s) research qualifications (including successful competition for research support) and track record of mentoring appropriate for the proposed fellowship?
- Is there evidence of a match between the research interests of the fellow and the sponsor (including an understanding of the applicant's research training needs)?
- Is there a demonstrated ability and commitment of the sponsor to assist in meeting the applicant's research training needs?

19.1.7.4 3. Research training plan

The subsection on **research training plan** on the NIH critique form asks reviewers to consider the following questions:

- Is the proposed research plan of high scientific quality, and does it relate to the fellow's training plan?

- Is the training plan consistent with the fellow's stage of research development?
- Will the research training plan provide the fellow with individualized and supervised experiences that will develop research skills needed for his or her independent and productive research career?

19.1.7.5 4. Training potential

The subsection on **training potential** on the NIH critique form asks reviewers to consider the following questions:

- Does the proposed research training plan have the potential to provide the fellow with the requisite individualized and supervised experiences that will develop his or her research skills?
- Does the proposed research training have the potential to serve as a sound foundation that will lead the fellow to an independent and productive career?

19.1.7.6 5. Institutional environment and commitment to training

The subsection on **institutional environment and commitment to training** on the NIH critique form asks reviewers to consider the following questions:

- Are the research facilities, resources, and training opportunities adequate and appropriate?
- Is there appropriate institutional commitment to fostering the fellow's training as an independent and productive researcher?

19.1.8 During the Study Section Meeting

Based on the reviewers and discussants' submitted written comments and preliminary scores, if all the reviewers agree in advance that an application for a Research Award (R series) is noncompetitive, the study section may choose not to discuss the application. These applications typically have preliminary scores in the bottom half of the applications. This process is termed **streamlining** or **triaging**. In general, approximately half of the applications reviewed by a study section are streamlined and therefore not discussed at the study section meeting.

In contrast, all applications for Career Development Awards (K series) and Fellowships (F series) are discussed, although this may change in the future.

For applications that are discussed at the meeting, the assigned reviewers will lead the discussion, presenting their impressions of the strengths and weaknesses of the application in terms of the review criteria. The discussion is then opened up to comments from all the study section members (without conflicts of interest). After this discussion (generally limited to 10–20 min), each study section member including the assigned reviewers provides an overall impact score.

Again, it is important to note that this overall impact score is not necessarily the arithmetic mean of the scores for each individual review criteria. Instead, reviewers are instructed to consider each of the review criteria but are not told how to *weigh* them. Other factors may affect the score (e.g., a human subject concern).

The **final overall impact score** for each discussed application is determined by calculating the mean score from all the study section members' (without conflicts of interest) impact scores and multiplying the average by 10. Thus, the final overall impact scores range from 10 (high impact) to 90 (low impact).

Numerical impact scores are not reported for applications that are not discussed (e.g., streamlined applications). Although not discussed, you will receive the written critiques of your assigned reviewers/discussants as well as their individual criterion scores.

Rarely, an application may be designated Not Recommended for Further Consideration (NRFC) by the study section if it lacks significant and substantial merit, presents serious ethical problems in the protection of human subjects from research risks, or in the use of vertebrate animals, biohazards, and/or select agents. Applications designated as NRFC do not proceed to the second level of peer review (the institute).

19.1.9 Common Reasons for Low Scores

- Lack of original idea and/or scientific rationale
- Diffuse, superficial, or unfocused research plan
- Questionable methodology
- Lack of important details
- Lack of experience in methodology
- Lack of generalizability of findings or methods
- No attention to human subjects issues
- Unrealistically large amount of work
- No apparent translatability of research into practice or policy
- Insufficient statistical power
- No or insufficient statistical support

19.1.10 Tips for a Successful Review

Tip #1: Volunteer to Serve on a Study Section
One of the best ways to get a sense for how a review is conducted is to volunteer to serve on a study section. You will learn firsthand which aspects of an application lead to a strong score and which lead to the application being triaged. In addition, you will be exposed to the experiences of senior reviewers on the panel.

Tip #2: Find Out Who the Study Section Members Will Be
If you know in advance to which study section you are targeting your application, it will be important to review the list of members in advance. In this way, you can obtain a sense of their expertise. It will also ensure that you do not omit to cite a relevant reference published by one of these members!

Tip #3: Be Kind to Your Reviewers: Subheadings Should Match Review Criteria
Reviewers on a study section are assigned a large number of applications to read and discuss. This task is in addition to their own responsibilities as a researcher themselves. So, a happy reviewer should be one of your top goals.

The most effective way to make a reviewer happy is to help them complete their review forms. As mentioned above, NIH reviewers are required to write bullet points on the strengths and weaknesses of overall impact, significance, investigators, innovation, approach, and environment. However, the formatting requirements of NIH grant applications do not require clearly labeled sections for each of these criteria. Therefore, the first way to be *kind* to your reviewers is by using these key terms as subheadings in your application.

Tip #4: The Abstract and Specific Aims Page Should Include a Synopsis of the Significance and Innovation
The reviewers assigned to your application will need to introduce it to the rest of the members of the study section. They have very limited time to do so. By including a synopsis of the significance and innovation of your proposal on the Abstract and Specific Aims pages, you increase the odds that the most important aspects of your application will be recognized by the entire panel.

Tip #5: Be Kind to Your Reviewers: Include a Brief Synopsis of Your Overall Study Design
Another way of being kind to the reviewers is by inserting a brief summary paragraph at the very beginning of the Methods section that encapsulates all the key features of the study design. This paragraph would give the sample size, study population, study design (e.g., prospective cohort case-control study, cross-sectional study), the key assessment tools to be used (e.g., self-reported questionnaire, plasma samples, medical record data), and any other key features of your study methods. This will help the reviewer to concisely present your study to the review panel. Examples of such summaries are provided in Chapter 9, *Study Design and Methods*.

19.2 PART II: AFTER YOUR APPLICATION IS REVIEWED

19.2.1 Step #1: Read the Summary Statement

Shortly after the study section meeting, your overall impact score or an indication that your application was streamlined (*not discussed* [*ND*]) will be posted on the NIH website (eRA Commons https://commons.era.nih.gov/). If you receive a numerical score, you are probably in the top half of applications reviewed by that section.

Wait for the summary statement from the study section meeting to also be posted—this usually occurs within 30 days or even sooner for new investigator applications. Do not call the program official at NIH until you receive this summary statement.

The summary statement will include the reviewers' critiques of your application and numerical scores for each of the individual review criteria. All discussed applications also include a *resume and summary of the discussion* written by the SRO that highlights the major factors in the discussion that drove the final scores.

Even an application that was not discussed (streamlined) at the review meeting will still receive a summary statement with the written critiques and preliminary criterion scores from each of the assigned reviewers.

19.2.2 If Your Application Was Streamlined (Unscored)

Do not despair because you are in good company. With the decrease in funding, applications that would have been funded are being resubmitted. So, the overall quality of applications continues to increase, but there will always be a bottom half. When your summary statement is available, read it quickly, then put it aside for a few days. Then, take it out and go through it carefully with your coinvestigators and mentors.

There are *two categories of streamlined applications*:

1. The most troubling is when there is a fatal flaw or other weaknesses, such as low perceived scientific importance, that may not be addressable. If there are, stand back and then decide the route to take next time.
2. However, usually there are weaknesses that are addressable. Revise the application as described in Chapter 20, *Resubmission of the Grant Proposal*, and resubmit when appropriate.

19.2.3 Step #2: Contact Your Program Official

Now that the review has been completed, the **program official at the assigned institute(s) becomes your NIH contact**. It is against NIH policy for a SRO to discuss your summary statement with you.

After reading the summary statement, make an appointment to discuss the critiques and your options with the program official assigned to your application. The program official can help you in interpreting your summary statement as he or she may have listened to or attended the review meeting.

The program official may also be able to provide guidance on the following issues:

- Further discussion and interpretation of the reviewers' comments
- The likelihood of NIH funding the application in light of your overall impact score and the institute's current funding payline
- What to address in your resubmission application, if this is your first submission
- How to develop a new application, if your resubmission was not successful
- The acceptable bases for appealing the peer review process

19.2.4 Appeal

Sometimes comments by reviewers in your summary statement might seem unfair or might indicate that the reviewer misunderstood your application. Usually, the best strategy is to diplomatically address all of the reviewers' comments in the Introduction of your resubmission application as described in Chapter 20, *Resubmission of the Grant Proposal*.

However, you may appeal the review process if there is evidence of bias or conflict of interest on the part of one or more of the reviewers, lack of appropriate expertise within the study section, and/or substantial factual errors made by one or more of the reviewers that could have altered the outcome of the review substantially. A difference in scientific opinion is not grounds for appeal. The decision to appeal should be discussed with your program official. However, while your appeal is making its way through the system, use the appeal memo you wrote as a basis for the Introduction section of the resubmission and start writing.

19.2.5 Funding: What Determines Which Awards Are Made?

After the study section meeting is complete, your priority scores and corresponding percentile rankings are transmitted to the assigned NIH institute, where the program official makes funding recommendations to the institute's National Advisory Council. The advisory council conducts this second level of review and makes final funding decisions.

You will see the date of the assigned NIH institute's Advisory Council Review on the NIH commons website. Generally, your application is likely to be funded if it receives an impact score or percentile ranking that is less than or equal to the payline of the assigned primary NIH institute.

The **payline** is the overall impact score or percentile ranking of this overall impact score at which the likelihood of funding goes from high to low. Having a score less than or equal to the payline is a good indication, but not a guarantee of funding. However, it is important to note that some institutes may choose not to fund some applications within their payline or, alternatively, may reach beyond the payline to fund an application to maintain mission focus, balance portfolios, or limit redundancy. However, these latter examples are unusual.

Some institutes publish their paylines and/or funding policies on their websites. However, if available, these apply only to the current fiscal year. If there is no published payline, the program official may be able to provide information on the likelihood (not a guarantee) of funding.

Issues that may impact the institute's funding decision are

- Program considerations
- Existing portfolio balance
- Anticipated impact of research
- Availability of funds

Resubmission of the Grant Proposal

20

Given today's economic challenges and the corresponding low NIH paylines, it is important to anticipate that your first grant submission will be rejected and to factor this into your overall timeline. Indeed, even the most famous scientists have had their grant proposals rejected. Therefore, this chapter goes on to describe the resubmission process along with strategic tips for how to be highly responsive to reviewer concerns—the key criteria in a successful resubmission. Part I describes the pathway to resubmitting your grant proposal. Part II goes on to provide strategic tips for the Introduction to the resubmission, the most critical aspect of the resubmission. Finally, Part III describes issues in revising the remainder of the body of the application.

20.1 PART I: PATHWAY TO RESUBMITTING

Put the summary statement away for a few days. Then, sit down with a glass of wine or the beverage of your choice and read the reviewers' comments. When you first read them, you are likely to feel sad and angry—sad regarding the amount of work that you put into the submission and angry at the reviewers for not understanding what you meant.

However, it is important to remember that the reviewers were selected due to their substantial track record of NIH funding as well as expertise in peer review. If, as scientists, they misinterpreted your writing, then it is likely that many more people would make a similar misinterpretation. Therefore, any errors in their comprehension are ultimately due to the need for you to more clearly convey your points.

Do not call the funding agency at this point in time. Wait a week to calm down and then reread the reviews as well as your application. Ask your coinvestigators and mentors to read the reviews as well. A senior investigator/mentor skilled in reading NIH reviews will be invaluable. She or he can read between the lines to assess whether the flaws should be considered *fatal* and whether the reviewers showed any enthusiasm for your study. They can assess whether the comments are largely addressable.

Consider the reviewers' suggestions for change and their requests for more preliminary data, if applicable. Determine what parts of your application might have confused them. Then decide in conjunction with your mentor whether your application is fatally flawed or fixable. More often than not, the latter is the most likely decision.

20.1.1 Whether to Resubmit

There should almost never be a question as to whether to resubmit your grant proposal. Rejection on the first submission is so common, almost the norm, that it should be planned for. Specifically, your overall grantsmanship timeline should take into account the time to revise and resubmit even before you first submit the proposal.

This is not to say that you should submit a version that is not perfect but that instead you should anticipate that the reviewers will want to make their mark on your proposal. Always remember that in the grant proposal process, grit and persistence may be more predictive (or just as predictive) of ultimate success than scientific intelligence.

20.1.2 Contact Your Program Official

Now that the review has been completed, the **program official at the assigned institute(s) becomes your NIH contact**. After reading the summary statement and discussing with your colleagues, make an appointment to discuss the critiques and your options with the program official assigned to your application. The program official can help you in interpreting your summary statement as he or she may have listened to or attended the review meeting.

The program official may be able to provide guidance on what to address in your resubmission application, if this is your first submission.

20.1.3 Timing of a Resubmission

Resubmitting as soon as possible after you receive the summary statement is preferable to ensure that you maximize your chances of obtaining the same review panel. Remember that reviewers like to make their mark on your proposals, and if your resubmission is reviewed by a new reviewer, this will be their first chance to make comments.

The primary reason for delaying a resubmission would be in response to a reviewer request that you provide additional pilot data. However, while your original submission was under review, you ideally already started a pilot study. If so, you will be well positioned to submit this new data as part of your resubmission.

> **eg** *example* Imagine a reviewer comment that you should conduct a small feasibility study prior to the proposed study. In the Introduction to the resubmission, you could state
>
> Since the time of the original submission, we have been in the field with a pilot feasibility study, "Healthy Heart Pilot" (Faculty Research Grant; PI: yourself). The goal of this pilot is to evaluate the feasibility and acceptability of the proposed intervention. The pilot has randomized 47 men to date and is on track for its goal of 66 men. Participants endorsed the interest and utility of the study materials (86%), ability to access a telephone for telephone interviews (100%), and the amount of time spent on the study (appropriate 86%, sometimes too much time 14%). Recruitment and retention rates were used to inform the revised power calculations.

20.1.4 Not All Reviewer Comments Are Equal

Remember the criteria for Research (R series) awards as presented in Chapter 19, *Review Process* (Table 20.1).

Weaknesses that fall under *Overall Impact* and *Significance* should be considered the most serious. However, before deciding to shift the grant's focus, consider whether these comments reflect a failure on your part to clearly convey the (1) research gap, (2) clinical significance, and (3) public health implications of your study findings.

In contrast, concerns about *approach* are typically more addressable as they may reflect logistic concerns about your ability to pull off the actual study.

Parts II and III of this chapter provide examples of responding to concerns pertaining to each of the review criteria.

TABLE 20.1 Review criteria for research awards

Overall impact
1. Significance
2. Investigators
3. Innovation
4. Approach
5. Environment

20.1.5 How Much Revision Is Necessary

A general rule of thumb is that the amount of revision should be **proportional** to the score of the application. In other words, significant revisions are required if your application was triaged. If the application was scored, the number of revisions should decrease as the score decreases. In fact, if you have a low score, be careful not to make dramatic revisions—just a few tweaks may be sufficient to respond to the reviewer comments.

This advice, however, assumes that the score is congruent with the content of the reviews. This is not always the case. While all reviewers are instructed to justify their numerical scores with appropriate text, variability exists among reviewers in the extent to which they describe the strengths and weaknesses of the scored criteria. If one of the critiques provided little justification for a low criterion score, try checking the corresponding comments on the other critiques. These can provide you with multiple viewpoints on that criterion.

In addition, check the *Resume and Summary of Discussion* section of the summary statement (included on all discussed applications). This resume may have additional information on the content and emphasis of the verbal discussion held by the reviewers about your proposal. Your NIH program official also can help you to interpret this summary, and he or she may have listened to or attended the review meeting.

20.1.6 Study Section Review of Resubmissions

For resubmissions, the study section will evaluate the application as now presented, taking into consideration the responses to comments from the previous study section and changes made to the project. The committee will consider whether the responses to comments from the previous study section are adequate and whether substantial changes are clearly evident.

20.2 PART II: INTRODUCTION TO THE RESUBMISSION

Just as the Specific Aims page was the most important page of your original application, the Introduction is the **most vital part** of the resubmission. Approximately half of your time revising your application should be spent on this **one-page** Introduction. Early drafts of the Introduction should be sent to your coinvestigators/mentors well in advance of the resubmission date.

In general, the scientific review officers will assign your revised application to the same reviewers who reviewed the first submission, given that they are still available. These reviewers will be reading your application for the second time and will **focus primarily on your responsiveness to their critique** as summarized in the Introduction. Specifically, they will cross-check each of their prior comments against your response in the Introduction as well as your marked changes in the body of the proposal.

Even new reviewers who are assigned to your resubmission will often defer to the expertise of the prior reviewers and therefore focus primarily on how responsive you are to these prior reviewers' comments.

Below are **strategic tips** for writing the Introduction. You will see that the **overall theme** is "If at all possible, try to take the advice of the reviewers."

20.2.1 General Format of the Introduction Page

Table 20.2 is a typical format for the Introduction page:

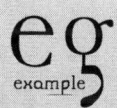

> **Example Paragraph #1:**
>
> This is a resubmission of DKxxxxx-01 "An Exercise Intervention to Prevent Diabetes" to test the hypothesis that an exercise intervention is an effective tool for preventing diabetes. The comments of the review panel were very helpful in revising this proposal. As the reviewers noted, "The application addresses a highly significant area in women's health that may have a lasting impact in a high-risk population for development of obesity and diabetes." "Using moderate intensity exercise to diabetes is innovative and could easily be translated into clinical practice." Changes made to the proposal are highlighted in italics throughout the text.

The majority of the remainder of the Introduction page will be made up by a point-by-point response to the major reviewer concerns.

How to determine which concerns are major?

- Concerns shared by more than one reviewer
- Concerns that were highlighted in the *Overall Impact* section
- Concerns that were highlighted in the *Resume and Summary of the Discussion* section

TABLE 20.2 Outline for the introduction page of a grant resubmission

1. Paragraph #1
   Specify the title and NIH assigned number of the grant proposal
   Thank the reviewers
   Quote several positive remarks from the reviews
   Clarify how revisions are highlighted in the body of the proposal
2. Point-by-point response to most important reviewer comments (bulk of the page)
3. Brief summary of response to more minor comments (one to two sentences)
4. Final positive summary (one to two sentences)

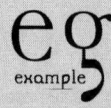

> **eg** **Example Final Positive Remark:**
>
> In summary, since the original submission, we have been in the field with three pilot studies. We have utilized information gleaned from these studies to make cultural modifications to our intervention materials, ensuring that the materials will be efficacious in Hispanics, the ethnic group with the highest rates of diabetes, as well as the other ethnic groups represented in the study population, while being sure to retain the integrity of our evidence-based intervention approach.

Examples of Introduction pages in their entirety are included at the end of this chapter.

20.2.2 Tip #1: Clearly Connect Your Responses to Specific Reviewer Concerns

While it is important to be brief in summarizing reviewer concerns to save space in the Introduction, be sure that the reviewer(s) can clearly find their concerns and your corresponding response in the Introduction.

How to Summarize Reviewer Concerns in the Introduction:

- List which reviewers share this concern according to reviewer number (i.e., R1, R2, R3).
- Repeat some of the identical phrasing used by the reviewers in your response.

Citing the reviewer number when listing the reviewer concern is a way of being kind to your reviewers. This will not only reassure the reviewers that you have covered their points but also help you to be sure that you have not missed any reviewer comments.

20.2.3 Tip #2: Resist the Urge to Defend Yourself

If you are a new investigator, your first instinct may be to try to *prove* yourself to the reviewers. The natural tendency is to defend yourself against their concerns by spending time justifying your original decisions.

In contrast, the reviewers' priority is to see that you have been **responsive** to their concerns. They don't want you to spend time showing that you are smart, well-educated, and/or never make errors. Instead, they will be going through each item in your Introduction and *checking off* in their notes whether or not you have made the changes they suggested.

Therefore, the most tactical approach is to set aside any need to prove yourself. Instead, if the suggested revision is feasible and does not seriously detract from your goals, then simply make the change. In the Introduction, simply state that you have made this change—there is no need to waste space by providing a rationale for why you originally did it another way.

20.2.4 Tip #3: Avoid Disagreeing with a Reviewer

It is almost never effective to not be responsive to a reviewer comment. Even a small revision is better than no revision. That is, you need to show that you are doing something in response to a reviewer concern.

If you are unable to be fully responsive to reviewer concerns,

1. Acknowledge the reviewer concern.
2. Describe the revision you made in response (even if it is a slight alternative to the reviewer's suggestion).
3. Describe what you are unable to address and why.

This approach avoids the common pitfall of starting your response by sounding nonresponsive or, at worst, argumentative. Instead, start out by saying that you recognize the reviewers' concern, followed by the positive change that you have made to the application in response to the reviewer comments (even if this is an alternative way to satisfy their concern), followed by any caveats regarding what you are unable to address.

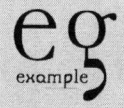

> *example*
>
> **Original Version**
> **R1. Recommend the addition of a 6-month follow-up study to ascertain if the effect persists after the structured intervention.**
> We chose not to conduct a follow-up study as our primary focus in this application was to determine whether the intervention could be effective in real time.
>
> **Improved Version**
> **R1. Recommend the addition of a 6-month follow-up study to ascertain if the effect persists after the structured intervention.**
> The reviewer raises an important point. Therefore, we have added a 3-month postintervention focus group that will assess whether the family continues to dance together, how often, and in what format. We are unable to follow the participants for 6 months due to the fact that recruitment is rolling over the first 2 years of the grant, leaving insufficient time to follow the last recruited family. However, we will also perform a 6-month focus group in a subgroup of the first 50 recruited families.

20.2.5 Tip #4: If You Must Disagree with a Reviewer, Focus on the Science

It is okay to disagree with reviewer concerns if you explain your decision in a way that will engage the reviewer scientifically. Do not write to the reviewers; write to the science. However, even in this situation, it is important to still try to be somewhat responsive to at least a part of their concern if at all possible.

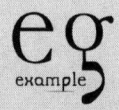

> *example*
>
> R2: **The investigators should consider defining physical activity using three cut points instead of two cut points.**
> In response to the reviewer's suggestion, we have added an additional analysis utilizing three cut points. However, because prior validation studies support the use of two cut points,[1,2] we also propose to retain our analysis using two cut points. This will facilitate comparisons with the prior literature that has, in general, utilized this approach. We will present findings from both approaches.

20.2.6 Tip #5: Avoid Using Cost or Logistics as a Rationale for Not Being Responsive to a Reviewer Comment

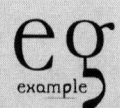

> *example*
>
> **Original Version**
> R1. **Concern that dropout rates may be high—monetary incentives should be considered.**
> The reviewer's valid point about possible attrition without monetary incentives concerns me also. However, our budget cannot afford such incentives.
>
> **Improved Version**
> R1. **Concern that dropout rates may be high—monetary incentives should be considered.**
> We agree with the reviewer. We have added a modest monetary incentive and will also partner with the school/community to incorporate nonmonetary ways to incentivize the participants.

> **Original Version**
> **R1: It is unclear why the proposed data analysis plan will only adjust for family history of diabetes and not history of preterm birth.** The dataset that we will be using does not include information on history of preterm birth.
>
> **Improved Version**
> **R1: It is unclear why the proposed data analysis plan will only adjust for family history of diabetes and not history of preterm birth.** While our dataset does not include information on history of preterm birth, we will address the threat of confounding by history of preterm birth by repeating the analysis among nulliparous women. We will compare the findings from this sensitivity analysis to the primary analysis to evaluate the degree of potential confounding by this variable.

20.2.7 Tip #6: Multiple-Bullet-Point Response to Major Concerns Is Highly Responsive

The space dedicated to each response should be in proportion to the importance of the reviewer concern. As mentioned earlier, concerns that fall under *Overall Impact* and *Significance* are often the most serious. In these situations, a bulleted list of multiple responses to this concern is recommended.

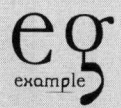

> **R1, R3 Need for data to demonstrate the efficacy of the physical activity intervention among pregnant Hispanic women.**
> In response to this important concern, our investigative team has been in the field with three pilot studies since the time of the original submission:
>
> - Pilot #1 is our focus group work among Latinas led by Dr. Smith (new coinvestigator). We have revised the intervention to address the themes from these six focus groups (Sections C.1 and D.3).
> - Pilot #2 is our ongoing exercise intervention among eight pregnant women that provides strong support for the efficacy of our exercise intervention (Section C.2).

- Pilot #3 is our completed pilot of acceptability/feasibility among 40 prenatal care patients that showed that the stage-matched manuals were feasible and acceptable in our population of multiethnic pregnant women (Section C.3).

Finally, since the time of original submission, a small vanguard pilot study has been published[1] supporting the efficacy of an exercise intervention in pregnant women at risk for GDM.

20.2.8 Tip #7: Acknowledge Your Mistakes or Lack of Clarity

At times, reviewers will make **basic errors of understanding** in their interpretation of your proposal. This may simply be due to the fact that they are facing a heavy load of proposals to review with a tight deadline, in combination with your proposal's failure to present something clearly.

In this case, it is important to be humble and apologize for your lack of clarity—even if you feel that the proposal was already clear and the reviewer was mistaken. Resist the temptation to point out that the first submission already described this point. Remember, you are not trying to prove to the reviewer that you are *smart*; instead, you are trying to prove to the reviewer that you are responsive to their comments.

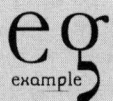

example: Imagine that you proposed to conduct a matched case-control study with age, race, and gender being your matching criteria. The reviewer missed the fact that you already included age as a matching criteria and asks you to do so in their comments.

While it will be tempting, **avoid saying** the following:

Original Version
We already included age as a matching criteria as noted on page 18 of the original application.

Improved Version
We apologize for our lack of clarity in describing the study design. We will include age as a matching criteria. Specifically, cases and controls will be matched on age <18, age ≥ 18 (see Section C.4. Study Design).

20.2.9 Tip #8: Don't Skip Any Reviewer Comments

Address each reviewer comment, if not individually, then at least in a summary paragraph near the end of the Introduction. The reviewers have each spent a lot of time reviewing your original application and will therefore carefully check whether you have addressed all their comments.

20.2.10 Tip #9: Avoid Collapsing Too Many Reviewer Concerns into One Bullet Point

This tip falls under the concept of being kind to your reviewer. In the example below, you can see how collapsing multiple concerns can lead to reviewer confusion.

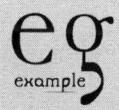

> *example*
>
> Imagine a proposal to conduct focus groups among girls.
>
> **Original Version**
>
> **R1. Aim 1 unclear; measurement of fun; control group.** The aim of the focus group is to determine whether the girls will find the activities fun and will want to participate; and to obtain advice from the mothers and daughters regarding potential barriers to the proposed intervention. Girls' enjoyment (fun) will be measured using the Facial Affective Scale. We have revised the methods to ensure that the control group will be seen as frequently as the other two groups.
>
> **Improved Version**
>
> **R1, R2: Aim 1 is unclear.** We apologize for our lack of clarity. Aim #1 is to conduct focus groups to (1) determine whether the girls will find the activities fun and will want to participate and (2) to obtain advice from the mothers and daughters regarding potential barriers to the proposed intervention.
>
> **R2, R3: Clarify how "fun" will be measured.** Girls' enjoyment (fun) will be measured using the Facial Affective Scale.
>
> **R1, R3: Concern that the control group has less contact time.** We have revised the methods to ensure that the control group will be seen as frequently as the other two groups.

20.2.11 Tip #10: Be Sure to Make Changes to the Body of the Proposal

In general, all responses to reviewer comments should refer to a section in the body of the proposal—so that the reviewer will be assured that you made the change to the protocol itself. The only exception would be items that reviewers suggested that you delete (however, sometimes even these are worth mentioning in the *Alternatives and Limitations* section).

Avoid the mistake of simply stating that you made a change in the Introduction and then leaving the body of the proposal unchanged. Reviewers will check this.

20.2.12 Stylistic Tip #1: Use Active (Not Passive) Voice

The use of the active voice in writing the Introduction to a resubmission further highlights your responsiveness to reviewer comments.

> **Original Version**
> R2. The intervention should incorporate a social support component based on recent findings supporting the efficacy of this approach.
> Changes were made to the proposal to incorporate a social support component.
> **Improved Version**
> R2. The intervention should incorporate a social support component based on recent findings supporting the efficacy of this approach.
> We agree with the reviewer and have now revised the intervention to incorporate a social support component.

20.2.13 Stylistic Tip #2: Avoid Use of the First Person

As with the body of the proposal, it is best to avoid use of the first person. You will almost always be submitting an application with a team of coinvestigators, collaborators, consultants, or mentors. The use of the term *we* always sounds more impressive than *I*, which can inadvertently come off as sounding like your own personal opinion.

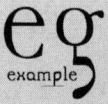

> **Original Version**
> R1, R3: Lack of rationale for choosing the Facial Affective Scale.
> I have selected the Facial Affective Scale in light of the lower validity which I believe the other scales face.
> **Improved Version**
> R1, R3: Lack of rationale for choosing the Facial Affective Scale.
> We selected the Facial Affective Scale based on published findings that show higher overall validity for this scale ($r = 0.75$–0.88) as compared to alternative scales ($r = 0.33$–0.66).

20.2.14 Stylistic Tip #3: Don't Waste Too Much Space Apologizing

Space in the Introduction is at a premium as you are limited to one page. Your primary emphasis will be on highlighting the changes you have made in response to reviewer concerns, as opposed to apologizing.

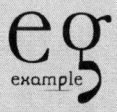

> **Original Version**
> **R1. Application fails to address alternatives if aim #1 is not successful.**
> We apologize for not explaining what will happen if we do not successfully establish the methodology. Since the time of the application, the methodology has been developed and validated as now described in Section C.3.
>
> **Improved Version**
> **R1. Application fails to address alternatives if aim #1 is not successful.**
> We apologize for this omission. Since the time of the application, the methodology has been developed and validated as now described in Section C.3.

20.3 PART III: BODY OF THE RESUBMISSION

20.3.1 How to Identify Revisions to a Grant Proposal

As noted in the current NIH guidelines for resubmissions, you should mark revisions in the body of the proposal by bracketing, indenting, or italicizing or changing the font (to one of the other acceptable fonts). The guidelines do not allow you to underline or shade the changes. Typically, *italics* are the easiest and clearest approach to take.

Be sure to cross-check the body of your revised proposal with your Introduction. Check that all revisions that you mentioned in the Introduction are not only made but also indicated by italics in the body of the proposal. Similarly, be sure that any changes to the body of the proposal are also summarized, even briefly, in the Introduction.

In the situation where the revisions are substantial, it is best not to mark them, as this would be distracting for the reviewer and make it difficult to read. Instead, the Introduction can state the following:

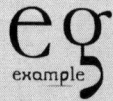

> *e.g. example* Over the past x months since the initial proposal submission, we have continued to develop the research outlined in the original proposal and hence can be more specific about the next steps that need to be undertaken. This has resulted in extensive changes in the proposal, including a change in the proposal's title to more appropriately reflect the central theme of the research. Every section of the proposal has been rewritten; new sections are not highlighted.

20.3.2 Rereview the Published Literature to Check for Recent Relevant Publications

This is a critical task in the resubmission process as there will be a time lag between your first submission and your resubmission during which new relevant findings may have been published. Assess whether the new data answer or inform your specific aims. If they do, refine your goals and specific aims and inform the reviewers about these new findings. At a minimum, add relevant citations to your Background and Significance section.

20.3.3 Obtain Revised Letters of Collaboration

Given the time lag between the original submission and the resubmission, it is important to obtain new letters of collaboration with a recent date for the purposes of the resubmission. The use of original letters will raise reviewer concerns that these collaborators may no longer be available to your proposed study.

20.3.4 Update Biosketches: Both Your Own and Those of Your Coinvestigators

Again, due to the time lag, be sure that all biosketches are revised to include any recent relevant publications as well as newly funded, or completed, grants.

20.4 EXAMPLES

20.4.1 Proposal to Conduct a Randomized Trial of a Postpartum Diabetes Prevention Program

Introduction to Revision

This is a resubmission of R03 DK12345 *"Randomized Trial of a Postpartum Diabetes Prevention Program for Hispanic Women"* (16th percentile score) to test the efficacy of a culturally and linguistically modified, individually tailored lifestyle intervention to reduce risk factors for type 2 diabetes and CVD among postpartum Hispanic women with a history of abnormal glucose tolerance during pregnancy. We thank the reviewers for noting, "Innovative proposal from an experienced team of investigators targeting a high risk population." "Finding effective, culturally relevant ways to reduce risk of developing T2D among Hispanic women with GDM or glucose intolerance has substantial public health significance." The comments of the review panel were very helpful in revising the proposal. Changes are highlighted in *italics* throughout the text.

R1: Weight loss not included as an intervention target. As recommended by the reviewer, we have revised the protocol to focus on weight loss as a key intervention target in addition to the exercise and dietary targets. Consistent with this revision, we now utilize dietary intervention materials found to be efficacious in our recent WIC Postpartum Pilot Study[102] that focused on *reduction in total caloric intake* (C.2. and Appendix II). We also provide our prior weight loss findings to support our ability to achieve these goals (C.2. Preliminary Studies).

R1. No expert in dietary assessment is included. We have added Dr. Taylor, professor of Nutritional Epidemiology and an expert in Hispanic dietary assessment, to lead the dietary assessment. Dr. Taylor and the PI have a track record of collaboration (C.1. *Progress Report* and Biosketches). We now describe the training and certification of the diet assessors in the Methods section (C.3. *Measure of Adherence with Diet*).

R1. Dietary intervention is not sufficiently developed nor described. We have revised the Methods section to carefully describe the dietary intervention in detail (C.3. and Appendix II). We now clarify how quality control procedures ensure that stage of change and social cognitive constructs are consistently represented in all intervention materials. Our systems-based pilot study ensures that all mailings of physical activity and dietary intervention materials are synchronized such that participants receive them at the same time (C.3. *Lifestyle Intervention*; Table 20.2). We provide revised power calculations for the expected reduction in total daily caloric intake based on prior postpartum interventions.[1]

R2. Conduct a small feasibility study prior to the evaluation study. Since the time of the original submission, we have been in the field with a pilot feasibility study, "Healthy Pilot" (Faculty Research Grant; PI: yourself). The goal of this pilot is to evaluate the feasibility and acceptability of the proposed intervention. The pilot has randomized 47 women to date and is on track for its goal of 66 women. Participants endorsed the interest and utility of the study materials (86%), ability to access a telephone for telephone interviews (100%), and the amount of time spent on the study (appropriate 86%, sometimes too much time 14%). Recruitment and retention rates were used to inform the proposed power calculations (C.3. *Power Calculations*).

R1: Initiate intervention during pregnancy after GDM diagnosis. We have revised the proposal to now initiate the intervention in pregnancy immediately after GDM diagnosis and the baseline assessment (randomization at ~29 weeks gestation) to capitalize on the fact that pregnant women with abnormal glucose tolerance receive counseling during that time period (C.3. *Usual Care*) and are motivated to make behavioral changes.

R1: Assessment of breastfeeding status is not well described. We have revised the protocol to now utilize a validated Infant Feeding Questionnaire[2] to assess history of breastfeeding and frequency and duration of current breastfeeding (i.e., exclusive breastfeeding, percentage of mixed breast and formula feeding, exclusive formula feeding), timing of introduction of solids, and other breastfeeding behaviors and beliefs.

R1: Comments on Budget/Appendix. We have revised the Methods section and budget to identify the participant incentive value. We have removed photos from the stage-matched manuals that depicted parents swinging toddlers and now use more appropriate photos (Appendix II).

R3: No concerns.

20.4.2 K Award Proposal to Conduct a Web-Based Intervention Study to Prevent Weight Gain in Men

Introduction to Resubmission

We are pleased that the reviewers noted several strengths of our original application including "a candidate with a good publication record and positive letters of support; an outstanding team of mentors with specific and varied expertise that is ideally suited to the proposed training and research plan; and an excellent research and training environment." We are also pleased that the reviewers recognized the importance of the research topic. We have carefully considered the reviewers' comments and have made significant revisions to the application. Specifically, we have refocused the research plan to develop and test the feasibility and acceptability of a theory-driven web-based intervention to prevent excessive weight gain that uses evidence-based strategies to help men achieve recommendations for weight gain, nutrition, and physical activity. We believe the application is significantly improved by our efforts to address the reviewers' comments. Major additions are *in italics* throughout the application and are summarized below.

R1, R2. Concern that characterization of weight gain patterns will not add to known determinants of excessive weight gain nor be a fruitful approach to intervening to prevent excessive weight gain. In response to these concerns, we have refocused the research and training plans on intervention development and testing feasibility and acceptability (Section APPROACH). We feel these changes have considerably strengthened the application and better reflect training and mentored research experiences needed to accelerate the candidate's research program in the area of weight gain and long-term cardiometabolic health.

R3. Suggest eliminating unwieldy stratification of focus groups. We have revised the application to conduct four focus groups of "all comers" as suggested by the reviewer (Section FGs).

R1, R3. Need for a more detailed description of proposed intervention including specific behavioral strategies. We now provide a more detailed description of our theory-driven web-based intervention to prevent excessive weight gain that uses evidence-based strategies to help men achieve the recommendations for weight gain, nutrition, and physical activity (Section INTERVENTION).

R2. Add a pilot randomized controlled trial (RCT) to evaluate intervention feasibility and acceptability. We have added a pilot trial to evaluate intervention feasibility and acceptability (Section RCT), which will provide critical data to support an R01 application to conduct a large RCT to evaluate efficacy (Section FUTURE).

R1, R2. The candidate does not list publications directly related to proposed research topic. Since the time of the original submission, the candidate now has two papers in the area of weight gain published or accepted for publication and an additional three under review (Sections CAND and PRELIM).

R1, 2, 3. Need for additional preliminary data. We now highlight the work we have done in direct support of this application since the time of the original submission (Section PRELIM).

R1. Replace the semester-long statistical courses with didactic training in obesity biology. We have added didactic training obesity biology and clinical shadowing; the revised training plan now better aligns with the revised research plan (Section TRAIN).

R2. Clarify how mentors will monitor progress, including yearly team meetings. See Section MENTORS.

R3. Clarify manuscripts and grant applications to be submitted during award period. See Section DISSEM.

Index

A

Abstracts and titles
  background section
    description, 291
    exposure–outcome relationship, 292–294
    public health impact, outcome, 292
  highlights, methodology, 295–297
  journal article abstract outline, 288
  methodology, 288–289
  NIH review, 290
  proposal abstract outline, 287–288
  proposal and book chapter, 289
  proposal title (*see* Proposal title)
  research aims, 294–295
  significance and innovation, 290, 297–299
  word count/line limitations, 291
Acid lowering agents (ALA), 248
AIDS awareness course, 45–46
ALA, *see* Acid lowering agents (ALA)
Alcohol awareness course, 42
Avoidance of synonyms, 76

B

Backup slides, 321
Behavioral intervention, feasibility study, 205
Behavioral Risk Factor Surveillance System (BRFSS), 39
Behaviors Affecting Adolescents (BAA) Study, 135
Best practices, data analysis plan
  bivariate analysis, 194
  case–control study, 195
  evidence, 192
  HIPAA protections, 194
  linear regression models, 193
  missing data, 193
  model diagnostics, 193
  multiple comparisons, 193–194
  participants *vs.* nonparticipants, 194
  respondents *vs.* nonrespondents, 194, 195
Bias, nondifferential/differential, 222
Biosketch
  coinvestigators, 374
  peer-reviewed publications, 373
  personal statement, 373
  positions and honors, 373
  research support, 373
Bivariate analysis plan
  categorical variables, 187
  confounding factors, 185
  covariates, 185, 186
  dichotomous variable, 185
  exposure and outcome variables, 185
  hemorrhage size and mortality, 185, 186
Bland–Altman plot, 277–278
BMI, *see* Body mass index (BMI)
Body mass index (BMI), 63, 163, 164
BRFSS, *see* Behavioral Risk Factor Surveillance System (BRFSS)

C

Candidate information, career development awards
  goals and objectives, 368
  independent research career, 368
  mentor, 367
  NIH reporter, accessing, 368
Cardiovascular risk factors, 42
Career development awards
  candidate, 388
  description, 387
  environment and institutional commitment, 389
  mentors, 389
  plan/career goals and objectives, 388
  research plan, 388
CDC, *see* Center for Disease Control and Prevention (CDC)
Center for Disease Control and Prevention (CDC), 110–111
Chalk-talk forum, 359
Chance
  possible study outcomes, 221
  random variability, 221
Classic limitations
  confounding, 256–260
  generalizability, 261
  information bias
    analysis techniques, 255–256
    design techniques, 254–255
    minimize nondifferential misclassification, 252–253
  selection bias
    analysis techniques, 254
    description, 253
    study design techniques, 254
  survivors bias, 260
  temporal bias, 260–261

Confounding
  causal pathway between high-fat diet and MI, 230
  confusion of effects, 229
  diagram, 230
  and effect modification, difference, 231–232
  information, confounders, 257
  inverse association, exposure and disease, 233
  known and unknown confounding factors, 231
  matched analysis, 259
  matching, 258
  multivariable regression, 259
  potential confounder, 230
  potential confounding factors, 231–233
  proxy variable, 260
  randomization, 258–259
  in randomized trials, 231
  sensitivity analysis, 260
  smoking, confounder, 231
  stratification, 258–259
  subject restrictions, 256–257
  uncontrolled confounding, impact, 232–233
Consortium/contractual arrangements, 379
Contractions, 78–79
Covariate assessment
  confounding factors, 168
  episiotomy, 168
  exposure–outcome relationship, 168
  modifiers, 169
  risk factors, 168
Critical reading
  case–control and cross-sectional studies, 241–242
  cohort studies, 239–240
  randomized trials, 240–241

D

DAGs, *see* Directed acyclic graphs (DAGs)
Data analysis plan
  alternate template, 180, 181
  best practices, 192–195
  bivariate analysis plan, 185–187
  dissertation proposal (*see* Dissertation proposal)
  exploratory data analyses, 191
  exposure variables, 180
  hemorrhage size and mortality, 183
  mock tables, 179, 183, 192
  multivariable analysis plan, 187–191
  parameterization, variables, 182
  proposed analyses
    exposure and outcome, interest, 179
    Lyme disease, 181
    tick-borne diseases, 182
  specific aims verbatim
    dissertation proposal, 179, 180
    hypotheses, 179
    univariate analysis plan, 183–185
Diabetes, postpartum, 105–107; *see also* Postpartum diabetes prevention program
Difference measures of association (continuous outcome variables)
  cohort and cross-sectional studies
    data, differences in means, 215
    mean difference in outcome, 215
    standard deviation, 215
  displaying power in proposal, 215
  sample t-test, 214
  strategic study design decision, 214
Directed acyclic graphs (DAGs), 189
Dissertation Committee
  adjunct faculty, 20–21
  and chair, responsibilities, 22
  contract, 23
  formulation, 19–20
  genetic and environmental risk factors, 20
  meetings, 21–22
  preproposal, recruitment tool, 20
  recommendation, 21
Dissertation proposal
  brainstorm session, 17
  chair, 19
  Committee Members (*see* Dissertation Committee)
  defense
    departmental faculty member, 24
    public health impact, 24
    public notification, 26
    questions of information, 24–25
  description, 15
  internship/practicum program, 18
  original data collection, 18
  pep talk, 19
  preliminary qualifying exams, 16–17
  psychosocial stress and hypertensive disorders of pregnancy
    bivariate analysis, 196, 199, 200
    gestational weight gain and BMI, 28
    multivariable analysis, 196, 201
    physical activity, 28
    response rates, 196, 198
    risk factors, 27–28
    sensitivity analysis, potential bias, 196, 202
    stress, 28
    univariate analysis, 196, 198–199
    variable categorization, 196–198
  purpose, 15–16
  research, conduct, 25
  secondary datasets, 18

submission, graduate school, 25, 26
timeline, 26–27
writing
    contract, 23
    format, 23–24
    structure, 22–23, 29–30

E

Early informal feedback, 81–82
Early-stage investigators (ESIs), 140
Epidemiology
    highlighted studies
        antioxidants and Alzheimer's disease, 114, 118–119
        key attributes, 118
        noncurrent articles, 118
        self-selection, 119
        statistical significance, 119
    laundry list, 113
    limitations, prior studies, 116–117
    literature reviews
        Alzheimer's disease, 55
        consistency, 55
        covariates, 62
        dissertation proposal, 63
        exposure and outcome assessment, 60
        organization, 60, 61
        postmenopausal hormone, 55
        potential confounding factors, 55
        research gaps, 62–63
        study design and population, 60
    prior literature, conflicting
        awareness, controversies, 117
        decision process, 117
    research gap, 115
    space requirements, 113
    study methods, 114–115
Epidemiology and preventive medicine, 339
ESIs, *see* Early-stage investigators (ESIs)
Exposure assessment
    attitudes, 162
    biomarkers, 162, 163
    case–control study, 165
    FG, 163
    food security and diabetes, 166
    gold standard, 166
    NIH, 162
    parameterization, 163–164
    plasma vitamin D levels, 165
    psychological distress, 165
    strengths and limitations, 165
    subjective measures, 164
    tools, 161, 162
    validation studies, 164

F

Fasting glucose (FG), 163
Fellowship awards
    applicant, 390
    institutional environment and commitment, 391
    overall impact/merit, 389–390
    research training plan, 390–391
    sponsors, collaborators and consultants, 390
    training potential, 391
Ferritin levels and type 2 diabetes, association, 210
FG, *see* Fasting glucose (FG)
First-person singular, 70
FOAs, *see* Funding opportunity announcements (FOAs)
Funding agencies, 3–4
Funding opportunity announcements (FOAs), 347–348

G

GDM, *see* Gestational diabetes mellitus (GDM)
General data-sharing plan, 376
Generalizability
    assuming causality, 235
    limit, reasons, 236–237
    physiological relationship, exposure and outcome, 235
    pitfalls, 236
    potential for funding, 234, 235
    potential public health impact, 234
Gestational diabetes mellitus (GDM)
    physical activity, 157, 158
    psychosocial stress and cortisol, 157, 158
    screening glucose, 157–159
Gestational weight gain (GWG)
    Latino community, 104
    lifestyle interventions, 103–104
    pregnancy, labor and delivery, 103
    primary aims, 105
Good diets, 41
Grant proposals, literature
    basic rational, 50
    dissertation proposals, 50
    journal articles, 50
    research gap, 50
Grant proposal submission
    appendices and supplemental materials, 377
    biosketch, 373–374
    budget justification, 374
    chalk-talk forum, 359
    collaborators, 355–356
    components
        bibliography and references, 369
        candidate information, 367–369
        human subjects protection/responsible conduct, 369–370

NIH, 360–361
    project narrative, 363
    project summary, 362
    research strategy, 363–365
    scientific, 361
    specific aims, 363
    training information, 365–366
    women, minorities and children, 370–371
consortium/contractual arrangements, 379
cover component, 377
cover letter, 371
description, 353
equipment, 372
facilities and resources, 371
graduate students, 354
letters of support, 377
mock study section, 359–360
modular budget guidelines, 374
multiple principal investigator model, 356–357
pre-award grants manager, 353–354
preparation process, 354–355
resource sharing plan, 376
time, external review, 358–359
timeline, 379–380
working relationship, coinvestigators, 356
writing steps, 357
GWG, *see* Gestational weight gain (GWG)

H

Hypertensive disorders, pregnancy
    depression, 128
    Estudio GDM, 130–131
    gestational hypertension and preeclampsia, 128–129
    inflammatory response, stress, 128
    job-related stress, 130
    Latina population, 128
    psychiatric diagnosis, 129
    psychosocial stress, 129
    work stressors, 129–130
Hypotheses
    AIDS awareness course, 45–46
    alcohol awareness course, 42
    "alternatives and limitations", 102
    background and significance section, 33–34
    biases, 44
    cardiovascular risk factors, 42
    courses in stress reduction, 45–46
    dependent and independent variables, 35–36
    diabetes, 36–37
    early-career investigators, 102
    exposed and *unexposed* groups, 37–38
    good diets, 41
    laundry list, 102
    mentors, outside readers and coinvestigators, 94
    midwives, 43

need, 31–32
original aims, 103
overall impact, 33
physical activity, stress and GDM risk, 95
population, 38–39
preterm birth, 44–45
prior literature
    advantage, 35
    measurement tool, 34
    protective effect, 34
    vitamin D supplementation programs, 34
qualitative and quantitative studies, 102
research questions, 47
significant and significance, 43–44
social class and *health literacy*, 40
statistical predictions, 40–41
to-do list, 32
unnecessary words, remove, 46–47
writing checklist, 47–48

I

ICD, *see* International Classification of Disease (ICD)
Information bias
    case–control or cross-sectional study, 227–228
    in a cohort study
        oral contraceptives (OCs), 229
        risk of venous thromboembolism (VTE), 229
        surveillance bias (detection bias), VTE and OCs, 228–229
International Classification of Disease (ICD), 175

L

Latin abbreviations, 77–78
Layperson's terms
    beta coefficient, 146–147
    description, 145
    effect modification, 147
    melanoma, 146
Limitations and alternatives
    ALA, 248
    analysis techniques, 250
    chance, bias and confounding, 220
    classic limitations (*see* Classic limitations)
    cross-sectional and case–control studies
        reverse causality, 234
        survivor bias, 234
        temporal bias, 234
    design techniques, 249–250
    dissertation committee, 245
    exposure/outcome, 246
    fourfold approach, 246

grant proposal
  approach section end, 251
  description, 250–251
  intermingled limitations sections, 251–252
  maternal heat exposure and congenital heart defects, 262–263
  positive impression, 250
  potential impact, 246–247
  professional jargon, 246
  prospective design, 248
  stress and risk of preeclampsia, 264–265
  threats to internal/external validity, 220
  transparency, 246
Literature reviews
  Alzheimer's disease, 52
  completeness, 59–60
  databases, 53
  description, 49
  dissertation proposal, 51
  effect modification hypothesis
    data dredging, 56
    interaction hypothesis, 57
    public health impact, outcome, 56
    synergistic effect, 56
  endometrial cancer, postmenopausal women, 65–67
  epidemiology (see Epidemiology)
  exposure–outcome relationship
    epidemiology, 54–55
    physiology, 54
  grant proposals, 50
  Hispanic women, 64–65
  iterative process, 51
  NSAIDS, postmenopausal women, 65–67
  organization, 49
  outline creation, 52
  Phoenix Health Study, 52
  postmenopausal hormone, 52
  pregnancy disorders, 64
  proposal writing, 49
  public health impact, outcomes, 53–54
  research gap, 49
  scan articles, 59
  search process
    coffee and bladder cancer, 57
    epidemiology, 57
    evolution, research technique, 58
    gestational diabetes, 58
    PubMed, 57
    research gap, 58
    retrieve articles, 59
    vein, 57
  specific aims/hypotheses, 51, 52
Loan repayment programs (LRPs), 345
LRPs, see Loan repayment programs (LRPs)

M

Maternal heat exposure and congenital heart defects, case–control study, 242–243
Mediterranean Observational Study (MOS), 176
Modular budget guidelines, 374
MOS, see Mediterranean Observational Study (MOS)
Multiple principal investigator model, 356–357
Multivariable analysis plan
  confounding factors
    bivariate analysis, 189
    covariate assessment, 188
    DAGs, 189
    hemorrhage size and mortality, 190
    logistic regression, 190
    rate ratio (RR), 190, 191
    regression model, 189
    risk factors, 188
    stratification, 188
  continuous outcomes, 188
  dichotomous outcome variables, 187
  linear regression model, 188
  logistic regression model, 187
  potential effect modifiers, 187, 190–191

N

National Heart, Lung and Blood Institute (NHLBI), 141
National Institutes of Health (NIH)
  ambitious, 100–101
  analytic/descriptive studies, 99
  career development awards, 343–344
  deal, one-page limitation, 97
  description, 89
  doctoral and postdoctoral fellowships, 341–342
  effect modification, methods, 102–103
  exercise intervention
    GWG, 103–105
    postpartum diabetes, 105–107
  existing dataset
    advantages and disadvantages, 98
    funding agencies, 98
    IRB approval, 98
    preterm birth, 99
  exploratory/secondary, 100
  FOAs, 347–348
  funding mechanism, 340
  hypotheses (see Hypotheses)
  innovation, 96–97
  institutes and centers, 340
  interdependent aims, 97
  investigator advantages, 347
  LRPs, 345
  purpose, 89–90

420 Index

research and training plan, 342
research awards, 346–347
researchers, training grants and
    fellowships, 342
research supplements, 345–346
RFAs, 348
significance, 95–96
study and research
    measurement tools and limitations, 92
    methodological weakness, 91–92
    physiological/behavioral
        mechanisms, 91
study methods, 93–94
training grants, 343
word of caution, 90
NHLBI, *see* National Heart, Lung and Blood
    Institute (NHLBI)
NIH, *see* National Institutes of Health (NIH)
Nondifferential misclassification
    of exposure
        alcohol consumption and laryngeal
            cancer, 223
        bias toward the null, 223
    of outcome
        case–control study of exercise and
            miscarriage, 224
        gold standard, 224

O

Oral proposal presentation
    background and significance section
        complex study design slide, 316
        description, 315
        improved study design slide, 316–317
        summary table slide, 317–318
    backup slides, 321
    critique, 326–327
    evaluation, 325–326
    guidelines
        aims slide, 312
        figures/tables, 311
        outline and slide titles, 310
        questionnaire excerpt, 313
        recommended slide aesthetics, 315
        results slide, 312–313
        study design slide, 313
        time, 310, 311
        user-friendly text slides, 314–315
    preliminary studies
        dense table slide, 319–320
        figure version, 318–319
        improved table slide, 320
        mock tables, dissertation
            proposal, 321
        table version, 318
        text version of slide, 318

speech, guidelines
    audience, relationship, 324
    audience's confidence, 325
    rehearsal, importance, 324–325
    tables/figures discussion, 322–324
    time limitation, 325
    transition phrases, 322
    words, 322

P

Parameterization, exposure assessment
    BMI, 163, 164
    categorical variable, 164
    continuous scale, 163
    dataset, 163
    dose–response relationship, 164
    study population, 164
Physiology, literature reviews
    causal pathway, 54
    postmenopausal hormone, 54
    potential mechanism, 54
Positive form, 77
Postpartum diabetes prevention program
    breastfeeding status, 412
    dietary assessment, 411
    dietary intervention, 411–412
    feasibility study, 412
    pregnancy, GDM diagnosis, 412
    weight loss, 411
Power and sample size
    adequacy, 216–217
    calculation
        analysis of existing dataset, 205
        pitfall, 205–208
        software packages, 207–208
    characteristics, 204–205
    definition, 204
    difference measures (*see* Difference measures
        of association (continuous outcome
        variables))
    final talk, 217
    influencing factors, 217
    outcome, exposed and unexposed group, 204
    power, definition, 203
    ratio measures (*see* Ratio measures of
        association (relative risks))
    sample size estimation
        basis, 206–207
        pilot study, 207
    timeline
        investigator's decision, 204
        possible study outcomes, 204
Preliminary data
    confidence intervals (CIs) and p-values,
        148–149
    contradict, hypotheses, 138–139

descriptions, 135–136
difficulties, 140
ESIs, 140
established relationships, coinvestigators, 136–137
existing datasets
    alcohol consumption and bladder cancer, 141–142
    efficient and economical, 141
    secondary data analysis, NHLBI, 141
    study population, 141
feasibility studies, 134
funding mechanisms, 137
layperson's terms, 145–147
lifestyle intervention, 138
management skills, 139
NIH grant proposal, 140
overweight/obese Hispanics, 151
pilot studies, 133–134
publications, 134–135
R01 application, 137–138
research team, 137
sentences and numbers, 148
tables/figures
    alcohol consumption, 144–145
    coffee drinking and melanoma risk, 142–143
    highlights, reviewer, 143–144
    numeric order, 147
    space-saving technique, 149
    titles, 150
    top to bottom, 147–148
tangential, 138
television, viewing, 139
Professional jargon, 75
Proposal, background and significance
    collective approach, 120–121
    comprehensive and complete, citations, 123–124
    description, 109–110
    epidemiology (see Epidemiology)
    historical context, 122
    hypothesis, 110
    innovation, 119–120
    NSAIDS and endometrial cancer
        HNPCC genes, 126
        in vitro evidence, 127
        inflammatory mechanisms, 126
        mortality rates, 125
        physiologic mechanism, 127
        risk factors, 126
        white and black women, disparities, 126
    opinions, limitations, 121
    physiology
        antioxidant nutrients, 112
        limited-space requirements, 111
        physical activity, stress and risk of GDM, 112
        theoretical model, dietary intervention, 112–113
    public health impact, disease, 110–111
    references, 124
    review article, 121
    statements, 123
    stress and hypertensive disorders, pregnancy, 128–131
    summary sentence, 122
    time frame, 125
Proposal title
    agency-friendly keywords, 300
    character limits, 299
    clever/provocative titles, 304
    exposure and outcome variables, 301
    features, 303
    journal article titles, 299
    question format, 304
    research goal and aims, 303–304
    results, proposed study, 301–302
    study design, 302
    study population, 302–303
Proposal writing
    abstract and specific aims
        mentors' and colleagues' feedback, 5–6
        NIH Reporter, 4–5
        review process, 5
        revising and rewriting, 4
        sample size, 5
    advantage, funding mechanisms, 1–2
    capitalization, coinvestigators, 6
    departmental colleagues, 12
    doctoral and postdoctoral granting mechanisms, 1
    figures and tables, 8
    funding agencies, 3–4
    grant mechanisms, 2
    interdependent aims, 6–7
    mock study section review, 9
    reviewers
        background and significance, 10
        innovation, 10
        methods section, 10–11
        risk factors, infertility, 11
    serving, coinvestigator, 12
    vice versa
        data analysis, 8
        mentored career award applications, 7
        seed grant, 7
    vision, early-career faculty, 2–3
Public health impact of outcomes (disease)
    Alzheimer's disease, 53
    postmenopausal hormone, 53–54
    risk factors, 53

R

Ratio measures of association (relative risks)
  chi-square test, 209
  cohort and cross-sectional studies
    data, RRs as measure of association, 209
    information, for statistical software packages, 210
    risk ratio (RR), 210
    sources, 210–211
  dichotomous outcomes, 208
  displaying power in proposal
    clinical significance, 212
    degree of observed power, 212
    fixed sample size, 212
    range of exposure distributions and outcome frequencies, 213
    range of RRs/ORs, 212
    statistical test, 212
  unmatched case–control studies
    data, ORs as measure of association, 211
    percent of controls, exposed, 211
    ratio of controls to cases, 211
Reconcile contradictory feedback, 83–84
Request for applications (RFAs), 348
Reproducibility and validity studies
  behavioral questionnaires, 271–272
  description, 267–268
  evaluation, 284–285
  interpret findings, 283–284
  measurements consistency, 268
  objective measures
    biomarkers, 273
    medical records/ICD codes, 273
    monitors, 273
  questionnaires
    advantages, 270
    disadvantages, 270–271
  relationship, 269–270
  sample size and power, 284
  statistical analysis, 285
  study design
    administrations number, comparison method, 276
    long intervals, 274
    objective comparison measures, 275–276
    short intervals, 274
    subjective comparison measures, 274–275
    time interval, 273
  study limitations, 286
  writing data analysis
    Bland–Altman plot, 277–278
    statistician consultation, 277
  writing limitations sections
    generalizability, 282–283
    observed validity scores, 281–282
    reproducibility scores observation, 279–281

Research gaps, epidemiology
  BMI, 63
  covariates, 63
  exposure assessment, 63
  study designs, 62
Resource sharing plan, 376
Resubmission, grant proposal
  active voice use, 408
  biosketches, 410
  collaboration, revised letters, 410
  collapse, avoidance, 407
  concern, responses, 405–406
  cost/logistics, avoidance, 404–405
  defending tendency, 402–403
  disagreeing, avoidance, 403
  first person, avoidance, 408
  introduction page format, 401–402
  mistakes/lack of clarity, acknowledgement, 406
  pathway
    grantsmanship timeline, 398
    program official, 398
    review criteria, research awards, 399
    reviewers' suggestions, 397–398
    revision, requirement, 400
    study section review, 400
    timing, 398–399
  postpartum diabetes prevention program, 411–412
  relevant publications, 410
  reviewer comments, 406
  reviewer concerns, 402
  revisions identification, 409–410
  space apologizing, 409
  specific aims page, 400
  web-based intervention study, 413–414
Review process
  approach, 386
  career development awards, 387–389
  environment, 386
  fellowship awards, 389–391
  innovation, 386
  investigators, 385–386
  low scores, 392
  NIH critique, significance, 385
  NIH 9-point rating scale, 384
  point rating scale, 384
  reviewed application
    appeal, 395
    funding, 395
    program official, 394
    streamlined applications, 394
    summary statement, 393–394
  scientific review group, 381–383
  SRO, 382–383
  study section meeting, 391–392
  study section reviewers, 383

RFAs, *see* Request for applications (RFAs)
Right funding source
    career faculty member, 351
    doctoral and postdoctoral training grants, 337
    epidemiology and preventive medicine, 339
    foundation grants, 338
    funding agencies, 339
    grantsmanship timeline, postdoctoral researcher, 339–340
    internal university funding, 337–338
    mentor, grantsmanship
        ambitious specific aims, 336–337
        coinvestigator, 335–336
        description, 331
        funding mechanisms, 334
        goal development, 332
        identification, 332
        pipeline, 335
        steady trajectory, 333–334
    NIH, 340–348
    resources, 338
    reviewers, 339

S

Scientific review group
    NIH, application, 381, 382
    study section, 381
    types, 382, 383
Scientific review officer (SRO)
    NIH, 382, 383
    roles and responsibilities, 382–383
Scientific writing
    acronyms, 78
    active voice, 70–71
    audience, 69
    the authors concluded, 73
    coinvestigators, 82
    contractions, 78–79
    direct quotations, 72–73
    early informal feedback, 81–82
    first-person singular, 70
    incorporating feedback, 82–83
    Latin abbreviations, 77–78
    needless words, omission, 74–75
    numbers, 79
    positive form, 77
    professional jargon, 75
    race and heat illnesses, military population, 84–85
    reconcile contradictory feedback, 83–84
    reference style, 79–80
    synonyms, avoidance, 76
    transitions, 71
    user-friendly draft, 80–81
    Writing Assistance Programs, 81

SEER Program, *see* Surveillance, Epidemiology and End Results (SEER) Program
Selection bias
    case–control study, 225, 226
    in Cohort Study, 226
    differential loss to follow-up, 226
    multiple sexual partners and HPV, 226
    overestimate or underestimate, 225
    potential, 226
Socioeconomic status, 72–73
SRO, *see* Scientific review officer (SRO)
Statistical predictions, hypotheses, 40–41
Stress and risk of preeclampsia, prospective cohort study, 242–243
Study design and methods
    benchmarks, 155–156
    covariate assessment, 168–169
    cross-sectional *vs.* case–control studies, 156
    data analysis, 154
    epidemiology, 156, 157
    exposure assessment (*see* Exposure assessment)
    FFQ, 176
    GDM, 155, 157
    gestational diabetes, 154, 155
    gestational hypertension, 175
    hypertensive disorders, pregnancy, 174
    ICD, 175
    logistic regression, 174
    melanoma, 176–177
    MOS, 176
    outcome assessment, 167–168
    parent study, 156
    preeclampsia, 175
    prenatal care, 154
    preventive medicine, 156, 157
    proposal, 153, 154
    psychosocial stress, pregnancy, 174
    retrospective cohort design, 156, 157
    strategy and methodology, 154
    stress scale, 175
    study population, 159–161
    timing, assessments, 157, 158
    variable categorization, 169–173
Study population
    case–control studies, 160
    episiotomy, 161
    exclusion criteria, 161
    inclusion criteria, 160
    matching, 160
    proposal, 159
    reference population, 159
    sociodemographic factors, 160
    subject ascertainment, 160

Study section meeting
    final overall impact score, 392
    streamlining/triaging, 391
Surveillance, Epidemiology and End Results (SEER) Program, 110–111
Survivors bias, 260

T

Talking skills, 220
Temporal bias, 260–261
Ten Top Tips for Successful Proposal Writing, 203, 207

U

Univariate analysis plan
    categorical variables, 183
    continuous variables, 184
    hemorrhage size, 184
    mortality, 185
    Project Health, 184, 185
    response rates, 184

V

Variable categorization
    doctoral proposal, 169, 172–173
    grant proposal, 169, 170
    hypertensive disorders, 169–170, 172–173
    organized plan, 169
    parameterization, 173

W

Writing assistance programs, 81